Respiratory Tract Infections: Advances in Diagnosis, Management and Prevention

Guest Editor

MICHAEL S. NIEDERMAN, MD

CLINICS IN CHEST MEDICINE

www.chestmed.theclinics.com

September 2011 • Volume 32 • Number 3

SAUNDERS an imprint of ELSEVIER, Inc.

W.B. SAUNDERS COMPANY
A Division of Elsevier Inc.

1600 John F. Kennedy Boulevard ● Suite 1800 ● Philadelphia, Pennsylvania 19103

http://www.theclinics.com

CLINICS IN CHEST MEDICINE Volume 32, Number 3
September 2011 ISSN 0272-5231, ISBN-13: 978-1-4557-1023-2

Editor: Sarah E. Barth

Clinics in Chest Medicine (ISSN 0272-5231) is published quarterly by Elsevier Inc., 360 Park Avenue South, New York, NY 10010-1710. Months of issue are March, June, September, and December. Periodicals postage paid at New York, NY and additional mailing offices. Subscription prices are $293.00 per year (domestic individuals), $475.00 per year (domestic institutions), $140.00 per year (domestic students/residents), $321.00 per year (Canadian individuals), $583.00 per year (Canadian institutions), $399.00 per year (international individuals), $583.00 per year (international institutions), and $195.00 per year (international and Canadian students/residents). International air speed delivery is included in all Clinics subscription prices. All prices are subject to change without notice. **POSTMASTER:** Send address changes to Clinics in Chest Medicine, Elsevier Health Sciences Division, Subscription Customer Service, 3251 Riverport Lane, Maryland Heights, MO 63043. **Customer Service: Telephone: 1-800-654-2452** (U.S. and Canada); **1-314-447-8871** (outside U.S. and Canada). **Fax: 1-314-447-8029. E-mail: journalscustomerservice-usa@elsevier.com** (for print support); **journalsonlinesupport-usa@elsevier.com** (for online support).

Reprints. For copies of 100 or more of articles in this publication, please contact the Commercial Reprints Department, Elsevier Inc., 360 Park Avenue South, New York, NY 10010-1710. Tel.: 212-633-3812; Fax: 212-462-1935; E-mail: reprints@elsevier.com.

Clinics in Chest Medicine is covered in *MEDLINE/PubMed (Index Medicus), Current Contents/Clinical Medicine, EMBASE/ Excerpta Medica, Science Citation Index,* and *ISI/BIOMED.*

Printed and bound by CPI Group (UK) Ltd, Croydon, CR0 4YY

Transferred to Digital Print 2011

Contributors

GUEST EDITOR

MICHAEL S. NIEDERMAN, MD
Chairman, Department of Medicine;
Department of Pulmonary and Critical Care
Medicine, Winthrop-University Hospital,
Mineola, New York; Professor and
Vice-Chairman, Department of Medicine,
SUNY at Stony Brook, Stony Brook, New York

AUTHORS

ROSANEL AMARO, MD
Servei de Pneumologia, Institut del Torax,
Hospital Clinic, IDIBAPS, Universitat de
Barcelona, Barcelona, Spain

ROSER ANGLES, MD, PhD
Quality Department, Vall D'Hebron Institut of
Research, Vall d'Hebron University Hospital,
CIBERES, Universitat Autonoma de Barcelona,
Barcelona, Spain

FOREST W. ARNOLD, DO
Assistant Professor of Medicine, Division of
Infectious Diseases, University of Louisville,
Louisville, Kentucky

STIJN BLOT, MNSc, PhD
General Internal Medicine and Infectious
Diseases, Ghent University Hospital,
Ghent, Belgium

SAMUEL M. BROWN, MD, MS
Assistant Professor, Pulmonary and Critical
Care Medicine; Division Associate, Medical
Ethics and Humanities, University of Utah;
Assistant Director, Critical Care
Echocardiography Service, Intermountain
Medical Center, Salt Lake City, Utah

JEAN CHASTRE, MD
Professor of Medicine, Service de Réanimation
Médicale, Institut de Cardiologie, Groupe
Hospitalier Pitié—Salpêtrière, Assistance
Publique—Hôpitaux de Paris, Faculté de
Médecine Paris 6—Pierre et Marie Curie,
Paris, France

ALAIN COMBES, MD, PhD
Professor of Medicine, Service de Réanimation
Médicale, Institut de Cardiologie, Groupe
Hospitalier Pitié—Salpêtrière, Assistance
Publique—Hôpitaux de Paris, Faculté de
Médecine Paris 6—Pierre et Marie Curie,
Paris, France

DONALD E. CRAVEN, MD
Centers for Infectious Diseases and
Prevention, Lahey Clinic Medical Center,
Burlington, Massachusetts; Tufts University
School of Medicine, Boston, Massachusetts

NATHAN C. DEAN, MD
Section Chief, Pulmonary and Critical Care
Medicine, Intermountain Medical Center and
LDS Hospital; Professor (Clinical) of Internal
Medicine, University of Utah, Salt Lake City, Utah

**CHARLES FELDMAN, MB, BCh, DSc, PhD,
FRCP, FCP(SA)**
Professor of Pulmonology and Chief Physician,
Division of Pulmonology, Department of
Internal Medicine, Faculty of Health Sciences,
Charlotte Maxeke Johannesburg Academic
Hospital, University of the Witwatersrand,
Johannesburg, South Africa

MIQUEL FERRER, MD, PhD
Servei de Pneumologia, Institut del Torax,
Hospital Clinic, IDIBAPS, Universitat de
Barcelona; Centro de Investigación Biomedica
En Red-Enfermedades Respiratorias,
Barcelona, Spain

THOMAS M. FILE Jr, MD, MSc,
Professor, Internal Medicine, Master Teacher, Head, Infectious Disease Section, Northeastern Ohio Universities College of Medicine, Rootstown, Ohio; Chief, Infectious Disease Service and Director, HIV Research, Summa Health System, Akron, Ohio

SETH T. HOUSMAN, PharmD, MPA
Infectious Diseases Pharmacotherapy Fellow, Center for Anti-Infective Research and Development, Hartford Hospital, Hartford, Connecticut

JANA HUDCOVA, MD
Department of Critical Care & Surgery, Centers for Infectious Diseases and Prevention, Lahey Clinic Medical Center, Burlington, Massachusetts; Tufts University School of Medicine, Boston, Massachusetts

MARIN H. KOLLEF, MD
Professor of Medicine, Division of Pulmonary and Critical Care, Washington University School of Medicine, St Louis, Missouri

JOSEPH L. KUTI, PharmD
Associate Director, Clinical and Economic Studies, Center for Anti-Infective Research and Development, Hartford Hospital, Connecticut

ANDREW LABELLE, MD
Fellow, Division of Pulmonary and Critical Care, Washington University School of Medicine, St Louis, Missouri

YUXIU LEI, PhD
Centers for Infectious Diseases and Prevention, Lahey Clinic Medical Center, Burlington, Massachusetts

THIAGO LISBOA, MD
Critical Care Department, Hospital de Clinicas, Porto Alegre, Brazil

CHARLES-EDOUARD LUYT, MD, PhD
Hospital Staff Physician, Service de Réanimation Médicale, Institut de Cardiologie, Groupe Hospitalier Pitié—Salpêtrière, Assistance Publique—Hôpitaux de Paris, Faculté de Médecine Paris 6—Pierre et Marie Curie, Paris, France

ROSARIO MENENDEZ, MD, PhD
Servicio de Neumologia, ISS Hospital Universitario La Fe, Valencia, Spain; Centro de Investigación Biomedica En Red-Enfermedades Respiratorias, Barcelona, Spain

MARK L. METERSKY, MD, FCCP
Professor, Division of Pulmonary and Critical Care Medicine, University of Connecticut School of Medicine, Farmington, Connecticut

DAVID P. NICOLAU, PharmD, FCCP, FIDSA
Director, Center for Anti-Infective Research and Development; Division of Infectious Diseases, Department of Medicine, Hartford Hospital, Hartford, Connecticut

MICHAEL S. NIEDERMAN, MD
Chairman, Department of Medicine; Department of Pulmonary and Critical Care Medicine, Winthrop-University Hospital, Mineola, New York; Professor and Vice-Chairman, Department of Medicine, SUNY at Stony Brook, Stony Brook, New York

LUCY B. PALMER, MD
Assistant Professor, Pulmonary, Critical Care and Sleep Division, SUNY at Stony Brook, Stony Brook, New York

PAULA PEYRANI, MD
Director of Clinical Research, Division of Infectious Diseases, University of Louisville, Louisville, Kentucky

KATHRYN A. RADIGAN, MD
Instructor, Division of Pulmonary and Critical Care Medicine, Northwestern University Feinberg School of Medicine, Chicago, Illinois

JULIO RAMIREZ, MD, FACP
Chief, Division of Infectious Diseases, University of Louisville, Louisville, Kentucky

JORDI RELLO, MD, PhD
Critical Care Department, Vall D'Hebron Institut of Research, Vall d'Hebron University Hospital, CIBERES, Universitat Autonoma de Barcelona, Barcelona, Spain

VASILIKI SOULOUNTSI, MD
Visiting Scholar, Department of Pulmonary and Critical Care Medicine, Winthrop-University Hospital, Mineola, New York; Attending Physician, Department of A-ICU, General Hospital G.Papanikolaou, Thessaloniki, Greece

ANTONI TORRES, MD, PhD
Servei de Pneumologia, Institut del Torax, Hospital Clinic, IDIBAPS, Universitat de Barcelona; Centro de Investigación Biomedica En Red-Enfermedades Respiratorias, Barcelona, Spain

JEAN-LOUIS TROUILLET, MD
Hospital Staff Physician, Service de Réanimation Médicale, Institut de Cardiologie, Groupe Hospitalier Pitié—Salpêtrière, Assistance Publique—Hôpitaux de Paris, Faculté de Médecine Paris 6—Pierre et Marie Curie, Paris, France

TIMOTHY WIEMKEN, PhD, MPH, CIC
Data Analyst, Division of Infectious Diseases, University of Louisville, Louisville, Kentucky

RICHARD G. WUNDERINK, MD
Director, Medical Intensive Care Unit, Division of Pulmonary and Critical Care Medicine, Northwestern University School of Medicine, Chicago, Illinois

Contents

broad-spectrum empiric therapy, which can represent antibiotic overuse and promote even more resistance. In an effort to combat this problem, de-escalation therapy has been proposed, with the goals of reducing the number of drugs, the spectrum of therapy, and the duration of therapy. This review examines the factors associated with an effective de-escalation strategy and ways to increase the rates of de-escalation in the future.

Non-cystic fibrosis (CF) bronchiectasis is a common, potentially serious, condition. Further investigations should be performed in an attempt to identify the underlying cause because it may lead to a change in therapy and have significant prognostic implications. MRI is being investigated as a radiation free alternative to high-resolution CT scan of the chest. Many of the treatment recommendations for non-CF bronchiectasis have not been studied in randomized controlled trials but have been extrapolated from the management recommendations for CF. Studies are beginning to inform decisions regarding the management of non-CF bronchiectasis, and an understanding of the best treatment options is beginning to emerge.

Intubated patients are at risk of bacterial colonization and ventilator-associated respiratory infection (VARI). VARI includes tracheobronchitis (VAT) or pneumonia (VAP). VAT and VAP caused by multidrug-resistant (MDR) pathogens are increasing in the United States and Europe. In patients with risk factors for MDR pathogens, empiric antibiotics are often initiated for 48 to 72 hours pending the availability of pathogen identification and antibiotic sensitivity data. Extensive data indicate that early, appropriate antibiotic therapy improves outcomes for patients with VAP. Recognizing and treating VARI may allow earlier appropriate therapy and improved patient outcomes.

This review summarizes recent clinical data examining the use of aerosolized antimicrobial therapy for the treatment of respiratory tract infections in mechanically ventilated patients in the intensive care unit. Aerosolized antibiotics provide high concentrations of drug in the lung without the systemic toxicity associated with the intravenous antibiotics. First introduced in the 1960s as a treatment of tracheobronchitis and bronchopneumonia caused by *Pseudomonas aeruginosa*, now, more than 40 years later, there is a resurgence of interest in using this mode of delivery as a primary therapy for ventilator-associated tracheobronchitis and an adjunctive therapy for ventilator-associated pneumonia.

Many regulatory bodies and payers measure the quality of care provided to patients admitted to the hospital with pneumonia. Some pneumonia quality measures were not based on high-level evidence, and there is also concern that public reporting of performance could drive excessive use of diagnostic testing and antibiotic treatment. There have been significant increases in the performance rate of several process of care recommended for patients hospitalized with pneumonia, accompanied by a decrease in 30-day mortality. To maximize the potential for improved patient outcomes, physicians and regulators must remain vigilant to detect unintended negative consequences related to performance measurement.

Infection prevention measures, specifically targeting ventilator-associated pneumonia (VAP), have been purposed as quality-of-care indicators for patients in intensive care units. The authors discuss some of the recent evidence of the prevention of nosocomial infections, with a particular emphasis on VAP. Moreover, there are several pitfalls in considering VAP rates as a safety indicator. Because of these limitations, the authors recommend the use of specific process measures, designed to reduce VAP, as the basis for interinstitutional benchmarking.

Clinics in Chest Medicine

THE CLINICS ARE NOW AVAILABLE ONLINE!

Access your subscription at:
www.theclinics.com

Preface

Respiratory Tract Infections: Advances in Diagnosis, Management and Prevention

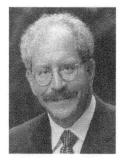

Michael S. Niederman, MD
Guest Editor

Respiratory tract infections are common and remain a major source of morbidity, mortality, and economic cost worldwide, despite advances in modern medicine. In fact, often as a consequence of progress in acute and chronic disease management, we have created patient populations at increased risk for immune impairment and for one specific respiratory infection, pneumonia. In 2004, pneumonia, along with influenza, was the eighth leading cause of death in the United States, the sixth leading cause of death in those over age 65, and the number one cause of death from infectious diseases. Patients at risk for pneumonia include not only previously healthy individuals, as well as the elderly with complex chronic illnesses, but also patients hospitalized for other illness, as well as those with novel forms of immunosuppressive illness as the result of new pharmacologic therapies, organ transplantation, or infection with the HIV virus. In addition to our need to face increasingly complex hosts, we must also confront organisms causing respiratory infection that continue to evolve, with new pathogens being recognized (particularly epidemic viruses) and many organisms that were previously easily managed with antimicrobial agents, now being resistant to commonly used therapies. At the same time, few new antibiotics are being developed, making it necessary to get the most from our current therapies. This can be done through a better understanding of pharmacokinetics and pharmacodynamics, more vigilant use of antimicrobial stewardship, application of new diagnostic methods employing molecular techniques and biomarkers, and by seeking novel routes of therapy, such as the delivery of aerosolized agents. In an effort to improve patient management and responsible antibiotic use, guidelines for managing respiratory infection have proliferated over the past 2 decades, and the value of this approach is now being documented. Prevention has become even more important in our current era of limited new therapies, but the benefits of such efforts may be overstated, as exemplified by the current belief that "zero ventilator-associated pneumonia" is a readily achievable goal.

This issue of *Clinics in Chest Medicine* has brought together an international group of experts to address the current challenges in respiratory infection management, highlighting the common forms of parenchymal disease, including community-acquired pneumonia, nosocomial pneumonia, and the recently defined and controversial entity of health-care-associated pneumonia. In addition, airway infections, including bronchiectasis and ventilator-associated tracheobronchitis, are discussed.

The monograph begins with a review of new diagnostic methods for pneumonia, highlighting the advances in molecular medicine and biomarker measurement that may eventually help us treat infections in a more targeted fashion, allowing for accurate therapy, without the overuse of our best

Clin Chest Med 32 (2011) xiii–xiv
doi:10.1016/j.ccm.2011.07.001

chestmed.theclinics.com

antimicrobials. The role of biomarkers to optimize the management of multidrug-resistant pathogens, particularly in critically ill patients, is also discussed. In an effort to optimize current therapy, the potential to get more from what we already have is highlighted by a discussion of optimizing drug dosing and infusion strategies, through a better understanding of pharmacokinetics and pharmacodynamics. In the setting of community-acquired pneumonia, we have recently learned much about the potential of epidemic viral infections, which are discussed, followed by an analysis of how to define and recognize, as soon as possible, severe forms of pneumonia that must be managed aggressively, usually in an ICU setting. In our efforts to better understand how to manage pneumonia, investigators have been able to glean useful insights from retrospective and prospective evaluation of large databases, and the insights from such studies are examined in a discussion written by several authors who have used this methodology. Then, a careful assessment of the impact of guidelines on the management of community and nosocomial pneumonia is presented. This discussion provides a framework for subsequent discussions of health-care-associated pneumonia, and how this entity fits into current guidelines for management, followed by an examination of de-escalation therapy, a management strategy that is now an integral part of nosocomial pneumonia guidelines.

Airway infections are also discussed, first with a review of bronchiectasis, which is primarily a chronic, outpatient disease, followed by an examination of ventilator-asscociated tracheobronchitis, a common illness in chronically ventilated patients, which may need therapy, and if managed successfully may prevent the subsequent development of pneumonia. In an effort to manage both airway infection and pneumonia due to drug-resistant pathogens, aerosolized antibiotics may be valuable, and the data from recent studies are examined to demonstrate the potential value of this therapy, which is often used as an adjunctive measure to systemic antimicrobial therapy. Finally, the monograph concludes by examining a modern consequence of our understanding of pneumonia, namely the measurement of processes of care in pneumonia management, as a tool to define the quality of care in a given hospital. This has become important in community-acquired pneumonia in the United States, with the development of "core measures" to evaluate inpatient care. In addition, in the management of ventilator-associated pneumonia, measurement of infection rates has become an important outcome, with the push to apply prevention strategies and achieve a zero rate of ventilator-associated pneumonia. While both of these approaches may be admirable, they have risen to a level of controversy with the public reporting of the results of these measurements.

I hope that you will find the discussions in this volume to be contemporary and stimulating. I want to thank all of the authors for their outstanding efforts to compile the most up-to-date information in their reviews and for all the efforts necessary to prepare their contributions. I also want to acknowledge the support provided by Sarah Barth of Elsevier and the support of my family for encouragement during work on this project.

Michael S. Niederman, MD
Department of Medicine
Winthrop University Hospital
222 Station Plaza North, Suite 509
Mineola, NY 11501, USA

E-mail address:
mniederman@winthrop.org

New Diagnostic Tests for Pneumonia: What is Their Role in Clinical Practice?

Thomas M. File Jr, MD, MSc[a,b,*]

KEYWORDS

• Pneumonia • Diagnosis • Molecular studies

The utility of diagnostic studies to determine the etiologic agents of community-acquired pneumonia (CAP) has been controversial in part because of the lack of rapid, accurate, easily performed, and cost-effective methods, which might allow results for most patients at the initial point of service (ie, the initial evaluation by a clinician in an office or acute care setting). Of note, except for the introduction of the urinary antigen tests for *Streptococcus pneumoniae* and *Legionella,* there has been slow advancement in diagnostic methods for determining the etiologic agent of CAP over the past century. For the most part, we have relied on techniques used since the time of Koch and Pasteur—standard microbiological stain and culture methods.

Recently, advancements in molecular testing methods have brought forth new potentials for diagnosis, and more rapid identification of pathogens is possible. In addition, recent studies have suggested that procalcitonin levels help to distinguish between bacterial and viral pneumonia, reduce antibacterial use, and can predict severity of CAP. This article explores new diagnostic tests (immunochromatographic antigen tests and molecular tests) and procalcitonin, and assesses their clinical utility.

PRESENT PROBLEMS WITH ETIOLOGIC DIAGNOSIS OF PNEUMONIA

Identification of the etiology of CAP in recent years has been minimal. From the results of most randomized clinical trials, the cause of CAP for patients admitted to a hospital is determined in approximately 20% to 40% of cases, and in observational studies has ranged from less than 10% for outpatients to approximately 20% for inpatients.[1] At present, several issues contribute to the difficulty with establishing an etiologic diagnosis in pneumonia, including (1) problems with currently available diagnostic tests, (2) recent trend toward empirical therapy without an emphasis on establishing an etiologic diagnosis, and (3) delays because of outsourcing of laboratory tests.

Traditional culture methods for detection of respiratory tract pathogens can be slow, are often insensitive, may not distinguish infection from colonization, and may be influenced by previous antibiotic therapy. Results of diagnostic laboratory tests may require several days (culture identification, serologic tests, in vitro susceptibility results), but timely administration of antibiotics is the pivotal factor in the recovery from severe infection, so empiric therapy has become the recognized

Disclosures: Recent research funding—Cempra, Pfizer; Boehringer Ingelheim, Gilead, Tibotec, The National Institutes of Health (contract # HHSN272201000040C); Scientific Advisory Board/Consultant—Astellas, Bayer, Cempra, Cerexa/Forest, Merck, Nabriva, Pfizer, Tetraphase.

[a] Infectious Disease Section, Internal Medicine Department, Northeastern Ohio Universities College of Medicine and Pharmacy, PO Box 95, Rootstown, OH 44272, USA

[b] Infectious Disease Service, HIV Research, Summa Health System, 75 Arch Street, Suite 506, Akron, OH 44304, USA

* Infectious Disease Service, Summa Health System, 75 Arch Street, Suite 506, Akron, OH 44304.

E-mail address: filet@summahealth.org

Clin Chest Med 32 (2011) 417–430

doi:10.1016/j.ccm.2011.05.011

and recommended practice. For culture of sputum, only a minority of patients expectorate adequate specimens, and if sputum is obtained, there is always the problem distinguishing colonization from true pathogen.

Over the past several decades, broad-spectrum empiric therapy had become the predominant approach to the management of CAP. Most studies found that once empiric therapy was given, the results of diagnostic laboratory tests did not affect management[2–6] because the spectrum of the empiric agents was so broad that regardless of whether or not the pathogen was identified, the clinical response was uniform and often was evident by the time the laboratory results were available to the physician. As a result, microbiological testing, including sputum cultures, Gram stains, and even blood cultures became deemphasized. According to the most recent Infectious Diseases Society of America–American Thoracic Society guideline, microbiological tests are presently universally recommended for high-risk patients intensive care unit (ICU) admitted to the hospital.[7] Although numerous reasons have been proposed for a decrease in microbiology testing, the most powerful influence by far has been the rise of empiricism.[8] With widespread use of broad-spectrum empiric therapy, antimicrobial resistance has increased.[8]

In addition, there has been a trend toward a significant decline in the role of the microbiology laboratory in the hospital setting.[9] In many hospitals, microbiology specimens are outsourced to other health care facilities or private laboratories, which may lead to delays in turnaround times, decreased communication for results, and loss of specimen viability. In addition, the Clinical Laboratory Improvement Amendments of 1988, which required that staff have credentials to interpret Gram stains, virtually eliminated house staff and attending laboratories located on the ward.[9]

A NEW ERA OF DIAGNOSTICS FOR MICROBIAL PATHOGENS

Recently there has been a rapid increase in technology for innovative molecular tests, most significantly associated with the use of nucleic acid amplification tests (NAATs), such as polymerase chain reaction (PCR). These new tests are becoming available with marked expansion of diagnostic capability for infectious diseases. Newer tests that may allow more rapid etiologic diagnosis include the newer generation of immunochromatographic urinary antigen tests as well as NAATs.

Urinary Antigen Tests

Immunochromatographic (ICT) tests that detect soluble pneumococcal antigen or *Legionella* antigen in urine have been an important advance in the diagnostic assessments of these 2 pathogens. These tests are much less influenced by prior antibiotic therapy than sputum or blood culture. The ease of performing the ICT card-type urine test makes it ideal for use in emergency departments, long-term care facilities, and even physician offices (although presently they are not waived by the Food and Drug Administration [FDA] for nonlaboratory, office use).

Pneumococcal urinary antigen

The ICT urinary antigen test is particularly attractive for detecting pneumococcal pneumonia when cultures cannot be obtained in a timely fashion or when antibiotic therapy has already been initiated. In serial specimens from known bacteremic cases, the pneumococcal urinary antigen detected by ICT assay was still positive in 83% of cases after 3 days of therapy.[10] This form of urinary antigen testing has the principal additional advantages of rapidity (about 15 minutes), simplicity, and reasonable specificity in adults. Studies in adults have shown a sensitivity of 50% to 80% and specificity exceeding 90%.[11–13] In one study, the use of the ICT pneumococcal urinary antigen test increased the yield of etiologic diagnosis of patients admitted for CAP from 39.1% to 53.1%.[11] Of 269 patients in this study who had no defined etiology using conventional methods, 69 (25.7%) had a positive pneumococcal urinary antigen test. The immunochromatography assay is also highly accurate in diagnosing pneumococcal meningitis (95% sensitivity with cerebrospinal fluid, 57% sensitivity with urine, and 100% specificity).[14]

The disadvantages of urinary antigen testing include the cost and the lack of an organism isolate for in vitro susceptibility tests. Notably, immunochromatography is not suitable for evaluation of therapeutic effect, because positive test results are obtained for several weeks to months after recovery. Moreover, the immunochromatographic assays are nonspecific for pneumococcal infections in children, particularly the very young, as nasopharyngeal carriage of *S pneumoniae* can cause false-positive results.[12] In one study, the presence of azotemia was an independent factor associated with a higher rate of a positive test for patients with bacteremia.[13] The investigators suggested this may have been because of increased concentration of urine for these patients, as most of the patients had reversible impaired renal function most likely caused by dehydration. Supporting the theory of the effect of concentrated urine, Gutierrez and colleagues[11] reported increased test sensitivity after urine concentration by centrifugation, and a study conducted by the manufacturer found that the test's ability to detect pneumococcal antigen decreased with serial dilution.[15] Thus, patients may be more likely to test positive after urine sample concentration or before intravenous fluid resuscitation. Of note, *pneumococcal* vaccine may cause false-positive results in urine in the Binax NOW *Streptococcus pneumoniae* test in the 48 hours following vaccination.[15]

Legionella urinary antigen

Presently the urinary antigen is the most used test in North America for detection of *Legionella*.[8] Although the test can reliably detect only one species, *Legionella pneumophila*, and only one serogroup, serogroup 1, it has significant advantages over previous "standard" tests (direct fluorescent antibody testing, serology, and culture), including its relatively low cost and rapid performance. Direct fluorescent antibody stains require substantial expertise for interpretation, and selection of reagents is critical. Culture on selective media detects all but very rare strains but is technically more demanding and requires 3 to 7 days.[16] Accurate interpretation of serologic tests requires comparison of acute and convalescent specimens, which is not relevant for clinical management. The *Legionella* urinary antigen test is 70% sensitive and greater than 90% specific for infections caused by *L pneumophila* serogroup 1 and should particularly be useful in the United States and Europe, as approximately 85% of community-acquired isolates are serogroup 1.[17,18] It may be less sensitive for nosocomial cases because of frequent involvement of serogroups other than serogroup 1. Urine is usually positive for antigen on day 1 of illness and continues to be positive for weeks.[19,20]

A recent meta-analysis by Shimada and colleagues[21] summarized the performance characteristics of the *Legionella* urinary antigen as having very good specificity but lower sensitivity for *L pneumophila* serogroup 1; thus, it is better for ruling in than ruling out disease. A positive urinary antigen test result, in the appropriate clinical setting, virtually rules in legionellosis, but a negative urinary antigen test result does not rule out the presence of disease, as 26% of patients with confirmed legionellosis have a negative urinary antigen test result. One potential "unintended" adverse consequence of the availability of the *Legionella* urinary antigen test is decreased use of *Legionella* culture.

All too often, clinicians order a urine antigen test without submitting or requesting a sputum culture. Both the urine antigen test and the *Legionella* culture should be performed for maximal effectiveness, especially if non–serogroup 1 *L pneumophila* is a consideration.

Nucleic Acid Amplification Tests

The development of NAATs has been a major advance in the understanding of respiratory infections.[8] PCR and related methodologies have revolutionized the field of molecular biology, and automated instrumentation has now been introduced successfully to the clinical laboratory setting. Molecular-based tests have moved from the research bench to the clinical diagnostic laboratory and now are becoming commercially available. Clinical application of these methods as comprehensive and rapid techniques may improve our ability to quickly and efficiently identify etiologic organisms associated with CAP. They may eventually have the potential to be point-of-care tests and allow pathogen-directed therapy at the time of initial administration of antimicrobial agents.

PCR directly detects microbial nucleic acid in clinical samples. The basic steps of PCR include DNA extraction from either a cultured pathogen or from a patient specimen sample and amplification of an established target gene.[22,23] Enzymes are used to copy this DNA via multiple rounds of replication, resulting in exponential amplification of the target sequence of interest. The PCR products can then be identified by gel electrophoresis and DNA sequencing.

Initially, PCR methods had several limitations, which included:

Requirement of adequate sample to detect DNA

Presence of PCR inhibitors in samples that can lead to false-negative results

Contamination, which can lead to false-positive results

Differentiation of colonization from true pathogens (eg, identification of S pneumoniae in a respiratory specimen; quantifying organisms may be helpful in this regard)

Equipment expense and requirement for trained personnel.

Lack of standardization of test methods (many hospital laboratories have their own methods that have not been validated in independent studies)

Only a few methods are presently approved by the FDA.

Many of these limitations have been addressed with advancements in methodology (see later in this article) or are expected to be resolved as technology improves. It is anticipated that molecular tests will be more available in the near future.

An important advance in NAAT technology has been the development of quantitative, real-time PCR.[24] With this method, amplification and detection of the DNA sequence occurs in a single tube, thus simplifying the procedure, as gel electrophoresis sequencing is not needed. The reaction is performed with fluorescent-labeled DNA probes, which allow the number of gene copies to be determined. This increases the speed and efficiency of testing and reduces the risks of operator error and cross contamination. This process can be performed with faster turnaround times, allowing results to be used in a more prominent role in direct patient management. Another advancement has been the development of multiplex PCR systems, in which multiple DNA targets are assessed in one reaction without increasing the required amount of technician time.[22,23] Some commercially available assays can measure more than a dozen respiratory pathogens. These assays may also have the ability to recognize potential dual or triple infections in the same patient. Several commercial assays, which are based on automated extraction instruments, are available (but few are FDA approved at the time of this writing) and these vary according to methodology. Specifications for commercially available real-time PCR (including gene targets) are beyond the scope of this article, but readers are referred to other reviews for greater details.[22–24] Presently FDA-approved tests are listed in **Table 1**.

Although PCR methods have been developed for several pneumonia pathogens, the clinical utility of these tests varies.[25–29] There are several advantages of PCR testing methods as compared with standard microbiological culture methods in the detection of pneumonia pathogens (**Box 1**). PCR is a potentially attractive diagnostic tool for rapid diagnosis because it does not rely on bacterial growth or the viability of the organism. Many pathogens, including Chlamydophila pneumoniae, Mycoplasma pneumoniae, and respiratory viruses, can be difficult to culture because of special growth requirements and slow growth. The time required for a final result is often too long to be clinically useful in the acute management of a patient. Real-time PCR has been shown to be as effective as culture methods for detecting these pathogens.[24]

PCR for specific pathogens–bacteria

Streptococcus pneumoniae, the most common pathogen associated with CAP, is easily detected by PCR in respiratory specimens. PCR techniques based on amplification of the pneumolysin or autolysin genes are applicable for the diagnosis of pneumonia, otitis media, and meningitis. Autolysin and pneumolysin PCR using sputum have shown a high sensitivity (more than 80%) but a low specificity (30%–40%).[30,31] Interpretation of sputum PCR is limited by the difficulty in differentiating between pneumococcal colonization and true infection. On the other hand, in pleural fluid, PCR detects the pneumolysin gene with a sensitivity of 78% and a specificity of 93%.[32] One approach that may help to resolve the problem of colonization versus infection is quantification of the target organism by real-time PCR. Yang and colleagues[33] evaluated the utility of a real-time pneumolysin gene PCR test using sputum samples from patients admitted with CAP. Of 129 patients, 23% had S pneumoniae isolated from blood or sputum. The sensitivity and specificity using real-time quantitative PCR were 90% and 80%, respectively. Of note, PCR of blood samples from patients with S pneumoniae infection does not appear to be useful. One study compared the ICT S pneumoniae urine antigen test to PCR of blood in patients with bacteremic pneumococcal infections.[34] The urinary antigen test was positive in 51 of 58 bacteremic pneumococcal cases (sensitivity, 88%; 95% confidence interval [CI], 77% to 95%), whereas PCR was positive in only 31 cases (sensitivity, 53.5%; 95% CI, 40% to 67%; P<.0001), and all of these had detectable urinary antigens. Both tests gave positive results in 2 of 51 control patients (referred to as other-organism septicemia), giving a specificity of 96% (95% CI, 86.5% to 99.5%). In 77 patients with nonbacteremic CAP, urinary antigen was detected significantly more often (in 21 patients [27%]) than a positive result by the PCR protocol (6 [8%]) (P<.002).[34] A recent meta-analysis concluded that currently available PCR methods using blood samples for the diagnosis of invasive pneumococcal diseases lack the sensitivity and specificity necessary for clinical practice.[35] To date there are no FDA-approved PCR tests for S pneumoniae.

There are several commercially available and/or institutionally developed NAATs for the atypical pathogens.[26,36–41] However, none of these are officially FDA approved or available at the present time in the United States. Despite this, PCR is increasingly being recognized as a method of choice for detection of M pneumoniae and C pneumoniae. For both of these pathogens, diagnosis has usually relied on serology, which, as indicated previously, is usually not useful to the clinician during acute medical management. One large study examined the use of real-time PCR to detect M pneumoniae in children with CAP and found that

Table 1
FDA-cleared/approved molecular tests for respiratory pathogens

Bacteria	Manufacturer	Test Name	Method
Francisella tularensis	Idaho Technology, Inc Salt Lake City, UT	Joint Biologic Agent Identification and Diagnostic System Tularemia Detection kit	Real-time PCR
Mycobacterium tuberculosis	Gen-Probe, Inc San Diego, CA	AMPLIFIED Mycobacterium tuberculosis Direct Test	Transcription-mediated amplification
Virus			
Adenovirus	Gen-Probe, Inc (Prodesse)	ProAdeno + Assay	Multiplex Real-time RT-PCR
Avian Flu	Centers for Disease Control and Prevention	Influenza A/H5	Real-time RT-PCR
Influenza virus panel	Centers for Disease Control and Prevention	Human Influenza virus Real-time RT-PCR Detection and Characterization Panel	Real-time RT-PCR
	Focus Diagnostics, Cypress, CA	Simplexa Influenza test	Real-time RT-PCR
Respiratory virus panel	Luminex Molecular Diagnostics, Toronto, Canada	xTAG Respiratory Viral Panel(Luminex LX 100/200) [includes Influenza A/H1, A/H3, A/2009 H1N1; Influenza B; Adenovirus; RSV A&B; Metapneumovirus, Parainfluenza 1,2,3; Rhinovirus]	RT-PCR
	Nanosphere, Inc Northbrook, IL	Verigene Respiratory Virus Nucleic Acid test and Verigen Respiratory Virus Test	Multiplex Gold Nanoparticle Probes
	Gen-Probe, Inc (Prodesse)	ProFlu + Assay (Influenza A/B, RSV); ProFast + Assay (Seasonal A/H1, A/H3, 2009 H1N1; ProParaFlu + Assay (+Parainfluenza virus)	Multiplex Real-time RT-PCR

Since the submission of this paper, the U.S. Food and Drug Administration has issued a clearance for the FilmArray instrument and the FilmArray Respiratory Panel from Idaho Technologies. The FilmArray Respiratory Panel (RP) is a multiplexed nucleic acid test designed for the simultaneous detection of 15 respiratory viruses in 1 hour (http://www.idahotech.com/pdfs/mediakit/PRESS%20RELEASE%20-%20FA_FDA.pdf).

Abbreviation: RT-PCR, Reverse transcriptase-polymerase chain reaction.

Data from FDA Office of In vitro Diagnostic Evaluation and Safety. Available at: www.fdagov/MedicalDevices/ProceduresandMedicalProcedures/DeviceApprovalsandClearance. Accessed December 16, 2010.

PCR detected more cases than standard diagnostic techniques, which included culture.[42] Of significance, PCR results were available within 2 hours—a major improvement over the 2 to 6 weeks usually required for serologic diagnosis. For *C pneumoniae*, culture on cell lines has traditionally been considered as a gold standard for diagnosis. However, cell cultivation is technically complex, and is associated with limited viability and slow growth such that it is restricted to specialized laboratories and is, therefore, not often used. For these reasons, PCR has become an option for diagnosis. There are numerous assays described (again non-FDA approved) but with various results of test performances and significant interlaboratory discordance of detection rates.[26,36,37]

For tuberculosis (TB), molecular techniques have been valuable.[27] Because the organism can require 3 to 8 weeks to grow in culture, molecular techniques can be useful, allowing appropriate isolation, treatment, and disease control. FDA-approved PCR assays are available, which are

---

Box 1
Advantages of molecular techniques compared with conventional diagnostic techniques

Advantages

Rapid

Greater sensitivity

Possibility to identify drug resistance

Ability to identify specific clones for epidemiologic assessment

Possibility to test for multiple pathogens simultaneously

Less affected by prior antimicrobial therapy

Able to detect organisms unable to be cultured

Data from Chan YR, Morris A. Molecular diagnostic methods in pneumonia. Curr Opin Infect Dis 2007;20:157–64.

---

most useful in patients with positive acid-fast smears. A positive PCR in a smear-positive patient is extremely likely to signal TB. Conversely, a negative PCR in a smear-positive patient likely signals infection with another species. Importantly, a negative PCR in a smear-negative patient does not rule out TB.

PCR for viruses

Perhaps the area where PCR can have the greatest impact on pathogen detection has been for respiratory viruses.[43–47] The gold standard for viral identification has been conventional cell culture. However, even in specialized laboratories many viruses cannot be readily cultivated. Thus, many cases of viral illness go undetected and the exact incidence of viruses in CAP has remained uncertain. PCR offers the potential to significantly improve viral detection. For many respiratory viruses, PCR is now the most sensitive diagnostic approach. Most clinical microbiology laboratories use reverse transcriptase PCR (RT-PCR) assays to detect RNA viruses from clinical specimens.[22] This technique is very sensitive and can detect transcript from a single cell. The method uses a reverse transcriptase enzyme to synthesize a complementary strand of DNA from an RNA template. The resulting complementary DNA is then used as the template in a PCR assay.

PCR was vital for epidemiology during the recent influenza H1N1 pandemic because commercially available rapid influenza detection tests (RIDTs) were found to be relatively insensitive (sensitivity ranging from 10%–70% depending in part on the method used).[48] Several recent studies have demonstrated that when

PCR methods are used for viral detection, there is a high frequency of viral identification from patients with lower respiratory tract infection. In a prospective study during a 12-month period (2004–2005) of adult patients admitted for CAP, etiology was assessed using molecular methods (PCR for viruses, *Legionella*, *Mycoplasma*, *Mycobacterium tuberculosis*, and *S pneumoniae*; urinary antigen assay for *S pneumoniae* and *Legionella pneumophila*, serogroup 1) in addition to conventional studies (blood, respiratory culture, serology) for 184 patients.[49] A microbial etiology could be identified for 67% of all the patients. However, in 38 patients for whom all diagnostic methods were applied, a pathogen was identified for 89% of cases. The most frequently detected pathogens were *S pneumoniae* and respiratory viruses (**Table 2**). Another study using NAATs for the identification of respiratory viruses in adult patients with CAP evaluated 183 adult patients with CAP, 450 control subjects, and 201 patients with nonpneumonic lower respiratory tract infection.[47] At least one respiratory virus was identified in 58 patients with CAP (31.7%) compared with 32 (7.1%) in control subjects and 104 (51.7%) in patients with nonpneumonic lower respiratory tract infections ($P<.01$ and $P<.01$, respectively) (**Table 3**). Of interest, the proportion of viruses identified in healthy subjects was not zero and this should be considered when interpreting corresponding proportions among patients.

Thus, by supplementing traditional diagnostic methods with new PCR-based techniques, it is now apparent that viruses are becoming increasingly recognized as important causes of CAP in adults, but in standard practice, except for influenza virus, respiratory viruses are not often identified. However, as stated in a recent editorial commentary by Niederman, "This may change once these new diagnostic tools become more widely available, especially if they help us define an etiologic role of these pathogens and if they encourage the development of new and effective antiviral therapies."[50]

UTILITY OF NEW METHODS FOR DIAGNOSIS

There are good reasons for establishing an etiologic diagnosis of CAP: (1) to permit optimal antibiotic selection of agents against a specific pathogen and limit the consequences of antibiotic misuse; (2) to identify pathogens of potential epidemiologic significance such as *Legionella* and TB; (3) to reduce overuse of broad-spectrum antimicrobials, which hopefully will reduce selection pressure antimicrobial resistance; and (4) to potentially reduce

Table 2
Etiology of community-acquired pneumonia using molecular and conventional diagnostic methods

Pathogen	No. (%) N = 184	Blood Culture	Respiratory Culture	Urinary Antigen	PCR	Serology
Streptococcus pneumoniae	70 (38)	27	17	16	10	—
Mycoplasma pneumoniae	15 (8)	—	—	—	8	7
Haemophilus influenzae	9 (5)	—	7	—	—	—
Moraxella catarrhalis	7 (4)	—	7	—	—	—
Staphylococcus aureus	4 (2)	2	2	—	—	—
Legionella pneumophila	3 (1)	—	1	2	—	—
Streptococcus milleri group	1 (0.5)	1	—	—	—	—
Nocardia sp	1 (0.5)	—	1	—	—	—
Fusobacterium necrophorum	1 (0.5)	1	—	—	—	—
Mycobacterium tuberculosis	2 (1)	—	2	—	—	—
Viruses	54 (29)	—	8	—	26	20
Influenza virus	14 (8)	—	3	—	4	7
Rhinovirus	12 (7)	—	—	—	12	—
RSV	7 (4)	—	1	—	1	5
Parainfluenza virus	7 (4)	—	1	—	1	5
Coronavirus	4 (2)	—	—	—	4	—
Metapneumovirus	3 (2)	—	1	—	3	—
Adenovirus	3 (2)	—	—	—	—	3
HSV 1	2 (1)	—	2	—	—	—
Enterovirus	1 (0.5)	—	—	—	1	—

Abbreviations: HSV, Herpes simplex virus; PCR, polymerase chain reaction; RSV, respiratory syncytial virus.
   Data from Ref.[49]

Table 3
Respiratory viruses associated with community-acquired pneumonia in adults

Virus	CAP (n = 183)	Controls (n = 450)	NPLRTI (n = 201)
Coronavirus	24 (13.1)	17 (3.8)	21 (10.4)
RSV	13 (7.1)	4 (0.2)	7 (3.5)
Rhinovirus	9 (4.9)	9 (2.0)	15 (7.5)
Influenza A	8 (4.4)	2 (0.4)	62 (30.8)
Influenza B	0	0	1 (0.5)
Adenovirus	3 (1.6)	0	0
Human metapneumovirus	2 (1.1)	0	0
Parainfluenza virus (2 or 3)	0	0	3 (1.5)
TOTAL			
Viruses	59 (32.2)	32 (7.1)	110 (54.7)
Positive subjects	58 (31.7)	32 (7.1)	104 (51.7)

Abbreviations: CAP, community-acquired pneumonia; NPLRTI, nonpneumonic lower respiratory tract infection; RSV, respiratory syncytial virus.
   Data from Lieberman D, Shimoni A, Shemer-Avni Y, et al. Respiratory viruses in adults with community-acquired pneumonia. Chest 2010;138:811–6.

adverse events. Thus, diagnostic testing to determine pneumonia etiology can have an essential role for patient care by ensuring appropriate and effective therapy for an individual. It can also play a vital role in disease surveillance and in defining etiologic spectrum and epidemiology characteristics of pneumonia cases and deaths. With the development of rapid antigen and molecular testing methods, the clinical laboratory is no longer reliant solely on traditional culture methods for detection of pathogens in clinical specimens and more rapid etiologic diagnoses may be achievable. However, the clinical impact of the use of molecular tests and the potential for point-of-care diagnosis remains to be clearly defined.

Clinical Impact of Pneumococcal Urinary Antigen Testing

A few studies have evaluated the clinical utility of urinary antigen testing for S pneumoniae in patients with CAP. Guchev and colleagues[51] prospectively assigned patients with mild pneumonia to 2 groups. Those with positive urinary antigen test results were treated using pneumococcal-directed therapy with amoxicillin. Those with negative urinary antigen test results were treated with clarithromycin, based on perceived likelihood of infection by atypical pathogens. Of 219 evaluable patients, 22% had a positive urinary antigen test result. There was no difference in the clinical outcomes of the 2 groups. Notably, 47 (62%) of 71 patients in whom an atypical pathogen was identified were in the urinary antigen–negative arm, whereas 24 (38%) were in the urinary antigen–positive arm, indicating that they had S pneumoniae in association with an atypical pathogen. However, since the atypical pathogens were determined by serologic methods, these latter cases might have represented a primary atypical infection followed by secondary infection by S pneumoniae. In such cases, it is probable that the clinical manifestations of infection that were treated were attributable to S pneumoniae, and this may explain the good response to amoxicillin alone. The investigators concluded that the urinary antigen test allowed them to administer targeted therapy with a penicillin-class antibiotic rather than a broader-spectrum agent, and added that such narrow-spectrum therapy can be more cost effective and can allow broad-spectrum agents, such as macrolides or fluoroquinolones, to be reserved for patients whose urinary antigen test result is negative. Potential cost reductions are likely to be influenced by price differences between the targeted and broad-spectrum agents and by the proportion of positive test results. Also, it should be noted that at the time of this study in Russia, there was little beta-lactam or macrolide resistance of S pneumoniae. In addition, the study was performed in military trainees who were young (mean age, 19 years) and generally healthy. The investigators suggested that additional trials are needed for other clinical settings.

In another study, Stralin and Holmberg[52] evaluated the urinary antigen test in 215 hospitalized patients with CAP, all of whom received initial beta-lactam monotherapy. The median age was 74 years, and approximately 45% of patients had a pneumonia severity index of class IV or V. Thus, these patients were more severely ill than those in the previously described study. Thirty-eight patients had a positive urinary antigen result for S pneumoniae, and 92% of these had a successful outcome; 114 had a negative urinary antigen result, and 78% of these had a successful outcome. There were no patients with a positive PCR sputum test result for an atypical pathogen in the urinary antigen–positive group, whereas 6 patients had a positive PCR result for Mycoplasma spp or Chlamydophila spp in the urinary antigen negative group. The investigators suggested that a positive urinary antigen test result supports treatment with narrow-spectrum beta-lactam antibiotics and that additional coverage for atypical pathogens is needed more frequently in patients with negative test results.

A more recent study purported to show no significant clinical benefit for "targeted treatment" based on the pneumococcal urinary antigen.[53] For a 2-year period (2006–2008), patients admitted for CAP to a hospital in Spain were randomly assigned to receive either empirical antimicrobial therapy according to international guidelines or to receive targeted treatment based on the urinary antigen test: 177 patients were randomized (89/88 for each arm); most cases of CAP were Pneumonia Severity Class IV–V. According to the investigators, targeted therapy was associated with a nonsignificant, slightly higher overall cost (primarily because of the cost of the antigen test), reduction in adverse events, and lower exposure to broad-spectrum antimicrobials. The investigators observed no significant clinical differences in outcomes (such as mortality, clinical relapse, or length of stay in the hospital). In fact, they observed more relapses in the targeted arm. The problem with this study, however, is that the investigators did not "target" therapy until 2 to 6 days after initial intravenous broad-spectrum therapy was initiated. Thus, this study really did not assess the potential for point-of-care decision. Indeed, the investigators acknowledge in their discussion that if there had been earlier introduction of targeted therapy, there may have been an economic benefit, and they indicate that targeted therapy has the potential to lead to *less resistance*.

Clinical Impact of Molecular Diagnostic Testing

Rapid identification of viral and bacterial pathogens is now possible with the use of PCR methods. An open randomized clinical trial was conducted to evaluate the clinical impact of PCR use for detection of etiologic pathogens in patients hospitalized with lower respiratory tract infections.[54] Between November 2002 and March 2004, 107 patients were included (55 had CAP, 22 had exacerbation of chronic obstructive pulmonary disease, and 30 had "other respiratory infections"). Patients were randomized to an intervention group, whereby results of PCR analyses (respiratory viruses and atypical pathogens) were reported ($\leq$48 hours), or a control group, which relied on conventional diagnostic tests (although PCR was run but not reported). Real-time PCR increased the diagnostic yield from 21% to 43% of patients compared with conventional tests and this was primarily because of an increase in the detection of respiratory viruses. This led to cessation of antibiotic treatment for 6 (11%) patients, but overall antibiotic use was comparable in the intervention groups and the control groups. Use of PCR was associated with an increase in cost (because of the cost of the PCR test). Clinical outcomes (mortality, length of therapy) were not significantly different. As pointed out in an accompanying editorial, the lack of a change in antibiotic use was not unexpected, given the study design.[55] Most additional diagnoses in the intervention group were of viral pathogens. Many clinicians would not be brave enough to stop antibacterial agents solely on the basis of discovery of a viral pathogen, especially given the possibility of bacterial co-pathogens in adults. Furthermore, the results were not available at the point of initial antimicrobial decision when directed therapy might be most effective. As the investigators indicate, "to mimic real-life situations, decisions regarding treatment changes after results of PCR analysis were left at the discretion of the physician." Thus, there was no standardized approach using this information by the clinician. One wonders if there had been an educational process to provide strategies for directed therapy there might have been a different result. Certainly with the present influence of antimicrobial stewardship programs, the knowledge of earlier diagnosis might be better

suited for directed point-of-care therapy. As stated by the investigators in the discussion, "real-time PCR might have been more cost-effective if clinicians would have been less reluctant to change clinical management on the basis of test results. Studies with protocol-based and more-rigorous patient management are needed to address this issue." Such a protocol is now under way, funded by the National Institutes of Health.[56]

PROCALCITONIN

Biologic markers have been used in an attempt to distinguish between bacterial and nonbacterial causes of pneumonia. The most promising marker is procalcitonin (PCT). PCT is a peptide precursor of calcitonin that is released by parenchymal cells in response to bacterial toxins and certain bacterial-specific proinflammatory mediators (ie, interleukin [IL]-1b, tumor necrosis factor-α, and IL-6), leading to elevated serum levels in patients with bacterial infections.[57,58] PCT shows a prompt increase upon initial infection within 6 to 12 hours and reduces rapidly when the bacterial infection is controlled by the host immune system and antimicrobial therapy. In contrast, PCT is downregulated in patients with viral infections because of release by cytokines typically associated with viral infections (interferon-γ). The 2 most commonly available tests are the Kryptor assay and the (Lumiphore; Brahms Aktiengesellschaft, Hennigsdorf, Germany) assay; the former is preferred because of higher sensitivity.[57]

PCT has been studied prospectively to facilitate the decision of whether to use antibacterial agents in patients with pneumonia. Using diagnosis-specific clinical algorithms, highly sensitive PCT measurements have been shown to markedly reduce the overuse of antimicrobial therapy without increasing risk to patients in 11 randomized clinical trials including more than 3500 patients.[58] These studies have been performed mostly in European countries and primarily in primary care or emergency department settings. In 2 trials, clinicians were strongly recommended not to prescribe antibacterials in patients with a PCT level lower than 0.1 μg/L, but were encouraged to use antibacterials in patients with levels higher than 0.25 μg/L.[59,60] Subsequent analysis suggested the correct decision in 83%.[60]

Several trials have shown that using PCT results to help determine whether antibiotics are necessary results in lower rates of antibiotic exposure.[59–61] A large (1359 patients), randomized noninferiority trial compared guideline-directed usual care with use of a rapid PCT assay to guide antibiotic use in a group of patients with lower respiratory symptoms presenting to an emergency room in Switzerland.[61] Patients were randomized to administration of antimicrobials based on a PCT algorithm with predefined cutoff ranges for initiating or stopping antimicrobials (PCT group; **Table 4**) or according to standard guidelines (control group). Use of PCT testing among the 150 patients with acute bronchitis halved the percentage of patients who received antibiotic therapy (50.0% for usual care vs 23.2% for PCT-guided treatment) with no difference in rates of adverse outcomes. Antimicrobial prescribing rates in patients with CAP (n = 925) remained appropriately high at 91%. In addition, the mean duration of antimicrobials in the PCT groups was lower (7 days) than in the control groups (10 days). Furthermore, the adverse effect rate for antimicrobials was also lower in the PCT group (23.5%) versus the control group (33.1%; 95% CI, −15.4 to −3.8). In another study, PCT testing led to a 72% decrease in antibiotic use in primary care for patients presenting with a variety of respiratory infections, including acute bronchitis, with no difference in ongoing symptoms or relapse at 28 days between groups.[62] Findings were similar in another randomized noninferiority trial of 550 patients with acute respiratory symptoms presenting to primary care.[63] There was no difference in the number of days with health impairment after day 14, comparing those who were assigned to PCT testing and controls, but there was a 42% decrease in antibiotic prescriptions in the intervention group.

Other studies have shown that PCT levels correlate with the severity of pneumonia.[64,65] In one study, PCT levels increased over time in nonsurvivors but decreased in survivors.[65] However, the prognostic value of PCT levels to predict mortality and other adverse events in CAP remains undefined. In a large prospective randomized clinical trial, Schuetz and colleagues[66] assessed the performance of PCT stratified into 4 predefined procalcitonin tiers (<0.10, 0.10–0.25, >0.25–0.50, >0.50 μg/L) and stratified by Pneumonia Severity Index (PSI) and CURB-65 (confusion, urea nitrogen, respiratory rate, blood pressure, 65 years and older) score to predict all-cause mortality and adverse events within 30 days of follow-up in patients with CAP. Initial PCT levels only moderately predicted mortality; however, PCT was helpful during follow-up and for prediction of adverse events and, thereby, improved the PSI and CURB-65 scores.

Clinical Impact of Procalcitonin

There is accumulating evidence that PCT testing can be useful in helping to identify patients with acute respiratory infection who do not warrant antibacterial therapy. If a practitioner has the capability of obtaining the results of a valid test in a timely manner at the point of care, the result can be useful for assessment of patients presenting with manifestations of acute respiratory infection, including pneumonia. PCT-guided initiation and termination of antibiotic therapy is a novel

---

Table 4
Use of procalcitonin for antimicrobial stewardship for respiratory tract infections based on PCT level

PCT <0.1 μg/L	Bacterial infection very unlikely	NO antimicrobials	Consider repeat in 6–24 hours; reassess based on clinical status and new result
PCT 0.1–0.25 μg/L	Bacterial infection unlikely	NO antimicrobials	Use of antimicrobials should be considered despite low PCT level if: Respiratory or hemodynamic instability; Life-threatening condition; Need for ICU admission; Evidence of empyema; Positive microbiological test (eg, pneumococcal or *Legionella* urinary antigen)
PCT >0.25–0.5 μg/L	Bacterial infection likely	YES antimicrobials	Consider clinical course and repeat PCT at days 3, 5, 7:
PCT >0.5 μg/L	Bacterial infection very likely	YES antimicrobials	Stop antimicrobial using the cutoffs above If peak PCT was very high, consider stopping antimicrobials when 80%–90% decrease If PCT remains high, consider treatment failure

Abbreviations: ICU, intensive care unit; PCT, procalcitonin assay.

approach to reduce antibiotic overuse and guide duration of therapy. This is essential to decrease the risk of side effects and emerging bacterial multidrug resistance. Interpretation of PCT levels must always account for the clinical setting and knowledge about assay characteristics. When PCT is used to guide diagnostic and therapeutic decisions in patients with CAP, the functional assay sensitivity and cutoff ranges need to be considered. The most sensitive assay, and the one with which most of the data are derived, is the Kryptor assay, from which results can be obtained within 1 hour.

Recommendations for antimicrobial stewardship have used specific PCT cutoffs (see **Table 4**). These specify 1 of 4 recommendations, ranging from "strongly discourage" and "discourage" to "recommend" and "strongly recommend," respectively.[58] The utility of this approach has been validated in multiple randomized controlled trials, as indicated previously. Thus, using the Kryptor method, initiation or continuation of antimicrobials is discouraged (<0.10 and <0.25, respectively) or encouraged (>0.50 or 0.25, respectively) (see **Table 4**). In case antimicrobials are initially withheld, clinical reevaluation and repeat PCT are recommended after 6 to 24 hours; if PCT has increased, a decision to initiate antimicrobials can be appropriate at that time. As with any guideline and to ensure patient safety, specific "overruling" criteria have been established such that the PCT-based recommendation should be bypassed based on associated factors and clinical judgment (see **Table 4**).

SUMMARY

Over the past decade, diagnostic tests for detection of respiratory pathogens are rapidly evolving. Immunochromatographic-based urinary antigen tests are rapid, simple-to-perform assays that can be easily developed as point-of-care patient tests. Further development is dependent on defining new antigens that can be readily detected. Molecular diagnostic techniques are becoming increasingly popular in clinical microbiology laboratories. Many of these combine sensitivity, specify, and rapid turnaround time to allow timely patient care. With the development of these methods, the clinical microbiology laboratory is no longer reliant solely on the conventional culture methods for detection of pathogens. Molecular methods have created new opportunities for the clinical microbiology laboratory to affect patient care in the areas of initial diagnosis and therapy. Over time, the methods have become more automated and the potential for clinical utility

increased. In addition to providing excellent new tools for diagnosis, molecular tests will also serve useful roles in infection control and public health.[55]

A critical issue regarding the clinical utility of the molecular tests will be the turnaround time. If we are to be able to use these tests for point-of-care diagnosis, it will be optimal to have results within 1 or 2 hours. However, even if the turnaround time is longer, they can still be useful for more appropriate antimicrobial therapy by allowing earlier pathogen-directed or discontinuation of therapy. Moreover, there will be the question of 24/7 availability. Will smaller community hospitals be able to rationalize the added cost of equipment and personnel to run these tests in a timely manner? In addition, the issue of laboratory reimbursement needs to be addressed, as the current reimbursement by CPT code does not adequately cover the cost of many molecular tests (of course if the test results can result in downstream lower total cost of care by shortening illness and length of stay, these costs can be justified).

As more molecular tests become available, more studies will be necessary to evaluate the real clinical value: Can use of these tests result in real improvement in patient care and outcomes, be cost effective, and reduce adverse events and antimicrobial resistance? Until results of such studies are available, the controversy concerning targeted therapy and empirical therapy will remain.

Finally, many studies (mostly from Europe) show that PCT levels help to distinguish between bacterial and viral pneumonia, reduce antibacterial use, predict severity based on the magnitude of the result, and may predict survival. As with the molecular tests, the timing of availability of results will determine to a great extent the utility as to a point-of-care test. Ongoing studies will further substantiate the utility of PCT.

ACKNOWLEDGMENTS

The author thanks Joseph DiPersio, PhD, and Victor Yu, MD, for their input and review of this article.

REFERENCES

1. Fine MJ, Stone RA, Singer DE, et al. Processes and outcomes of care for patients with community-acquired pneumonia: results from the Pneumonia Patient Outcomes Research Team cohort study. Arch Intern Med 1999;159:970–80.
2. Read RC. Evidence-based medicine: empiric antibiotic therapy in community-acquired pneumonia. J Infect 1999;39:171–8.

3. van der Eerden MM, Vlaspolder F, de Graaff CS, et al. Comparison between pathogen directed antibiotic treatment and empirical broad spectrum antibiotic treatment in patients with community acquired pneumonia: a prospective randomized study. Thorax 2005;60(8):672–8.

4. File TM Jr, Niederman MS. Antimicrobial therapy of community-acquired pneumonia. Infect Dis Clin North Am 2004;18:993.

5. Sharuatzadeh MR, Marrie TJ. Does sputum culture affect the management and/or the outcome of community-acquired pneumonia? East Mediterr Health J 2009;15:792–9.

6. Campbell SG, Marrie TJ, Anstey R, et al. The contribution of blood cultures to the clinical management of adult patients admitted to the hospital with community-acquired pneumonia: a prospective observational study. Chest 2003;123:1142–50.

7. Mandell LA, Wunderink RG, Anzueto A, et al. Infectious Diseases Society of America/American Thoracic Society consensus guidelines on the management of community-acquired pneumonia in adults. Clin Infect Dis 2007;44(Suppl 2):S27.

8. Yu VL, Stout JE. Rapid diagnostic testing for community acquired pneumonia: can innovative technology for clinical microbiology be exploited? Chest 2009;136:1618–21.

9. Bartlett JG. Decline in microbial studies for patients with pulmonary infections. Clin Infect Dis 2004;39: 170–2.

10. Smith MD, Derrington P, Evans P, et al. Rapid diagnosis of bacteremic pneumococcal infections in adults by using the Binax NOW *Streptococcus pneumoniae* urinary antigen test: a prospective, controlled clinical evaluation. J Clin Microbiol 2003; 41:2810–3, 92.

11. Gutierrez F, Masia M, Rodriguez JC, et al. Evaluation of the immunochromatographic binax NOW assay for detection of *Streptococcus pneumoniae* urinaryantigen in a prospective study of community-acquired pneumonia. Clin Infect Dis 2003;36:286–92.

12. Dominguez J, Blanco S, Rodrigo C, et al. Usefulness of urinary antigen detection by an immunochromatographic test for diagnosis of pneumococcal pneumonia in children. J Clin Microbiol 2003;41:2161–3.

13. Selickman J, Paxos M, File TM Jr, et al. Performance measure of urinary antigen in patients with *Streptococcus pneumoniae* bacteremia. Diagn Microbiol Infect Dis 2010;67(2):129–33.

14. Samra Z, Shmuely H, Nahum E, et al. Use of the NOW *Streptococcus pneumoniae* urinary antigen test in cerebrospinal fluid for rapid diagnosis of pneumococcal meningitis. Diagn Microbiol Infect Dis 2003;45(4):237–40.

15. Binax, Portland (ME). Binax NOW *Streptococcus pneumoniae* urinary antigen test package insert.

16. Available at: http://binax.com. Accessed November 1, 2011.

16. Doern GV. Detection of selected fastidious bacteria. Clin Infect Dis 2000;30:166–73.

17. Stout JE, Yu VL. Legionellosis. N Engl J Med 1997; 337:682–7.

18. Waterer GW, Baselski VS, Wunderink RG. *Legionella* and community-acquired pneumonia: a review of current diagnostic tests from a clinician's viewpoint. Am J Med 2001;110:41–8.

19. Helbig JH, Uldum SA, Luck PC, et al. Detection of *Legionella pneumophila* antigen in urine samples by the Binax NOW immunochromatographic assay and comparison with both Binax *Legionella* Urinary Enzyme Immunoassay (EIA) and Biotest *Legionella* Urinary Antigen EIA. J Med Microbiol 2001;50: 509–16.

20. Murdoch DR, Laing RT, Mills GD, et al. Evaluation of a rapid immunochromatographic test for detection of *Streptococcus pneumoniae* antigen in urine samples from adults with community-acquired pneumonia. J Clin Microbiol 2001;39:3495–8.

21. Shimada T, Noguchi Y, Jackson JL, et al. Systematic review and meta-analysis: urinary antigen tests for legionellosis. Chest 2009;136:1576–85.

22. Mahlen SD. Applications of molecular diagnostics. In: Mahon CR, Lehman DC, Manuselis G, editors. Textbook of diagnostic microbiology. 3rd edition. St Louis (MO): Saunders Elsevier; 2007. p. 272–302.

23. Nolte FS, Caliendo AM. Molecular detection and identification of microorganisms. In: Murray PR, Baron EJ, Jorgensen JH, et al, editors. Manual of clinical microbiology. 9th edition. Washington, DC: ASM Press; 2007. p. 218–44.

24. Espy MJ, Uhl JR, Sloan LM, et al. Real-time PCR in clinical microbiology: applications for routine laboratory testing. Clin Microbiol Rev 2006;19:165–256.

25. Nolte FS. Molecular diagnostics for detection of bacterial and viral pathogens in community-acquired pneumonia. Clin Infect Dis 2008;47(Suppl 3):S123–6.

26. teWitt R, van Leeuwen WB. Specific diagnostic tests for atypical respiratory tract pathogens. Infect Dis Clin North Am 2010;24:229.

27. Chan YR, Morris A. Molecular diagnostic methods in pneumonia. Curr Opin Infect Dis 2007;20:157–64.

28. Murdoch DR, Jennings LC, Bhat N, et al. Emerging advances in rapid diagnostic of respiratory infections. Infect Dis Clin North Am 2010;24:791–807, 112, 713–727.

29. Murdoch DR, O'Brien KL, Scott JA, et al. Breathing new life into pneumonia diagnostics. J Clin Microbiol 2009;47:3405–8.

30. Butler JC, Bosshardt SC, Phelan M, et al. Classical and latent class analysis evaluation of sputum polymerase chain reaction and urine antigen testing for diagnosis of pneumococcal pneumonia in adults. J Infect Dis 2003;187:1416–23.

31. Saukkoriipi A, Palmu A, Kilpi T, et al. Real-time quantitative PCR for the detection of *Streptococcus pneumoniae* in the middle ear fluid of children with acute otitis media. Mol Cell Probes 2002;16:385–90.

32. Falguera M, Lopez A, Nogues A, et al. Evaluation of the polymerase chain reaction method for detection of *Streptococcus pneumoniae* DNA in pleural fluid samples. Chest 2002;122:2212–6.

33. Yang S, Lin S, Khalil A, et al. Quantitative PCR assay using sputum samples for rapid diagnosis of pneumococcal pneumonia in adult emergency department patients. J Clin Microbiol 2005;43:3211–26.

34. Smith MD, Sheppard CL, Hogan A, et al. Diagnosis of *Streptococcus pneumoniae* infections in adults with bacteremia and community-acquired pneumonia: clinical comparison of pneumococcal PCR and urinary antigen detection. J Clin Microbiol 2009;47:1046–9.

35. Avni T, Mansur N, Leibovici L, et al. PCR using blood for diagnosis of invasive pneumococcal disease: systematic review and meta-analysis. J Clin Microbiol 2010;48:489–96.

36. She RC, Thurber A, Hymas WC, et al. Limited utility of culture for *Mycoplasma pneumoniae* and *Chlamydophila pneumoniae* for diagnosis of respiratory tract infections. J Clin Microbiol 2010;48:3380–2.

37. Kerdsin A, Uchida R, Verathamjamrus C, et al. Development of triplex SYBR green real-time PCR for detecting *Mycoplasma pneumoniae, Chlamydophila pneumoniae*, and *Legionella* spp. without extraction of DNA. Jpn J Infect Dis 2010;63:173–80.

38. Kim NH, Lee JA, Eun BW, et al. Comparison of polymerase chain reaction and the indirect particle agglutination antibody test for the diagnosis of *Mycoplasma pneumoniae* pneumonia in children. Pediatr Infect Dis J 2007;26:897–903.

39. Liu FC, Chen PY, Huang FL, et al. Rapid diagnosis of *Mycoplasma pneumoniae* infection in children by polymerase chain reaction. J Microbiol Immunol Infect 2007;40:507–12.

40. Cloud JL, Carroll KC, Pixton P, et al. Detection of *Legionella* species in respiratory specimens using PCR with sequencing confirmation. J Clin Microbiol 2000;38:1709–12.

41. Diederen BM, Van Der Eerden MM, Vlaspolder F, et al. Detection of respiratory viruses and *Legionella* spp. by real-time polymerase chain reaction in patients with community acquired pneumonia. Scand J Infect Dis 2009;41(1):45–50.

42. Morozumi M, Ito A, Murayama SY, et al. Assessment of real-time PCR for diagnosis of *Mycoplasma pneumoniae* pneumonia in pediatric patients. Can J Microbiol 2006;52:125–9.

43. van Elden LJ, van Kraaij MG, Nijhuis M, et al. Polymerase chain reaction is more sensitive than viral culture and antigen testing for the detection of respiratory viruses in adults with hematological cancer and pneumonia. Clin Infect Dis 2002;34(2):177–83.

44. Fox JD. Nucleic acid amplification tests for detection of respiratory viruses. J Clin Virol 2007;40(Suppl 1):S15–23.

45. Mahony JB. Detection of respiratory viruses by molecular methods. Clin Microbiol Rev 2008;21:716–47.

46. Templeton KE, Scheltinga SA, Beersma MF, et al. Rapid and sensitive method using multiplex real-time PCR for the diagnosis of infections by influenza a, influenza b, respiratory syncytial virus, parainfluenza viruses 1, 2, 3, and 4. J Clin Microbiol 2004;42:1564–9.

47. Lieberman D, Shimoni A, Shemer-Avni Y, et al. Respiratory viruses in adults with community-acquired pneumonia. Chest 2010;138:811–6.

48. Barry MA. Review of influenza diagnosis and treatment. JAMA 2010;304:671–8.

49. Johansson N, Mats K, Tiveljung-Lindell A, et al. Etiology of community-acquired pneumonia: increased microbiological yield with new diagnostic methods. Clin Infect Dis 2010;50:202–9.

50. Niederman MS. Viral community-acquired pneumonia. If we do not diagnose it and do not treat it, can it still hurt us? Chest 2010;138:767–9.

51. Guchev IA, Yu VL, Sinopalmikov A, et al. Management of nonsevere pneumonia in military trainees with urinary antigen test for *Streptococcus pneumoniae*: an innovative approach to targeted therapy. Clin Infect Dis 2005;40:1608–16.

52. Stralin K, Holmberg H. Usefulness of the *Streptococcus pneumoniae* urinary antigen test in the treatment of community-acquired pneumonia. Clin Infect Dis 2005;41:1209–10.

53. Falguera M, Ruiz-Gonzalez A, Schoenenberger JA, et al. Empirical treatment versus targeted treatment on the basis of the urine antigen results in hospitalized patients with community-acquired pneumonia. Thorax 2010;65:101–6.

54. Oosterheert JJ, van Loon AM, Schuurman R, et al. Impact of rapid detection of viral and atypical bacterial pathogens by real-time polymerase chain reaction for patients with lower respiratory tract infection. Clin Infect Dis 2005;41:1438–44.

55. Murdoch DR. Impact of rapid microbiological testing on the management of lower respiratory tract infection. Clin Infect Dis 2005;41:1445–7.

56. Yu V. Comparing narrow-spectrum antimicrobial therapy to standard of care in patients with community-acquired pneumonia [Press release]. Available at: www.nih.gov/news/health/oct2010/niaid-19.htm. Accessed January 13, 2011.

57. Niederman MS. Biological markers to determine eligibility in trials for community-acquired pneumonia: a focus on procalcitonin. Clin Infect Dis 2008;47:S127–32.

58. Schuetz P, Albrich W, Christ-Crain M, et al. Procalcitonin for guidance of antibiotic therapy. Expert Rev Anti Infect Ther 2010;8:575–87.

59. Christ-Crain M, Jaccard-Stolz D, Bingisser R, et al. Effect of procalcitonin-guided treatment on antibiotic use and outcome in lower respiratory tract infections: cluster-randomised, single-blinded intervention trial. Lancet 2004;363:600.

60. Christ-Crain M, Stolz D, Bingisser R, et al. Procalcitonin guidance of antibiotic therapy in community-acquired pneumonia: a randomized trial. Am J Respir Crit Care Med 2006;174:84.

61. Schuetz P, Christ-Crain M, Thomann R, et al. Effect of procalcitonin-based guidelines vs standard guidelines on antibiotic use in lower respiratory tract infections: the ProHOSP randomized controlled trial. JAMA 2009;302:1059.

62. Briel M, Schuetz P, Mueller B, et al. Procalcitonin-guided antibiotic use vs a standard approach for acute respiratory tract infections in primary care. Arch Intern Med 2008;168:2000–7.

63. Burkhardt O, Ewig S, Haagen U, et al. Procalcitonin guidance and reduction of antibiotic use in acute respiratory tract infection. Eur Respir J 2010;36:601.

64. Masiá M, Gutiérrez F, Shum C, et al. Usefulness of procalcitonin levels in community-acquired pneumonia according to the patient's outcome research team pneumonia severity index. Chest 2005;128:2223.

65. Boussekey N, Leroy O, Alfandari S, et al. Procalcitonin kinetics in the prognosis of severe community-acquired pneumonia. Intensive Care Med 2006;32:469.

66. Schuetz P, Suter-Widmer I, Chaudri A, et al. Prognostic value of procalcitonin in community-acquired pneumonia. Eur Respir J 2011;37(2):384–92.

Biomarkers to Optimize Antibiotic Therapy for Pneumonia Due To Multidrug-Resistant Pathogens

Charles-Edouard Luyt, MD, PhD*, Alain Combes, MD, PhD,
Jean-Louis Trouillet, MD, Jean Chastre, MD

KEYWORDS

- Procalcitonin • Ventilator-associated pneumonia
- Hospital-acquired infection • Antibiotics
- Resistant pathogen

Ventilator-associated pneumonia (VAP) is the most common nosocomial infection in patients on mechanical ventilation (MV), and is associated with prolonged hospital stays and higher mortality.[1,2] Of note, the rate of VAP due to multidrug-resistant (MDR) pathogen(s) reaches 79% in some countries.[3–6] This high frequency is due, in part, to the dramatically different profiles of patients admitted to and treated in intensive care units (ICU) over the past 20 years: patients are now older with more severe comorbidities, and medical care is more likely to include invasive devices, major surgery, prolonged antimicrobial treatment, and/or immunosuppressants, which enhance host susceptibility to bacterial infections with MDR pathogens and increase mortality. In addition, many outbreaks result from cross-contamination by health care personnel.

Key issues in the management of MDR VAP are rapid and accurate identification of patients with true VAP so that antibiotics can be started as soon as possible while avoiding their overuse, isolation of the responsible microorganism(s), and determination of its (their) susceptibility pattern(s) to optimize antimicrobial therapy and shorten its duration. Although pathogen isolation and its (their) susceptibility determination require microbiologic sampling of the lower respiratory tract,[1,2] concerns about the inaccuracy of conventional VAP-management strategies incited some investigators to explore whether use of biologic markers could improve identification of patients with true VAP and facilitate the decision about whether to treat, monitor the response to antibiotics, and shorten treatment duration.

This review focuses on the potential contribution of biomarkers to guide antibiotic use in patients with VAP caused by MDR pathogens.

PROCALCITONIN

One of the precursors of the hormone calcitonin, procalcitonin (PCT), is a 116-amino-acid peptide devoid of known hormonal activity.[7–9] It is normally produced by thyroid C cells and then cleaved into 3 distinct molecules: calcitonin, katacalcin, and an

Conflicts of interests: C-E.L. received lecture fees from Brahms, BioMérieux, and MSD. J.C. received lecture fees from Brahms, Nektar–Bayer, Pfizer, Wyeth and Astellas. The other authors have nothing to disclose.

Service de Réanimation Médicale, Institut de Cardiologie, Groupe Hospitalier Pitié-Salpêtrière, Assistance Publique–Hôpitaux de Paris and Faculté de Médecine Paris 6–Pierre et Marie Curie, 47–83 boulevard de l'Hôpital, 75651 Paris Cedex 13, France

* Corresponding author.

E-mail address: charles-edouard.luyt@psl.aphp.fr

Clin Chest Med 32 (2011) 431–438
doi:10.1016/j.ccm.2011.05.004

N-terminal fragment. In healthy individuals, circulating PCT levels are very low (<0.1 ng/mL). However, microbial infections, through the actions of their own toxins and certain bacterium-specific proinflammatory cytokines (eg, interleukin [IL]-1β, tumor necrosis factor [TNF]-α, and IL-6), ubiquitously stimulate calcitonin-gene expression and constitutive PCT release from all parenchymal tissues and differentiated cell types throughout the body.[7–9] In this context, because enzymatic cleavage of calcitonin is circumvented, PCT levels may increase without any concomitant calcitonin level increase. Although the precise role of PCT during sepsis remains unclear, results obtained with animal models of sepsis demonstrated that PCT administration increased mortality, whereas antibody neutralization of PCT prolonged survival.[10–12] Of note, interferon-γ and other cytokines generated by viral infections attenuated PCT induction, meaning that PCT might serve as valuable biomarker able to distinguish between bacterial and viral infections.[9,13,14]

Using PCT to Diagnose VAP and Start Antibiotics

Although PCT has been established as a good marker of community-acquired infection, this finding does not seem to hold true for hospital-acquired infections. The results of several studies showed that PCT, measured in the blood or bronchoalveolar lavage (BAL) fluid of VAP patients, was not a good marker of this pneumonia. Incorporating its value into a clinical score (eg, the clinical pulmonary infection score) did not improve its diagnostic performance.[15–20] Several reasons can explain why PCT fails to indicate nosocomial infection. First, pneumonia may be a localized infection, with only local PCT synthesis and no systemic release (as in other such infections), thereby explaining its low blood level or apparent decline in patients with true pulmonary infections.[21] Second, during the same hospitalization, ICU patients may be suffering from preexisting severe sepsis or septic shock or multiorgan failure, or may have developed a systemic inflammatory response syndrome after surgery or trauma, all conditions known to raise the circulating levels of biomarkers, including PCT, in the absence of infection. Thus, a high PCT concentration the day VAP is suspected is not useful, because it is not possible to know whether that elevated level results from a prior noninfectious condition or an active infection. Third, knowing that a time lag of 24 to 48 hours can exist between onset of bacterial infection and peak PCT release might also explain the apparently low PCT level the day of VAP onset.[22]

Crude PCT values have proved not to be reliable markers of infection in the ICU.[17,23] When severe infection, especially one caused by an MDR microorganism, is suspected, intensivists are understandably reluctant to rely exclusively on biologic markers. Thus, PCT provides no guiding light for clinicians to start antibiotics, as confirmed by the PRORATA trial results.[24] One of the primary outcome measures of this trial was the usefulness of applying a PCT-guided algorithm to start antibiotics when ICU patients were suspected of having bacterial infections. Among the 307 patients randomized to algorithm-guided management, only 10.4% were not given antibiotics at inclusion; despite having PCT concentrations of less than 0.5 ng/mL, 65 patients received antibiotics because their treating physicians considered that the presence of a true infection could not be excluded.[24]

Using PCT to Shorten Duration of Antimicrobial Treatment

The antibiotic duration for patients with MDR VAP remains controversial. In the PNEUMA trial,[25] which enrolled 401 patients, 127 had VAP caused by nonfermenting gram-negative bacilli (NF-GNB), mostly *Pseudomonas aeruginosa*. Compared with patients who received antibiotics for 15 days, patients with NF-GNB VAP given antibiotics for 8 days did not have poorer outcomes, even though the latter group had a slightly higher percentage of recurrent pulmonary infections. Although the results of more recent studies showed that the shorter antibiotic treatment of NF-GNB VAP was not associated with higher recurrence and mortality rates,[26,27] clinicians remain hesitant about prescribing fewer days of antibiotic treatment for this patient subset.[1]

The notion of using a biomarker to tailor antibiotic-treatment duration relies on the inflammatory response being most often proportional to infection severity. When that response is absent or low, it could be logical to discontinue antibiotics earlier. Moreover, it is well known that PCT levels reflect the inflammatory response intensity and are related to outcome.[28] Thus, adapting antimicrobial-treatment duration to PCT kinetics seems reasonable.

A prospective, observational study examined the value of PCT kinetics as a prognostic factor during VAP.[28] Sixty-three consecutive patients with microbiologically proven VAP who survived 3 days after its diagnosis were included and grouped according to clinical outcome: favorable or unfavorable, defined as death, VAP recurrence, or extrapulmonary infection requiring antibiotics before day 28. Between days 1 and 7, serum PCT and

C-reactive protein (CRP) concentrations declined in both groups but were significantly higher in patients whose outcomes would be unfavorable than in those with subsequent favorable outcomes. To predict an unfavorable outcome, a PCT threshold of 0.5 ng/mL on day 7 had 90% (95% confidence interval [CI], 80%–96%) sensitivity and 88% (95% CI, 77%–94%) specificity,[28] thereby confirming data obtained in patients with severe sepsis. Other clinical or biological factors, for example, white blood cell counts or CRP, were unable to discriminate between patients who would have unfavorable or favorable outcomes. On day 7, the overlap of PCT levels was small and the area under the receiver-operating characteristics (ROC) curve was 0.9, leading the investigators[28] to postulate that day-7 PCT could be useful when combined with clinical factors, such as PaO_2/FiO_2, radiologic assessment, and sequential organ failure assessment (SOFA) scores, to predict which patients are likely to fail. Thus, serum PCT levels might provide an opportunity to modify the treatment strategy early during the course of VAP: either to intensify treatment when PCT levels stay "high" or to avoid unnecessarily prolonged antibiotics when PCT levels decline rapidly.

Several studies tested the ability of PCT-based algorithms to shorten antimicrobial-treatment duration: 6 were conducted in the community setting,[29–34] and all showed that algorithm use led to fewer antibiotic prescriptions, compared with an empiric strategy–based antimicrobial-treatment duration.

So far, 6 trials implementing a PCT-based algorithm have been conducted in surgical or mixed ICU,[24,35–39] 5 of which concerned specific or general populations.[24,36–39] All investigators concluded that antibiotic exposure in critically ill, septic patients could be reduced without compromising clinical outcomes. Those trials were included in the recently published meta-analysis, which confirmed that conclusion.[40] Moreover, the latter

investigators found that using PCT-guided algorithms to manage severely ill septic patients was associated with less antibiotic consumption, and similar mortality rates and ICU or hospital lengths of stay, and comparable superinfection and persistent or relapsed infection rates. Furthermore, for patients managed with a PCT-guided algorithm, antibiotic-treatment duration for the first infectious episode and total antibiotic-therapy duration were shorter, and they had more antibiotic-free days, hence confirming less antibiotic use.

Three of the 6 ICU studies included VAP patients, either specifically[36] or not.[24,35] Their findings were similar when a PCT-guided algorithm was applied: the shorter duration of antibiotic use did not affect survival,[24,35,36] compared with patients managed with a conventional strategy (**Table 1**). Nobre and colleagues[35] showed that a PCT-guided algorithm reduced antimicrobial-treatment duration in patients with severe sepsis or septic shock. In this study, some patients had VAP. Stolz and colleagues[36] managed 101 randomized VAP patients either according to guidelines for discontinuing antibiotics (controls) or based on serum PCT concentrations (PCT group). In their study, one-third of the patients had VAP due to MDR pathogen: 36 patients had VAP due to NF-GNB and 10 to methicillin-resistant *Staphylococcus aureus*. After 72 h of treatment, physicians received the following PCT-level recommendations for PCT-group patients: when serum PCT was less than 0.5 ng/mL or decreased by 80% or more compared with the first day, they were encouraged to withdraw antibiotics or diminish their dose; when serum PCT was 0.5 ng/mL or greater or decreased by less than 80% compared with the first day, they were incited not to terminate antibiotics or lower their dose. When this decision tree was applied, the PCT group had significantly more antibiotic-free days alive during the 28 days after VAP diagnosis than the controls (respective medians [IQR], 13 days[2–21] vs 9.5 days [1.5–17]). This shorter antibiotic use pertinently was not associated with poorer outcomes;

Table 1
Studies evaluating PCT-based algorithms to stop antibiotics in patients with VAP

Study	No. of Patients		Days of Treatment for the First Episode[a]		Antibiotic-Free Days from Day 1 to Day 28[a]		Mortality Rate (%)	
	PCT	Control	PCT	Control	PCT	Control	PCT	Control
Bouadma et al,[24] 2009	75	66	6 (4–10)	8 (7–12)	13 (6–19)	11 (2–16)	31	33
Stolz et al,[36] 2009	51	50	9 (5–16)	12 (7–18)	14 (1–21)	7 (0–13.5)	20	28

Abbreviations: PCT, procalcitonin; VAP, ventilator-associated pneumonia.
[a] Values are expressed as medians (interquartile range). The shorter treatment durations observed for both PCT groups were statistically significant.

moreover, the 2 groups had comparable ventilator-free days, ICU-free days, lengths of hospital stay, and 28-day mortality and hospital mortality rates.

In the PRORATA trial,[24] 621 ICU patients suspected of having developed infections were randomized to be treated according to a conventional strategy (antimicrobial-treatment duration decided by the treating physician's judgment, based on international and local guidelines) or to a PCT-level–based algorithm. In this study, 15% of the patients had an infection due to MDR pathogens. Bouadma and colleagues[24] used 2 interventions to manage antibiotics: the decisions to initiate and terminate antibiotics were based on serial serum PCT concentrations. Physicians were encouraged to start antibiotics when PCT was 0.5 ng/mL or greater, or discouraged from prescribing them when PCT was less than 0.5 ng/mL. Nevertheless, regardless of the PCT concentration and in all cases, the treating physician made the final decision to start antibiotics. Patients receiving antibiotics had their PCT levels measured daily until the end of treatment. When the PCT concentration was less than 80% of the first peak concentration or had reached an absolute concentration of less than 0.5 ng/mL, treating physicians were encouraged to stop antibiotics, even as early as day 3. Again, regardless of the PCT concentration, the final decision was the prerogative of the physician. This PCT group of patients benefited from significantly more antibiotic-free days than the controls (respective means ± standard deviation: 14.3 ± 9.1 vs 11.6 ± 8.2 days; absolute difference, 2.7 days; 95% CI, 1.4–4.1; $P<.0001$). Again, this PCT group's diminished antibiotic use was not associated with poorer outcomes, as the PCT group and controls, respectively, had comparable day-28 (21.2% [65/307] vs 20.4% [64/314]; absolute difference 0.8%; 95% CI −4.6 to 6.2) and day-60 mortality rates (30% [92/307] vs 26.1% [82/314]; absolute difference 3.8%; 95% CI −2.1 to 9.7).

In the PRORATA trial, 141 patients had VAP (75 in the PCT group and 66 controls). Analyses of these subgroup data yielded the same results, with more antibiotic-free days for the PCT group than controls (12.8 ± 7.8 vs 9.7 ± 7.0 days, respectively; absolute difference, 3.1 days; 95% CI 0.7–5.6; $P = .01$). Moreover, the PCT group benefited from a significantly shorter duration of antibiotic administration (for the first episode) than the controls (respective medians [IQR]: 6 [4–10] vs 8 [7–12] days; $P = .02$). Again, this shorter length of antibiotic use was not associated with poorer outcomes; comparing PCT-group patients to controls, respectively, they had comparable rates of recurrence (12% vs 12.1%, $P>.99$), superinfection (48% vs 42%, $P = .51$), 28-day mortality (18.7% vs 25.8%,

$P = .31$), and 60-day mortality (30.7% vs 33.3%, $P = .73$).

These findings strongly support that the antibiotic-treatment duration can probably be safely shortened for patients with MDR VAP provided that, once antibiotics are stopped, physicians remain extremely vigilant and are willing to perform fiberoptic bronchoscopy as soon as a potential relapse is suspected. Because low PCT values are associated with favorable outcomes,[24,28] using serial PCT determinations to guide antimicrobial administration and to discontinue their use as soon as its concentration falls below the 0.5 ng/mL threshold or has decreased by 80% or more compared with the first day seems to be a viable option for these patients.

USEFULNESS OF OTHER BIOMARKERS
C-Reactive Protein

CRP, a pentameric protein synthesized by hepatocytes, comprises 5 noncovalently bound identical subunits, and has with an overall molecular mass of approximately 118,000 Da. Infection or tissue inflammation generates cytokine release, particularly IL-6, IL-1, and TNF which, in turn, stimulate CRP. The investigators of numerous studies concluded that CRP contributes to diagnosing invasive bacterial infection, implying that it might have a role in the emergency department or ICU.[41–44] However, CRP use for diagnostic purposes has yielded widely conflicting data. Some argue that because CRP is, by definition, a nonspecific indicator of inflammation, it cannot accurately differentiate among the many sources of potential tissue destruction. Moreover, in the ICU, consistently conclusive data have not been obtained.[15,28,45]

Nonetheless, observations made in several studies suggested the usefulness of CRP to diagnose VAP. Povoa and colleagues[42] found that, for a threshold of 9.6 mg/dL, CRP had 87% sensitivity and 88% specificity for VAP diagnosis. These same investigators also reported that daily CRP measurements in ICU patients enabled early diagnosis of sepsis.[44] However, their findings were not confirmed by others.[15,20,46] Povoa and colleagues[41] also claimed that CRP was a prognostic marker of VAP resolution, but no data are available on the potential contribution of CRP for starting, pursuing, or terminating antibiotics in septic patients and, thus, it has no established role in patients with MDR VAP.

Soluble Triggering Receptor Expressed on Myeloid Cells 1

Triggering receptor expressed on myeloid cells 1 (TREM-1) was identified as a molecule involved in the inflammatory response.[47] Expressed on the surfaces of neutrophils, mature monocytes, and macrophages, it belongs to the immunoglobulin superfamily.[48] TREM-1 engagement acts in synergy with the Toll-like receptor signaling pathway by amplifying the inflammatory response mediated by several microbial components. By contrast, TREM-1 is not upregulated in samples from patients with noninfectious inflammatory disorders, for example, psoriasis, ulcerative colitis, or vasculitis caused by immune complexes.[48] In mice, TREM-1 binding to agonist monoclonal antibodies stimulated the production of proinflammatory cytokines and chemokines, for example, IL-8, monocyte chemoattractant proteins 1 and 3, and macrophage inflammatory protein 1a, and rapid neutrophil degranulation and oxidative burst.[47,48] The ability of TREM-1 amplification of the inflammatory response to reduce mortality was confirmed in animal models of septic shock in which TREM-1 signaling was blocked.[47,48]

In addition to its membranous form, soluble TREM-1 (sTREM-1) is known to be specifically released during several infectious processes.[15] sTREM-1 measurement in biologic fluids might prove to be a promising diagnostic test for severe sepsis and pneumonia, especially when patients have already received antibiotics, because it can be assessed rapidly at low cost in individual or small batches of samples.[9]

The potential value of sTREM-1 measurement in BAL fluid for VAP diagnosis remains unclear: although it was apparently a reliable marker of pneumonia, especially VAP,[15,49,50] more recent studies obtained contradictory findings, thereby raising doubt as to its usefulness for VAP patients.[51–53] The same controversy exists concerning its prognostic value in patients with infection. According to Gibot and colleagues,[54] sTREM-1 kinetics in blood were associated with death for patients with septic shock. Giamarello-Bourboulis and colleagues[55] reported that initial sTREM-1 levels were higher in survivors of VAP than in nonsurvivors. However, observations differed for patients with community-acquired pneumonia[56] and patients with septic shock.[57]

To date, mostly because this marker is not routinely available and because data on it in patients with MDR VAP are lacking, sTREM-1 cannot be used as an indicator to guide antibiotic use in such situations.

Other Potential Useful Markers of Infection in VAP

GNB cause more than 80% of VAP episodes and are associated with higher mortality. Because GNB pneumonia might be diagnosed more rapidly by endotoxin measurement in BAL fluid, several investigators tested this hypothesis.[58–61] In 1992 Pugin and colleagues[58] reported that an endotoxin concentration of greater than 6 endotoxin units (EU)/mL in BAL fluid could accurately identify patients with GNB VAP. Three other studies confirmed the potential contribution of this tool. Kollef and colleagues[60] used quantitative cultures of 71 BAL to diagnose 63 hospitalized adults suspected of having lung infection. Applying a threshold of greater than 5 EU/mL in BAL fluid yielded the best operating characteristics for GNB-pneumonia diagnosis (100% sensitivity; 75% specificity; area under the ROC curve: 0.88). Moreover, elevated endotoxin concentrations in BAL fluid and microbiologically confirmed GNB pneumonia had good diagnostic agreement (kappa statistic: 0.64; 83% concordance). Similar results were obtained by Nys and colleagues[59] in their 2-part study on a total of 170 patients with clinically suspected VAP. Their threshold of greater than 4 EU/mL to distinguish between patients with significant GNB counts ($>10^4$/mL) and those merely colonized achieved 82% to 93% sensitivity, 81% to 95% specificity, and 85% to 90% correct classifications. Gram staining of BAL fluid for GNB identification yielded slightly inferior operating characteristics. These findings suggest that endotoxin determination in BAL fluid could become an acceptable adjunct for the rapid diagnosis of GNB pneumonia in the near future.

The ability of other biologic markers to predict VAP prognosis was assessed in only a few studies. Froon and colleagues[62] studied 42 patients with microbiologically proven VAP and found that bactericidal/permeability-increasing protein (BPI, an inflammatory protein released by killed or activated neutrophils) and soluble E-selectin were higher early during the course of VAP in patients who would die, compared with survivors, but that systemic levels of inflammatory mediators did not predict clinical severity or patient outcome better than daily Simplified Acute Physiology Score II.[62] Evaluating oxidative stress indicators in the plasma and BAL samples of 36 patients with VAP and 42 without VAP,[63] Duflo and colleagues[63] found that VAP patients had higher thiobarbituric acid–reactive substances in both samples, and higher alveolar concentrations of glutathione peroxidase than those without VAP, but failed to demonstrate a plasma or BAL oxidative stress-factor difference between survivors and nonsurvivors.

SUMMARY

The performance of biomarkers tested so far to diagnose VAP has been poor and their true prognostic value remains unclear. PCT is the biomarker with the most convincing data: a rapid serum PCT-level decline is associated with good outcomes, whereas its increase or stabilization is associated with poor outcomes (death, multiorgan failure), inappropriate antibiotic regimen, or super-infection.[28,64] Using the PCT concentration to individually tailor antibiotic-treatment duration in the ICU has been thoroughly evaluated in 6 studies, all of which demonstrated significantly less antibiotic use when a PCT-based algorithm was applied, with no detrimental impact on outcomes.[24,35–39] Therefore, for MDR VAP patients whose serum PCT concentrations are less than 0.5 ng/mL or decreased by 80% or more, compared with the first peak concentration, terminating antibiotics may be considered as early as day 3 after their initiation. Because other biomarkers (CRP, sTREM-1, endotoxin, or oxidative stress indicators) have not yet been sufficiently evaluated in this subset of patients, their use to guide the withdrawal of antibiotics cannot be recommended. VAP caused by MDR pathogens occurs frequently and its rate has been increasing. The use of biomarkers to guide its management was proposed recently, particularly to improve identification of patients with true VAP, to facilitate the decision about whether to treat, to monitor the response to antibiotics, and to shorten treatment duration. Among the 3 most studied biomarkers (procalcitonin, CRP, and the sTREM), none can be used as a diagnostic marker to help clinicians know when to start antibiotics. However, procalcitonin's good prognostic value can provide guidance to stop antibiotics in VAP patients as early as day 3 after their initiation, even for those whose pneumonia is due to a multidrug-resistant microorganism, when its concentration is less than 0.5 ng/mL or has decreased by at least 80% compared with the peak concentration. With this strategy, extreme vigilance must be maintained after terminating antimicrobial therapy, and microbiologic sampling of the distal airways must be performed as soon as possible when relapse is suspected. The other 2 biomarkers have not yet been evaluated for this indication.

REFERENCES

1. American Thoracic Society, Infectious Diseases Society of America. Guidelines for the management of adults with hospital-acquired, ventilator-associated, and healthcare-associated pneumonia. Am J Respir Crit Care Med 2005;171:388–416.
2. Chastre J, Fagon JY. Ventilator-associated pneumonia. Am J Respir Crit Care Med 2002;165:867–903.
3. Dey A, Bairy I. Incidence of multidrug-resistant organisms causing ventilator-associated pneumonia in a tertiary care hospital: a nine months' prospective study. Ann Thorac Med 2007;2:52–7.
4. Joseph NM, Sistla S, Dutta TK, et al. Ventilator-associated pneumonia in a tertiary care hospital in India: role of multi-drug resistant pathogens. J Infect Dev Ctries 2010;4:218–25.
5. Markogiannakis H, Pachylaki N, Samara E, et al. Infections in a surgical intensive care unit of a university hospital in Greece. Int J Infect Dis 2009;13:145–53.
6. Burgess DS. Curbing resistance development: maximizing the utility of available agents. J Manag Care Pharm 2009;15:S5–9.
7. Muller B, Becker KL. Procalcitonin: how a hormone became a marker and mediator of sepsis. Swiss Med Wkly 2001;131:595–602.
8. Muller B, White JC, Nylen ES, et al. Ubiquitous expression of the calcitonin-I gene in multiple tissues in response to sepsis. J Clin Endocrinol Metab 2001;86:396–404.
9. Chastre J, Luyt CE, Trouillet JL, et al. New diagnostic and prognostic markers of ventilator-associated pneumonia. Curr Opin Crit Care 2006;12:446–51.
10. Nylen ES, Whang KT, Snider RH Jr, et al. Mortality is increased by procalcitonin and decreased by an antiserum reactive to procalcitonin in experimental sepsis. Crit Care Med 1998;26:1001–6.
11. Wagner KE, Martinez JM, Vath SD, et al. Early immunoneutralization of calcitonin precursors attenuates the adverse physiologic response to sepsis in pigs. Crit Care Med 2002;30:2313–21.
12. Becker KL, Nylen ES, Snider RH, et al. Immunoneutralization of procalcitonin as therapy of sepsis. J Endotoxin Res 2003;9:367–74.
13. Christ-Crain M, Muller B. Procalcitonin in bacterial infections—hype, hope, more or less? Swiss Med Wkly 2005;135:451–60.
14. Schuetz P, Albrich W, Christ-Crain M, et al. Procalcitonin for guidance of antibiotic therapy. Expert Rev Anti Infect Ther 2010;8:575–87.
15. Gibot S, Cravoisy A, Levy B, et al. Soluble triggering receptor expressed on myeloid cells and the diagnosis of pneumonia. N Engl J Med 2004;350:451–8.
16. Duflo F, Debon R, Monneret G, et al. Alveolar and serum procalcitonin: diagnostic and prognostic value in ventilator-associated pneumonia. Anesthesiology 2002;96:74–9.
17. Luyt CE, Combes A, Reynaud C, et al. Usefulness of procalcitonin for the diagnosis of ventilator-associated pneumonia. Intensive Care Med 2008;34:1434–40.
18. Charles PE, Kus E, Aho S, et al. Serum procalcitonin for the early recognition of nosocomial infection in the critically ill patients: a preliminary report. BMC Infect Dis 2009;9:49.
19. Jung B, Embriaco N, Roux F, et al. Microbiological data, but not procalcitonin improve the accuracy of

the clinical pulmonary infection score. Intensive Care Med 2010;36:790–8.

20. Ramirez P, Garcia MA, Ferrer M, et al. Sequential measurements of procalcitonin levels in diagnosing ventilator-associated pneumonia. Eur Respir J 2008; 31:356–62.

21. Brunkhorst FM, Al-Nawas B, Krummenauer F, et al. Procalcitonin, C-reactive protein and APACHE II score for risk evaluation in patients with severe pneumonia. Clin Microbiol Infect 2002;8:93–100.

22. Meisner M. Procalcitonin: experience with a new diagnostic tool for bacterial infection and systemic inflammation. J Lab Med 1999;23:263–72 [in German].

23. Tang BM, Eslick GD, Craig JC, et al. Accuracy of procalcitonin for sepsis diagnosis in critically ill patients: systematic review and meta-analysis. Lancet Infect Dis 2007;7:210–7.

24. Bouadma L, Luyt CE, Tubach F, et al. Use of procalcitonin to reduce patients' exposure to antibiotics in intensive care units (PRORATA trial): a multicentre randomised controlled trial. Lancet 2010;375:463–74.

25. Chastre J, Wolff M, Fagon JY, et al. Comparison of 8 vs 15 days of antibiotic therapy for ventilator-associated pneumonia in adults: a randomized trial. JAMA 2003;290:2588–98.

26. Pugh RJ, Cooke RP, Dempsey G. Short course antibiotic therapy for Gram-negative hospital-acquired pneumonia in the critically ill. J Hosp Infect 2010; 74:337–43.

27. Hedrick TL, McElearney ST, Smith RL, et al. Duration of antibiotic therapy for ventilator-associated pneumonia caused by non-fermentative gram-negative bacilli. Surg Infect (Larchmt) 2007;8:589–97.

28. Luyt CE, Guerin V, Combes A, et al. Procalcitonin kinetics as a prognostic marker of ventilator-associated pneumonia. Am J Respir Crit Care Med 2005;171:48–53.

29. Christ-Crain M, Jaccard-Stolz D, Bingisser R, et al. Effect of procalcitonin-guided treatment on antibiotic use and outcome in lower respiratory tract infections: cluster-randomised, single-blinded intervention trial. Lancet 2004;363:600–7.

30. Christ-Crain M, Stolz D, Bingisser R, et al. Procalcitonin guidance of antibiotic therapy in community-acquired pneumonia: a randomized trial. Am J Respir Crit Care Med 2006;174:84–93.

31. Briel M, Schuetz P, Mueller B, et al. Procalcitonin-guided antibiotic use vs a standard approach for acute respiratory tract infections in primary care. Arch Intern Med 2008;168:2000–7 [discussion: 7–8].

32. Schuetz P, Christ-Crain M, Thomann R, et al. Effect of procalcitonin-based guidelines vs standard guidelines on antibiotic use in lower respiratory tract infections: the ProHOSP randomized controlled trial. JAMA 2009;302:1059–66.

33. Stolz D, Christ-Crain M, Bingisser R, et al. Antibiotic treatment of exacerbations of COPD: a randomized, controlled trial comparing procalcitonin-guidance with standard therapy. Chest 2007;131:9–19.

34. Kristoffersen KB, Sogaard OS, Wejse C, et al. Antibiotic treatment interruption of suspected lower respiratory tract infections based on a single procalcitonin measurement at hospital admission–a randomized trial. Clin Microbiol Infect 2009;15:481–7.

35. Nobre V, Harbarth S, Graf JD, et al. Use of procalcitonin to shorten antibiotic treatment duration in septic patients: a randomized trial. Am J Respir Crit Care Med 2008;177:498–505.

36. Stolz D, Smyrnios N, Eggimann P, et al. Procalcitonin for reduced antibiotic exposure in ventilator-associated pneumonia: a randomised study. Eur Respir J 2009; 34:1364–75.

37. Schroeder S, Hochreiter M, Koehler T, et al. Procalcitonin (PCT)-guided algorithm reduces length of antibiotic treatment in surgical intensive care patients with severe sepsis: results of a prospective randomized study. Langenbecks Arch Surg 2009;394:221–6.

38. Svoboda P, Kantorova I, Scheer P, et al. Can procalcitonin help us in timing of re-intervention in septic patients after multiple trauma or major surgery? Hepatogastroenterology 2007;54:359–63.

39. Hochreiter M, Kohler T, Schweiger AM, et al. Procalcitonin to guide duration of antibiotic therapy in intensive care patients: a randomized prospective controlled trial. Crit Care 2009;13:R83.

40. Kopterides P, Siempos II, Tsangaris I, et al. Procalcitonin-guided algorithms of antibiotic therapy in the intensive care unit: a systematic review and meta-analysis of randomized controlled trials. Crit Care Med 2010;38:2229–41.

41. Povoa P, Coelho L, Almeida E, et al. C-reactive protein as a marker of ventilator-associated pneumonia resolution: a pilot study. Eur Respir J 2005;25:804–12.

42. Povoa P, Coelho L, Almeida E, et al. C-reactive protein as a marker of infection in critically ill patients. Clin Microbiol Infect 2005;11:101–8.

43. Povoa P, Coelho L, Almeida E, et al. Pilot study evaluating C-reactive protein levels in the assessment of response to treatment of severe bloodstream infection. Clin Infect Dis 2005;40:1855–7.

44. Povoa P, Coelho L, Almeida E, et al. Early identification of intensive care unit-acquired infections with daily monitoring of C-reactive protein: a prospective observational study. Crit Care 2006;10:R63.

45. Clyne B, Olshaker JS. The C-reactive protein. J Emerg Med 1999;17:1019–25.

46. Oppert M, Reinicke A, Muller C, et al. Elevations in procalcitonin but not C-reactive protein are associated with pneumonia after cardiopulmonary resuscitation. Resuscitation 2002;53:167–70.

47. Bouchon A, Dietrich J, Colonna M. Cutting edge: inflammatory responses can be triggered by TREM-1, a novel receptor expressed on neutrophils and monocytes. J Immunol 2000;164:4991–5.

48. Bouchon A, Facchetti F, Weigand MA, et al. TREM-1 amplifies inflammation and is a crucial mediator of septic shock. Nature 2001;410:1103–7.

49. Determann RM, Millo JL, Gibot S, et al. Serial changes in soluble triggering receptor expressed on myeloid cells in the lung during development of ventilator-associated pneumonia. Intensive Care Med 2005;31:1495–500.

50. Horonenko G, Hoyt JC, Robbins RA, et al. Soluble triggering receptor expressed on myeloid cell-1 is increased in patients with ventilator-associated pneumonia: a preliminary report. Chest 2007;132:58–63.

51. Phua J, Koay ES, Zhang D, et al. Soluble triggering receptor expressed on myeloid cells-1 in acute respiratory infections. Eur Respir J 2006;28:695–702.

52. Oudhuis GJ, Beuving J, Bergmans D, et al. Soluble triggering receptor expressed on myeloid cells-1 in bronchoalveolar lavage fluid is not predictive for ventilator-associated pneumonia. Intensive Care Med 2009;35:1265–70.

53. Anand NJ, Zuick S, Klesney-Tait J, et al. Diagnostic implications of soluble triggering receptor expressed on myeloid cells-1 in BAL fluid of patients with pulmonary infiltrates in the ICU. Chest 2009;135:641–7.

54. Gibot S, Cravoisy A, Kolopp-Sarda MN, et al. Time-course of sTREM (soluble triggering receptor expressed on myeloid cells)-1, procalcitonin, and C-reactive protein plasma concentrations during sepsis. Crit Care Med 2005;33:792–6.

55. Giamarellos-Bourboulis EJ, Zakynthinos S, Baziaka F, et al. Soluble triggering receptor expressed on myeloid cells 1 as an anti-inflammatory mediator in sepsis. Intensive Care Med 2006;32:237–43.

56. Muller B, Gencay MM, Gibot S, et al. Circulating levels of soluble triggering receptor expressed on myeloid cells (sTREM)-1 in community-acquired pneumonia. Crit Care Med 2007;35:990–1.

57. Phua J, Koay ES, Zhang D, et al. How well do serum sTREM-1 measurements prognosticate in septic shock? Anaesth Intensive Care 2008;36:654–8.

58. Pugin J, Auckenthaler R, Delaspre O, et al. Rapid diagnosis of gram negative pneumonia by assay of endotoxin in bronchoalveolar lavage fluid. Thorax 1992;47:547–9.

59. Nys M, Ledoux D, Canivet JL, et al. Correlation between endotoxin level and bacterial count in bronchoalveolar lavage fluid of ventilated patients. Crit Care Med 2000;28:2825–30.

60. Kollef MH, Eisenberg PR, Ohlendorf MF, et al. The accuracy of elevated concentrations of endotoxin in bronchoalveolar lavage fluid for the rapid diagnosis of gram-negative pneumonia. Am J Respir Crit Care Med 1996;154:1020–8.

61. Flanagan PG, Jackson SK, Findlay G. Diagnosis of gram negative, ventilator associated pneumonia by assaying endotoxin in bronchial lavage fluid. J Clin Pathol 2001;54:107–10.

62. Froon AH, Bonten MJ, Gaillard CA, et al. Prediction of clinical severity and outcome of ventilator-associated pneumonia. Comparison of simplified acute physiology score with systemic inflammatory mediators. Am J Respir Crit Care Med 1998;158:1026–31.

63. Duflo F, Debon R, Goudable J, et al. Alveolar and serum oxidative stress in ventilator-associated pneumonia. Br J Anaesth 2002;89:231–6.

64. Seligman R, Meisner M, Lisboa TC, et al. Decreases in procalcitonin and C-reactive protein are strong predictors of survival in ventilator-associated pneumonia. Crit Care 2006;10:R125.

Optimizing Antibiotic Pharmacodynamics in Hospital-acquired and Ventilator-acquired Bacterial Pneumonia

Seth T. Housman, PharmD, MPA[a], Joseph L. Kuti, PharmD[a], David P. Nicolau, PharmD[a,b],*

KEYWORDS

- Hospital-acquired pneumonia
- Ventilator-acquired pneumonia • Pharmacodynamics
- Monte Carlo simulation

Nosocomial pneumonia, the second most common type of hospital-acquired infection in the United States, can be further classified by when and where it was acquired.[1–3] The American Thoracic Society (ATS) and the Infectious Diseases Society of America (IDSA) define hospital-acquired bacterial pneumonia (HABP) as the presence of an acute infection with clinical signs and symptoms in a patient hospitalized for more than 48 hours or within 7 days after discharge from the hospital.[1] Ventilator-acquired bacterial pneumonia (VABP) can be defined by patients ventilated for 48 hours or more or who have been extubated for less than 48 hours and display clinical symptoms.[1] The incidence of nosocomial pneumonia is approximately 5 to 10 cases per 1000 hospital admissions, represents approximately 25% of all infections in intensive care units (ICUs), and increases in frequency in patients who have prolonged intubation periods.[1,4,5] The development of HABP/VABP is associated with an attributable mortality of 33% to 50% and further increases the length of hospital stay by 7 to 9 days and adds greater than $40,000 in excess cost to each patient's cost of care.[1,4–6] This is particularly true for those patients with late-onset symptoms, 5 days or more from admission into the hospital. Along with community-acquired bacterial pneumonia (CABP), HABP/VABP accounts for a substantial burden on health care use and approximately $10 billion in health care cost.[7]

The ATS and the IDSA have supported recommendations for specific antimicrobials and dosing regimens based on infecting organism and risk of multidrug resistant (MDR) organisms but also recognize there is a consistent period of 48 to 72 hours in which therapy is empiric. As such, the ATS and IDSA have also provided recommendations for empiric selection of agents to be used before knowing the pathogen or susceptibility.

An understanding of local epidemiology is necessary to create appropriate empiric regimens. The guidelines use risk stratification to determine which pathogen is most likely. Risk factors include prior receipt of antibiotics and onset of disease in relation to length of hospitalization, among others.[1] Those patients with risk factors have

Disclosures: S.T. Housman has nothing to disclose. J.L. Kuti and D.P. Nicolau are involved with Speaker bureau and received research grants from AstraZeneca and Ortho McNeil.
[a] Center for Anti-Infective Research and Development, Hartford Hospital, 80 Seymour Street, Hartford, CT 06102, USA
[b] Department of Medicine, Division of Infectious Diseases, Hartford Hospital, 80 Seymour Street, Hartford, CT 06102, USA
* Corresponding author.
E-mail address: dnicola@harthosp.org

Clin Chest Med 32 (2011) 439–450
doi:10.1016/j.ccm.2011.05.006

a higher likelihood of an infection caused by MDR organisms including *Pseudomonas aeruginosa*, methicillin-resistant *Staphylococcus aureus* (MRSA), *Acinetobacter* spp, and drug resistant Enterobacteriaceae. For those patients without such risk factors, less drug resistant organisms such as *Streptococcus pneumoniae*, methicillin-susceptible *S aureus*, *Haemophilus influenzae*, and drug-susceptible Enterobacteriaceae are more commonly implicated, although resistant organisms are still possible.[8–10] Surveillance studies routinely report the top pathogens. **Table 1** shows the pathogens isolated from patients hospitalized in the last 5 years of the SENTRY Antimicrobial Surveillance Program.[10] *P aeruginosa* and *S aureus* are the 2 most common pathogens isolated. Empiric selection should be based on institution-specific or even unit-specific information whenever possible and should cover for these common organisms. This approach allows for the greatest likelihood of providing appropriate antibiotic therapy early and then de-escalation once the infecting organism and susceptibility are known.

Once identification of the organism has been made, most microbiology laboratories report susceptibility of the organism as susceptible (S), intermediate (I), or resistant (R). Although these categorical interpretations are helpful, they do not always provide clinicians with adequate information to choose appropriate therapy and never guide the best regimen to choose. The question must always be asked, given the high rate of resistance, "What happens when microbiology reports show nothing susceptible?" Combined with S, I, R, minimum inhibitory concentrations (MICs) are particularly useful to interpret the antibiotic's relative potency and provide important information about which dosage regimens are most likely to be successful against a pathogen. This interaction between drug and bug is the basis for antibiotic pharmacodynamics, and allows for the selection of optimal therapy, or antibiotic regimens (dose, infusion time, and interval) selected to obtain the maximal bactericidal exposure.[11] Optimal therapy through the use of pharmacodynamics is an important concept given the high incidence of infection, the rising resistance rates seen especially in critical care areas, and poor outcomes. It also helps a clinician to choose optimal dosing regimens when there are multiple to choose from. This article reviews the concepts of optimal therapy based on pharmacodynamic properties of specific antibiotics for the treatment of HABP/VABP and expands on the role of antibiotic MICs and alternative dosing, including high-dose strategies and extended-infusion intervals given alterations in pharmacokinetic parameters among these critically ill patients.

PHARMACOKINETICS AND PHARMACODYNAMICS

Pharmacokinetics describes the change in drug concentration throughout the body over time. Pharmacokinetics can vary in patients with different infections, particularly pneumonia, because many patients are critically ill and admitted to the ICU during treatment.[12] Two pharmacokinetic parameters, clearance (CL) and volume of distribution (V_d), can change substantially in critically ill patients.[13–15] A review by Varghese and colleagues[12] presents an in-depth description of antimicrobial pharmacokinetic and pharmacodynamic issues in the critically ill. In general, CL can change rapidly given the fluctuating hemodynamic state and renal function of patients with critical illness.[12,16–19] V_d is often larger, with the likelihood of fluid boluses and capillary leakage. Protein binding can also vary dramatically, given it is an acute-phase reactant, which can affect both CL and V_d.[20] Capillary leakage causes fluid to enter the interstitial space from the intravascular space and large fluid boluses to correct hypotension cause an increase in V_d.[21] Given all of the changing parameters, studies have observed inadequate concentrations of antibiotics during critical illness, necessitating the need for optimal doses in these specific patients.[22,23]

Table 1
Incidence of pathogens isolated from patients hospitalized with pneumonia in the United States in the last 5 years of the SENTRY Antimicrobial Surveillance Program

Pathogen	Incidence (%) n = 31,346
S aureus	36.3
P aeruginosa	19.7
Klebsiella spp	8.5
Enterobacter spp	6.5
Acinetobacter spp	4.8
Escherichia coli	4.6
Serratia spp	4.1
Stenotrophomonas maltophilia	3.1
S pneumoniae	2.5
H influenzae	2.5

Data from Jones RN. Microbial etiologies of hospital-acquired bacterial pneumonia and ventilator-associated bacterial pneumonia. Clin Infect Dis 2010;51(S1):S81–7.

The therapeutic effect of antibiotics (ie, inhibiting growth of and killing bacteria) can qualitatively be described as time dependent or concentration dependent.[13] Quantitatively, 3 predominant pharmacodynamic parameters predict antimicrobial efficacy: the time in which the free concentration of the drug is more than the MIC ($fT > MIC$), the ratio of maximum free drug concentration of drug to the MIC ($fCmax/MIC$), and a combination of time and concentration known as the ratio of the area under the curve (AUC) to the MIC.[13–15] Among antibiotics commonly used to treat HABP/VABP, β-lactams, oxazolidinones, and vancomycin are the most common time-dependent antibiotics.[14,24–26] Of these, β-lactams follow the $fT > MIC$ parameter. AUC/MIC is the best predictor of efficacy for oxazolidinones and vancomycin. Aminoglycosides, fluoroquinolones, and polymixins typically display concentration-dependent killing and are best predicted by the ratio $fCmax/MIC$.[13,27–29] A strong understanding of pharmacokinetic changes in patients with critical illness and HABP is necessary to understand dosing implications. By using specific pharmacodynamic properties of antibiotics, it is then possible to optimize therapy for patients with HABP/VABP.

OPTIMAL PHARMACODYNAMIC ATTAINMENT

Not all antibiotics are created equal. Among the β-lactams, penicillins, cephalosporins, and carbapenems do not require the same $fT > MIC$ for maximal killing efficacy. Penicillins, including piperacillin/tazobactam, require the $fT > MIC$ by at least 50% to reach maximal bactericidal activity.[13,14] Cephalosporins require $fT > MIC$ of at least 50% to 70%.[13,14] One recent article studied cefepime concentrations in patients infected with *P aeruginosa* to determine the optimal $fT > MIC$.[30] Their results from 56 patients found that, when the $fT > MIC$ by at least 60%, microbiological failure was only 36.2% compared with 77.8% when the $fT > MIC$ did not reach 60%. Carbapenems have also been shown to have bacteriostatic and bactericidal activity when achieving an $fT > MIC$ of 20% and 40%, respectively.

Linezolid and vancomycin are time-dependent antibiotics for which AUC/MIC is the best predictor of efficacy, as mentioned earlier. For linezolid, animal models of infection have demonstrated $fT > MIC$ and AUC/MIC as predictors of efficacy.[31] This was correlated with a retrospective pharmacodynamic study done in critically ill patients that also found that AUC/MIC was a better predictor than % $fT > MIC$.[32] Pharmacodynamic parameter breakpoints were identified in lower respiratory

tract infections at 99 and, overall, the investigators suggest AUC/MIC values of 80 to 120.[32] Vancomycin has shown predictive efficacy given the AUC/MIC greater than or equal to 400.[33] In one study involving patients with lower respiratory tract infections caused by *S aureus*, clinical improvement and microbiological eradication time were significantly better when the AUC/MIC was greater than or equal to 400, as opposed to less than 400.[34]

Aminoglycosides have maintained impressive activity against Gram-negative organisms over time.[1] As a concentration-dependent antibiotic, the predominant pharmacodynamic property needed for efficacy is C_{max}/MIC.[28,35–37] In one single-center study, it was determined that those patients who received an aminoglycoside dosed to a C_{max}/MIC of greater than or equal to 10 for nosocomial pneumonia within the first 48 hours had a 90% probability of fever resolution and leukocyte reduction by day 7.[38]

Fluoroquinolone pharmacodynamics have been studied extensively in animal models and in humans. Levofloxacin has been studied against *S pneumoniae* in patients. Given a free drug concentration AUC/MIC ratio of greater than 33.7, 100% of patients had microbiological response, compared with only 64% when the ratio of AUC/MIC was less than 33.7.[39] In patients infected with Gram-negative organisms including *P aeruginosa*, a higher AUC/MIC ratio of 125 has been found to be optimal.[40–42] This AUC/MIC ratio of greater than 125 for ciprofloxacin significantly prolonged the time to development of resistance and was shown by Forrest and colleagues[40] to significantly decrease the time to bacterial eradication.[40]

OPTIMIZING ANTIBIOTIC THERAPY

Few data have been published to support specific dosing recommendations in critically ill patients. With a multitude of dosing regimens available for each antibiotic, choosing an appropriate dose can be difficult, let alone optimizing the regimen. Cefepime is recommended to be given as 1 to 2 g intravenously (IV) every 8 to 12 hours for HABP/VABP.[1] With this wide range of dosing schemes, it can be difficult for the clinician to decide. It has been published numerous times, but currently recommended dosing strategies do not achieve appropriate pharmacodynamic properties ($fT > MIC$ or $fCmax/MIC$).[30,43–47] Furthermore, large clinical trials can produce evidence to support specific dosing regimens, but are inherently difficult given the acuity of illness, small patient population, and difficulty of obtaining consent.[48] However, Monte

Carlo simulations produce hypothetical patient simulations given a small set of pharmacokinetic parameters collected in the identified patient population. These simulations produce the probability of target attainment (PTA), the probability that a given dosing regimen will achieve its pharmacodynamic target at a given MIC in a specific patient population. PTAs and cumulative fraction of response (CFR), a representation of the in vivo efficacy of dosing regimens when applied to MIC distribution of selected organisms, can be used to determine optimal regimens given an organism and MIC. The value of Monte Carlo simulations is ideal because multiple regimens can quickly be evaluated instead of conducting large and extremely expensive clinical trials. Large multinational surveillance studies like OPTAMA (Optimizing Pharmacodynamic Target Attainment using the MYSTIC [Meropenem Yearly Susceptibility Test Information Collection] Antibiogram) Program provide insight into common causal organisms for HABP. Using this data set, Monte Carlo simulations of multiple regimens allow for comparison of multiple drug and dosing regimens. **Table 2** summarizes results from 4 recent surveillance studies using Monte Carlo simulations to develop theoretic pharmacodynamic exposures against common pathogens isolated in HABP/VABP.[49–52]

Optimization of time-dependent antibiotics requires the concentrations of the drug to remain at more than the MIC for longer durations of the dosing interval. Two ways to accomplish this are through extended-infusion and continuous-infusion strategies. Piperacillin-tazobactam dosing regimens were identified using Monte Carlo simulations to predict higher probabilities of target attainment given a range of MICs for *P aeruginosa*.[53] Simulations showed that, when 3.375 g was given as a 4-hour infusion every 8 hours, the probability of reaching optimal target attainment, defined as greater than 90%, was achieved with MICs up to 16 μg/mL. Recommended regimens of 3.375 g IV every 6 hours and 3.375 g IV every 4 hours decreased to less than the optimal target attainment at MICs of 8 μg/mL.

Cefepime dosing regimens have been extensively studied to determine optimal dosing strategies.[22,25,30,44,54] In one study, multiple intermittent-infusion regimens were compared with continuous-infusion regimens using a Monte Carlo simulation based on pharmacokinetic data from 11 patients in ICUs.[55] The simulation found that at the highest dose per day given as an intermittent infusion, 2 g IV every 8 hours, the PTA was greater than 90% up to and including an MIC of 2 μg/mL. Continuous infusion of 6 g cefepime per day was able to achieve PTA up to 8 μg/mL. A continuous infusion of 2 g cefepime per day was able to achieve similar PTA to the intermittent infusion of 2 g IV every 8 hours with optimal PTA at an MIC of 2 μg/mL. This result shows the ability of continuous infusion to be used for more resistant isolates with higher MICs, and the possibility of using less drug to achieve the same PTA.

Similar results can be found for meropenem. The PTA values of meropenem in critically ill patients receiving meropenem were calculated using a 5000-patient Monte Carlo simulation.[56] Multiple regimens were used and are displayed in **Fig. 1**. As the regimen (1 g IV every 8 hours) is manipulated from a 0.5-hour infusion to a 3-hour infusion, the optimal PTA increases from an MIC of 1 μg/mL to 4 μg/mL. Subsequently, higher doses produce even further increases in PTA, with 2 g IV every 8 hours as a 3-hour infusion increasing the PTA from 4 μg/mL for the 1 g IV every 8 hours regimen to 8 μg/mL. By giving higher doses at prolonged infusion times, meropenem exposures would be optimal for an additional 22% of *P aeruginosa* isolates from 214 US hospitals collected from the 2009 CAPITAL (Carbapenem Antimicrobial Pseudomonas Isolate Testing at Regional Locations) Surveillance Program.

As mentioned previously, renal function in patients with critical illness can change dramatically because of poor perfusion to the kidneys. Crandon and colleagues[56] collected pharmacokinetic samples from patients admitted to their ICUs at Hartford Hospital, Hartford, CT, receiving meropenem for at least 3 consecutive doses. A Monte Carlo simulation was then performed to create 5000 concentration-time profiles. Simulations were run for 3 different creatinine clearance (CrCL) ranges including 50 to 120 mL/min, 30 to 49 mL/min, and 10 to 29 mL/min. From these profiles, the PTA assuming a pharmacodynamic target of at least 40% $fT > MIC$ was calculated for a range of MICs from 0.008 μg/mL to 64 μg/mL. Results of selected regimens given as a 0.5-hour and 3-hour infusion are described in **Table 3**. Given worsening renal function with a CrCL of 30 to 49 mL/min, meropenem doses of 1 g every 8 hours as a 0.5-hour or 3-hour infusion were sufficient to target an MIC up to 4 μg/mL; however, only the 3-hour infusion was able to meet optimal conditions at MICs of 8 μg/mL. Doses of 500 mg every 6 hours as a 0.5-hour infusion and 1 g every 12 hours both achieved optimal target attainment (≥95.1% and ≥96%, respectively) against MICs greater than or equal to 4 μg/mL. These results show that organisms with high MICs are still able to be treated with meropenem given an optimized dose and most likely the need for extended infusion.

Pharmacodynamic optimization of concentration-dependent antibiotics can be done through increases in doses. Through the use of high-dose, extended-interval dosing, aminoglycosides can achieve high C_{max}/MIC ratios, and can help to decrease the risk of toxicity, most commonly ototoxicity and nehprotoxicity.[35–37] After implementation of a once-daily aminoglycoside program, one study showed continued clinical efficacy and decreased rates of toxicity from a historical perspective.[37] Empiric dosing strategies based on the patient's weight and CrCL have been created. It is important to individualize the dosing regimen by manipulating the dose to increase or decrease the peak concentration and increase or decrease the interval between doses to change the trough concentration to achieve an optimal C_{max}/MIC of greater than or equal to 10. Given the high rate of success and decreased incidence of side effects, high-dose, extended-interval dosing is recommended in the guidelines for HABP/VABP.[1]

Fluoroquinolones are concentration-dependent antibiotics listed in the guidelines for the treatment of HABP in combination with an antipseudomonal β-lactam for patients with risk factors for MDR organisms.[1] Given dose-related toxicity, specifically central nervous system related toxicities, it has been difficult to obtain AUC/MIC ratios greater than 125.[57] One study of levofloxacin conducted in critically ill patients with ventilator-associated pneumonia found that the fAUC after being given a 1000-mg loading dose on day 1 and 500 mg daily thereafter was ~50 μg/mL.[58] The investigators concluded, based on their pharmacokinetic results, that a dose of 1000 mg daily would most likely result in treatment failures against pathogens with MICs of 2 μg/mL, pathogens that would be labeled as levofloxacin susceptible in microbiology sensitivity and susceptibility reports. Furthermore, a randomized, double-blind, retrospective study was conducted to determine the safety and efficacy of 2 regimens of levofloxacin for CABP: 500 mg daily for 10 days or 750 mg daily for 5 days.[59] Baseline characteristics between patients were similar, with the 500-mg group being slightly older (76 vs 72.5 years; $P = .029$) and having higher pneumonia severity index (PSI) scores (90.7 vs 83.1; $P = .017$). Results showed no difference between clinical efficacy and microbiological eradication even when controlling for age and PSI scores. The incidence of adverse events was not different either. This study shows the ability to decrease duration of therapy by optimizing therapy. Through the use of higher doses, this concentration-dependent antibiotic was able to be given in a shorter course.

CLINICAL APPLICATIONS OF PHARMACODYNAMIC OPTIMIZATION

Lodise and colleagues[53] adopted an extended-infusion strategy for piperacillin/tazobactam, the most common antipseudomonal β-lactam at their institution. After implementation, the investigators conducted a retrospective cohort study to identify differences between the historical intermittent-infusion group (3.375 g IV every 4–6 hours) and the extended-infusion group (3.375 g IV every 8 hours as a 4-hour infusion). Baseline characteristics between the groups were similar. Those in the historical control group predominately received 3.375 g IV every 6 hours, with only 4 patients (4.3%) receiving more frequent dosing every 4 hours. In those patients with an Acute Physiology and Chronic Health Evaluation (APACHE II) score greater than or equal to 17, 14-day mortality and median length of stay were both lower in patients who received extended-infusion regimens than the intermittent-infusion regimen. In those patients with APACHE II scores less than 17, there was no statistically significant reduction in either mortality or length of stay. This study identified a possible benefit when using extended-infusion piperacillin/tazobactam in critically ill patients with APACHE II scores greater than or equal to 17.

In one retrospective chart review, intermittent-infusion ceftazidime 2 g infused over 30 minutes every 12 hours was compared with continuous-infusion ceftazidime 2 g infused over 12 hours every 12 hours after a loading dose of 1 g over 30 minutes.[60] A total of 121 patients were enrolled, with similar baseline characteristics between groups. After logistic regression analysis, continuous-infusion ceftazidime was associated with a significantly greater clinical cure rate than intermittent infusion, 89.3% versus 52.3% respectively. Another retrospective study was designed to identify differences in clinical cure in patients with VABP between meropenem 1 g IV as a 30-minute infusion every 6 hours versus continuous-infusion meropenem 1 g IV over 6 hours every 6 hours.[61] There were no significant differences at baseline including microbiologic data between groups. Continuous-infusion meropenem showed a significantly better clinical cure rate than intermittent infusion. Against *P aeruginosa*, there was a clinical cure rate of 84.6% versus 40% with the intermittent infusion. When the MIC of the infecting organism was greater than or equal to 0.5, clinical cure was observed significantly more in the continuous-infusion group than with the intermittent infusion, 80.95% versus 29.41%, respectively.

Table 2
Summary of antibiotic drug regimens and cumulative fraction of response against common pathogens isolated in patients with HABP using Monte Carlo simulations from the OPTAMA and PASSPORT programs

Drug and Regimen[a]	CFR (%)				
	S aureus (MRSA Excluded)	P aeruginosa	Klebsiella spp	Acinetobacter spp	E coli
Cefepime					
1 g IV every 12 h	94.7	76.8–80.9	83.9–99.3	32.3–44.5	90.2–99.9
1 g IV every 8 h	98.1	86.2	88.0	46.3	92.5
1 g IV every 6 h	ND	93.6–94.9	93.7–100	ND	98.8–100
2 g IV every 12 h	98.0	83.6–91.1	90.9–99.8	52.9–65.5	94.4–100
2 g IV every 8 h	99.8	90.1–97.1	95–100	60.9–83.5	96.9–100
2 g IV every 8 h (3-h infusion)	100	93.2–98.0	96.4–100	64.0–82.7	97.7–100
Ceftazidime					
1 g IV every 8 h	83.6	78.8–86.9	72.3–97.2	26.8–53.1	90.1–99.5
2 g IV every 8 h	97.8	91.3–97.9	83.9–98.3	53.4–73.9	97.4–99.8
2 g IV every 8 h (3-h infusion)	99.5	93.3–98.2	92.4–99.8	55.2–80.7	99.1–99.9
Ciprofloxacin					
400 mg IV every 12 h (1-h infusion)	ND	56.1–63.5	79.8–93.6	43.6–44.5	73.2–91.6
400 mg IV every 8 h (1-h infusion)	75.8	61.9–67.0	58.3–95.6	20.8–46.3	46.8–78.6
Doripenem					
500 mg IV every 8 h (1-h infusion)	ND	82.8	96.4	60.3	99.0
500 mg IV every 8 h (4-h infusion)	ND	93.9	ND	67.5	ND
1 g IV every 8 h (1-h infusion)	ND	88.8	ND	66.4	ND
1 g IV every 8 h (4-h infusion)	ND	97.2	ND	72.8	ND
2 g IV every 8 h (1-h infusion)	ND	93.1	ND	73.7	ND
2 g IV every 8 h (4-h infusion)	ND	98.8	ND	80.6	ND

Ertapenem					
1 g IV every 24 h	99.8	14.0	80–97.9	2.9	99.3–99.9
Imipenem					
500 mg IV every 8 h	ND	63.2	91.9	41–60.2	95.5
500 mg IV every 6 h	99.1	61.8–86.3	78.6–99.4	63.7–76.7	97.7–100
1 g IV every 8 h	99.9	66.9–87.7	80.6–99.6	46.3–79.6	99.4–99.8
1 g IV every 8 h (3-h infusion)	100	74.0–93.9	83.6–100	58.2–71.6	100
Levofloxacin					
500 mg IV every 24 h	ND	40.4	90.3	46.7	78.3
750 mg IV every 24 h (1.5-h infusion)	82.3	40.4–55.8	50.2–91.8	18.1–48.2	39.6–78.6
Meropenem					
500 mg IV every 8 h	100	80.7	97.5	59.4	99.8
500 mg IV every 6 h	100	72.9–89.9	81.9–100	37.8–67.4	99.8–100
1 g IV every 8 h	100	76.7–91.7	83.0–100	42.0–70.6	99.9–100
1 g IV every 8 h (3-h infusion)	100	83.3–95	84.8–100	49.1–68.9	100
2 g IV every 8 h	100	86.0–94.9	86.4–100	53.1–69.6	100
2 g IV every 8 h (3-h infusion)	100	93.4–97.0	89.5–100	62.3–74.9	100
Piperacillin/tazobactam					
3.375 g IV every 6 h	ND	74.1–78.3	81.1–93.9	46.6	92.9–97.2
3.375 g IV every 4 h	ND	82.0	95.6	51.9	98.4
3.375 g IV every 8 h (3-h infusion)	ND	80.5–85.1	84.7–96.6	48.3	96.6–98.4
4.5 g IV every 6 h	93.2	76.6–82.0	55.3–95.1	20.1–49.0	78.5–97.6
4.5 g IV every 8 h	ND	69.3–72.5	91.3	44.3	95.2
4.5 g IV every 6 h (3-h infusion)	100	84.1–89.2	60.5–97.2	26.9–52.6	85.2–98.7

Abbreviation: ND, not done.
[a] All infusions are 0.5 hours unless noted.
Data from Refs. [49–52]

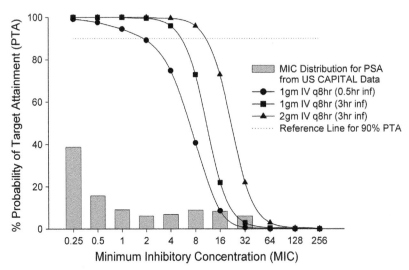

Fig. 1. Probability of attaining 40% $fT > MIC$ in doubling dilutions with varying meropenem dosing regimens used for HABP/VABP. The MIC distribution for *P aeruginosa* (PSA) against respiratory isolates collected from the CAPITAL (Carbapenem Antimicrobial Pseudomonas Isolate Testing at Regional Locations) data is plotted to explain the implication of the PTA curves.

Furthermore, Lorente and colleagues[62] conducted a historical cohort study to determine differences between continuous-infusion and intermittent-infusion piperacillin/tazobactam. Results from this study were similar to the 2 previous studies, identifying a statistically higher rate of clinical cure with continuous-infusion piperacillin/tazobactam given as a loading dose of 4.5 g IV over 30 minutes, then 4.5 g IV infused over 6 hours versus 4.5 g IV over 30 minutes every 6 hours. Clinical cure was statistically significant when MICs were 8 μg/mL

or greater, with clinical cures for the continuous-infusion regimen equal to ~88%, whereas the intermittent-infusion clinical cure rate was only 40% when the MIC was 8 μg/mL, and even less (16.7%)when the MIC was 16 μg/mL against piperacillin/tazobactam. Mortality, duration of mechanical ventilation, and ICU stay were not statistically significant in this study.

A study published by Nicasio and colleagues[63] created a pharmacodynamic-based clinical pathway for empiric antibiotic choice in patients with

Table 3
PTA of various meropenem regimens at varying degrees of renal function for an MIC range

CrCL Regimen	PTA, % MIC 1 μg/mL	PTA, % MIC 2 μg/mL	PTA, % MIC 4 μg/mL	PTA, % MIC 8 μg/mL	PTA, % MIC 16 μg/mL
50–120 mL/min					
1 g IV every 8 h (0.5-h infusion)	94.5	89.2	74.8	40.7	8.6
1 g IV every 8 h (3-h infusion)	97.6	94.5	89.2	74.8	40.7
2 g IV every 8 h (0.5-h infusion)	100	99.6	99.6	73	21.9
2 g IV every 8 h (3-h infusion)	100	100	99.8	95.9	73.0
30–49 mL/min					
1 g IV every 8 h (0.5-h infusion)	100	100	99.8	89.6	38.4
1 g IV every 8 h (3-h infusion)	100	100	99.8	89.6	38.4
10–29 mL/min					
1 g IV every 12 h (0.5-h infusion)	99.7	98.0	84.0	43.5	11.5
1 g IV every 12 h (3-h infusion)	100	99.9	96.0	61.3	17.6

Data from Crandon JL, Ariano RE, Zelenitsky SA, et al. Optimization of meropenem dosage in the critically ill population based on renal function. Intensive Care Med 2011;37(4):632–38.

VABP. A unique aspect of the development of this study was that the investigators used institution-specific information to develop empiric therapy for each of their ICUs. Monte Carlo simulations were designed and used to calculate the cumulative response given specific antibiotic regimens. In the surgical and neurotrauma ICU, cefepime 2 g IV infused over 3 hours every 8 hours was chosen given its best response rate. In the medical ICU, a meropenem regimen was chosen (2 g IV every 8 hours as a 3-hour infusion). High-dose, extended-interval tobramycin and vancomycin were also added to the empiric regimen. Patients were included in the study if admitted to the ICU and diagnosed with VABP based on clinical and radiologic criteria and compared with a historical control group. Baseline clinical characteristics were similar between groups with the exception of the historical group, which had a higher incidence of liver disease than the clinical pathway (17.6% vs 3.2%).

Triple-drug regimens recommended by the current ATS/IDSA guidelines were used in only 3 (4.1%) patients in the historical control and in 73 (77.7%) of the clinical pathway patients, a statistically significant result ($P<.001$). Combination therapy targeting *P aeruginosa* was also statistically higher in the pathway groups, whereas fluoroquinolone therapy, having some of the lowest cumulative responses against *P aeruginosa* in the Monte Carlo simulation, was lower in this group. Patients treated using the clinical pathway had lower infection-related mortality and more commonly received appropriate antibiotics within 24 hours, an important treatment strategy for sepsis and critically ill patients. Of the 94 patients treated on the clinical pathway, 9 patients had infections with MICs greater than or near the breakpoint. Of the 9 patients treated, 8 of them responded successfully, most with prolonged-infusion regimens. The clinical pathway also showed a lower rate of superinfections and infection-related length of stay. Implementation of the clinical pathway for empiric treatment of VABP, patient outcomes, including infection-related mortality and superinfections, were improved. The investigators not only showed improved patient outcomes but it was later determined that patients on the clinical pathway had shorter lengths of ICU and total hospital stay and lower hospital costs after the treatment of VABP when controlling for the differing baseline demographics and the length of stay before developing VABP.[64] The investigators also mention the increased cost of antibiotic use when giving higher doses and using empiric triple therapy, but this small cost was offset by the large savings associated with decreased duration of antibiotic use and length of hospital stay. The program implemented at Hartford Hospital, Hartford, CT, is the first known clinical pathway to use institution-specific information to choose empiric antibiotic choice and improve patient outcomes in patients with VABP while reducing costs.

SUMMARY

There is a high morbidity and mortality associated with hospital-acquired and ventilator-acquired pneumonia and costs associated with this type of treatment are substantial. Although prevention methods are necessary to decrease the risk and incidence, no program can eliminate these infections. Pharmacodynamic optimization of antibiotics is necessary given the high rates of resistance seen in nosocomial infections. ICUs and critical care units are seeing resistance rates increase to the point of complete resistance against all available antibiotics. Optimizing pharmacodynamics can increase the likelihood of obtaining adequate concentrations to achieve bactericidal concentrations and treat pathogens deemed nonsusceptible by conventional laboratory susceptibility panels. The use of extended-infusion and continuous-infusion strategies with time-dependent antibiotics has been implemented and shown to improve the probability of clinical cure. Furthermore, high-dose, extended-interval strategies have been used to optimize the pharmacodynamic profile while minimizing the potential toxicity of the aminoglycosides.

Specific programs using individual institution data like the one created at Hartford Hospital are ideal given that local and even regional resistance rates can be dramatically different. Enhancing patient outcomes by identifying and using optimal antibiotic therapies through the use of Monte Carlo simulation can be an effective tool in the management of infection. In addition to the noted clinical usefulness and better outcomes associated with this pneumonia pathway, the resulting improvements in the economics of care further support the feasibility of this management strategy.

REFERENCES

1. American Thoracic Society, Infectious Diseases Society of America. Guidelines for the management of adults with hospital-acquired, ventilator-acquired, and healthcare-associated pneumonia. Am J Respir Crit Care Med 2005;171:388–416.

2. Kieninger AN, Lipsett PA. Hospital-acquired pneumonia: pathophysiology, diagnosis, and treatment. Surg Clin North Am 2009;89:439–61.

3. Rello J, Sa-Borges M, Correa H, et al. Variations in etiology of ventilator-associated pneumonia across four treatment sites: implications for antimicrobial prescribing practices. Am J Respir Crit Care Med 1999;160:608–13.

4. Chastre J, Fagon JY. Ventilator-associated pneumonia. Am J Respir Crit Care Med 2002;165:867–903.

5. Rello J, Ollendorf DA, Oster G, et al. Epidemiology and outcomes of ventilator-associated pneumonia in a large US database. Chest 2002;122:2121.

6. Fagon JY, Chastre J, Hance AJ, et al. Nosocomial pneumonia in ventilated patients: a cohort study evaluating attributable mortality and hospital stay. Am J Med 1993;94:281–8.

7. AHRQ News and Numbers. Pneumonia most common reason for hospitalization 2008. Agency for healthcare research and quality, Rockville (MD). Available at: http://www.ahrq.gov/news/nn/nn070208. htm. Accessed December 12, 2010.

8. Kollef MH, Shorr A, Tabak YP, et al. Epidemiology and outcomes of health-care associated pneumonia: results from a large US database of culture-positive pneumonia. Chest 2005;128:3854–62.

9. Weber DJ, Rutala WA, Sickbert-Bennett EE, et al. Microbiology of ventilator-associated pneumonia compared with that of hospital-acquired pneumonia. Infect Control Hosp Epidemiol 2007;28(7):825–31.

10. Jones RN. Microbial etiologies of hospital-acquired bacterial pneumonia and ventilator-associated bacterial pneumonia. Clin Infect Dis 2010;51(S1):S81–7.

11. Gillespie EL, Kuti JL, Nicolau DP. When "S" doesn't mean success: the importance of choice of antibiotic and dose on clinical and economic outcomes of severe infections. Conn Med 2005;69:203–10.

12. Varghese JM, Roberts JA, Lipman J. Antimicrobial pharmacokinetic and pharmacodynamic issues in the critically ill with severe sepsis and septic shock. Crit Care Clin 2011;27:19–34.

13. Craig WA. Pharmacokinetic/pharmacodynamic parameters: rational for antibacterial dosing of mice and men. Clin Infect Dis 1998;26:1–10.

14. Turnidge JD. The pharmacodynamics of β-lactams. Clin Infect Dis 1998;27:10–22.

15. Drusano GL. Antimicrobial pharmacodynamics: critical interactions of "bug and drug". Nat Rev Microbiol 2004;2:289–300.

16. Bochud PY, Calandra T. Pathogenesis of sepsis: new concepts and implications for future treatment. BMJ 2003;326:262–6.

17. Glauser MP, Zanetti G, Baumgartner JD, et al. Septic shock. Pathogenesis Lancet 1991;338(8769): 732–6.

18. Buerger C, Plock N, Dehghanyar P, et al. Pharmacokinetics of unbound linezolid in plasma and tissue interstitium of critically ill patients after multiple dosing using microdialysis. Antimicrob Agents Chemother 2006;50(7):2455–63.

19. Joukhadar C, Frossard M, Mayer BX, et al. Impaired target site penetration of beta-lactams may account for therapeutic failure in patients with septic shock. Crit Care Med 2001;29(2):385–91.

20. Ulldemolins M, Roberts JA, Rellow J, et al. The effects of hypoalbuminemia on optimizing antibacterial dosing in critically ill patients. Clin Pharmacokinet 2011;50(2):99–110.

21. Fleck A, Raines G, Hawker F, et al. Increased vascular permeability: a major cause of hypoalbuminemia in disease and injury. Lancet 1985;1(8432): 781–4.

22. Taccone FS, Laterre PF, Dugernier T, et al. Insufficient β-lactam concentrations in the early phase of severe sepsis and septic shock. Crit Care 2010; 14(4):R126.

23. Roberts JA, Roberts MS, Roberston TA, et al. Piperacillin penetration into tissue of critically ill patients with sepsis-bolus versus continuous administration? Crit Care Med 2009;37(3):926–33.

24. Meagher AK, Forrest A, Rayner CR, et al. Population pharmacokinetics of linezolid in patients treated in a compassionate-use program. Antimicrob Agents Chemother 2003;47(2):548–53.

25. Ong CR, Tessier PR, Li C, et al. Comparative in vivo efficacy of meropenem, imipenem, and cefepime against Pseudomonas aeruginosa expressing MexA-MexB-OprM efflux pumps. Diagn Microbiol Infect Dis 2007;57:153–61.

26. Mattoes HM, Kuti JL, Drusano GL, et al. Optimizing antimicrobial pharmacodynamics: dosage strategies for meropenem. Clin Ther 2004;26:1189–98.

27. Li J, Turnidge J, Milne R, et al. In vitro pharmacodynamic properties of colistin methanesulfonate against Pseudomonas aeruginosa isolate from patients with cystic fibrosis. Antimicrob Agents Chemother 2001; 45:781–5.

28. Moore RD, Smith CR, Lietman PS. The association of aminoglycoside therapy: importance of the ratio of peak concentration to minimal inhibitory concentration. J Infect Dis 1987;155:93–9.

29. Preston SL, Drusano GL, Berman AL, et al. Pharmacodynamics of levofloxacin: a new paradigm for early clinical trials. JAMA 1998;279:125–9.

30. Crandon JL, Bulik CC, Kuti JL, et al. Clinical pharmacodynamics of cefepime in patients infected with Pseudomonas aeruginosa. Antimicrob Agents Chemother 2010;54(3):1111–6.

31. Andes D, van Ogtrop ML, Pen J, et al. In vivo pharmacodynamics of a new oxazolidinone (linezolid). Antimicrob Agents Chemother 2002;46(11):3484–9.

32. Rayner CR, Forrest A, Meager AK, et al. Clinical pharmacodynamics of linezolid in seriously ill patients treated in a compassionate use programme. Clin Pharmacokinet 2003;42(15):1411–23.

33. Liu C, Bayer A, Cosgrove SE, et al. Clinical practice guidelines by the Infectious Diseases Society of

America for the treatment of methicillin-resistant *Staphylococcus aureus* infections in adults and children. Clin Infect Dis 2011;52:1–38.

34. Moise-Broder PA, Forrest A, Birmingham MC, et al. Pharmacodynamics of vancomycin and other antimicrobials in patients with *Staphylococcus aureus* lower respiratory tract infections. Clin Pharmacokinet 2004;43(13):925–42.

35. Moore RD, Smith CR, Lietman PS. The association of aminoglycoside plasma levels with mortality in patients with gram-negative bacteremia. J Infect Dis 1984;149:443–8.

36. Freeman CD, Nicolau DP, Belliveau PP, et al. Once-daily dosing of aminoglycosides: review and recommendations for clinical practice. J Antimicrob Chemother 1997;39:677–86.

37. Nicolau DP, Freeman CD, Belliveau PP, et al. Experience with a once-daily aminoglycoside program administered to 2,184 adult patients. Antimicrob Agents Chemother 1995;39:650–5.

38. Kashuba AD, Nafziger AN, Drusano GL, et al. Optimizing aminoglycoside therapy for nosocomial pneumonia caused by gram-negative bacteria. Antimicrob Agents Chemother 1999;43(3):623–9.

39. Ambrose PG, Grasela DM, Grasela TH, et al. Pharmacodynamics of fluoroquinolones against *Streptococcus pneumoniae* in patients with community-acquired respiratory tract infections. Antimicrob Agents Chemother 2001;45(10):2793–7.

40. Forrest A, Nix DE, Ballow CH, et al. Pharmacodynamics of intravenous ciprofloxacin in seriously ill patients. Antimicrob Agents Chemother 1993;37: 1073–81.

41. Thomas JK, Forrest A, Bhavnani SM, et al. Pharmacodynamic evaluation of factors associated with the development of bacterial resistance in acutely ill patients during therapy. Antimicrob Agents Chemother 1998;42:521–7.

42. Shentag JJ. Clinical pharmacology of fluoroquinolones: studies in human dynamic/kinetic models. Clin Infect Dis 2000;31(Suppl 2):S40–4.

43. Zelenitsky SA, Ariano RE, Zhanel GG. Pharmacodynamics of empirical antibiotic monotherapies for an intensive care unit (ICU) population based on Canadian surveillance data. J Antimicrob Chemother 2011;66(2):343–9.

44. Nicasio AM, Ariano RE, Zelenitsky SA, et al. Population pharmacokinetics of high-dose, prolonged infusion cefepime in adult critically ill patients with ventilator-associated pneumonia. Antimicrob Agents Chemother 2009;53(4):1476–81.

45. Drusano GL. Prevention of resistance: a goal for dose selection for antimicrobial agents. Clin Infect Dis 2003;36(Suppl 1):S42–50.

46. Patel N, Scheetz MH, Drusano GL, et al. Identification of optimal renal dosage adjustments for traditional and extended-infusion piperacillin-tazobactam dosing regimens in hospitalized patients. Antimicrob Agents Chemother 2010;54(1):460–5.

47. Nicolau DP. Pharmacokinetic and pharmacodynamic properties of meropenem. Clin Infect Dis 2008;47:S32–40.

48. Roberts JA, Kirkpatrick CM, Lipman J. Monte Carlo simulations: maximizing antibiotic pharmacokinetic data to optimize clinical practice for critically ill patients. J Antimicrob Chemother 2011; 66:227–31.

49. Koomanachai P, Bulik CC, Kuti JL, et al. Pharmacodynamic modeling of intravenous antibiotics against gram-negative bacteria collected in the United States. Clin Ther 2010;32(4):766–79.

50. Sun HK, Kuti JL, Nicolau DP. Pharmacodynamics of antimicrobials for the empirical treatment of nosocomial pneumonia: a report from the OPTAMA program. Crit Care Med 2005;33(10):2222–7.

51. Kim A, Kuti JL, Nicolau DP. Probability of pharmacodynamic target attainment with standard and prolonged-infusion antibiotic regimens for empiric therapy in adults with hospital-acquired pneumonia. Clin Ther 2009;31(11):2765–78.

52. Crandon JL, Kuti JL, Jones RN, et al. Comparison of 2002–2006 OPTAMA programs for US hospitals: focus on gram-negative resistance. Ann Pharmacother 2009;43(2):220–7.

53. Lodise TP, Lomaestro B, Drusano GL. Piperacillin-tazobactam for *Pseudomonas aeruginosa* infection: clinical implications of an extended-infusion dosing strategy. Clin Infect Dis 2007;44:357–63.

54. Georges B, Conil JM, Cougot P, et al. Cefepime in critically ill patients: continuous infusion vs. an intermittent dosing regimen. Int J Clin Pharmacol Ther 2005;43:360–9.

55. Roos JF, Bulitta J, Lipman J, et al. Pharmacokinetic-pharmacodynamic rationale for cefepime dosing regimens in intensive care units. J Antimicrob Chemother 2006;58:987–93.

56. Crandon JL, Ariano RE, Zelenitsky SA, et al. Optimization of meropenem dosage in the critically ill population based on renal function. Intensive Care Med 2011;37(4):632–8.

57. Deryke CA, Kuti JL, Nicolau DP. Re-evaluation of current susceptibility breakpoints for gram-negative rods based on pharmacodynamic assessment. Diagn Microbiol Infect Dis 2007;58:337–44.

58. Benko R, Matuz M, Doro P, et al. Pharmacokinetics and pharmacodynamics of levofloxacin in critically ill patients with ventilator-associated pneumonia. Int J Antimicrob Agents 2007;30(2):162–8.

59. Shorr AF, Zadeikis N, Xiang JX, et al. A multi-center, randomized, double-blind, retrospective comparison of 5- and 10-day regimens of levofloxacin in a subgroup of patients aged >or = 65 years with community-acquired pneumonia. Clin Ther 2005; 27(8):1251–9.

60. Lorente L, Jimenez A, Palermo S, et al. Comparison of clinical cure rates in adults with ventilator-associated pneumonia treated with intravenous ceftazidime administered by continuous or intermittent infusions: a retrospective, nonrandomized, open-label, historical chart review. Clin Ther 2007;29(11):2433–9.

61. Lorente L, Lorenzo L, Martin MM, et al. Meropenem by continuous versus intermittent infusion in ventilator-associated pneumonia due to gram-negative bacilli. Ann Pharmacother 2006;40:219–23.

62. Lorente L, Jiminez A, Martin MM, et al. Clinical cure of ventilator-associated pneumonia treated with piperacillin/tazobactam administered by continuous or intermittent infusion. Int J Antimicrob Agents 2009;33(5):464–8.

63. Nicasio AM, Eagye KJ, Nicolau DP, et al. Pharmacodynamic-based clinical pathway for empiric antibiotic choice in patients with ventilator-associated pneumonia. J Crit Care 2010;25(1):69–77.

64. Nicasio AM, Eagye KJ, Kuti EL, et al. Length of stay and hospital costs associated with a pharmacodynamic-based clinical pathway for empiric antibiotic choice for ventilator-associated pneumonia. Pharmacotherapy 2010;30(5):453–62.

Epidemic Viral Pneumonia and Other Emerging Pathogens

Kathryn A. Radigan, MD[a],*, Richard G. Wunderink, MD[b]

KEYWORDS

- Pneumonia • Virus • Influenza • Epidemic

Viral respiratory tract infections are the most common cause of symptomatic human disease, accounting for more days lost from work than any other infection.[1] Viral respiratory infections can present in myriad ways but most commonly present as two different clinical syndromes: the common cold or the flu.[2] With the growing immunocompromised and elderly populations, viruses are now also recognized as major contributors to lower respiratory tract infections (LRTIs), including bronchitis, bronchiolitis, and, most importantly, viral pneumonia. In the past, viral pneumonia was classified as atypical pneumonia, a residual term from the beginning of the antibiotic era used for a pneumonia in which no bacterial pathogen could be identified and response to antibiotics was minimal.[3]

Traditionally, the lack of focus on viral pneumonia resulted from limited antiviral treatment availability, poor diagnostic tests, and an impression that viral pathogens play a minor role in community-acquired pneumonia (CAP). Principally because of the development of nucleic acid amplification tests for diagnosis, viral pneumonia is now recognized as a major cause of CAP, causing anywhere from 18% to 28% of cases.[4,5] CAP is a frequent and serious problem, contributing to significant morbidity and mortality in the United States. In patients on Medicare who are hospitalized with CAP, 1-year mortality may be as high as 40%.[6] The fraction of those deaths that is actually from viral pneumonia is unclear.

PATHOGENESIS OF VIRAL PNEUMONIA

To cause pneumonia, the virus must reach the lower respiratory tract. Droplet transmission is often limited by distance.[7] Airborne virus-containing droplets are initially deposited in the upper respiratory tract. Once the virus replicates and spreads within squamous epithelial cells, it eventually reaches the lower respiratory tract. Other viruses, including varicella and rubeola, are transmitted through aerosols deposited directly to the lower respiratory tract. Direct contact is the least common pathway of transmission.

The interferon signaling system may be one of the most critical pathways in antiviral defense.[8] The importance of Stat1, one activator of the transcription (JAK-STAT) pathway, has been verified with both human research and experimental models. For instance, Sendai virus, simian virus 5, and measles virus encode for V and C proteins that inhibit Stat1 expression and activation. Furthermore, respiratory syncytial virus (RSV) has developed three different mechanisms to block interferon signaling. Viruses may also be able to manipulate the relationship between the airway epithelial cells and lung macrophages. For example, RSV infection may provide an antiapoptotic signal to macrophages, which leaves viral replication and subsequent inflammation unchecked. This chain of events can potentially lead to lethal outcome from an otherwise controllable infection.

The authors have nothing to disclose.

[a] Division of Pulmonary and Critical Care Medicine, Northwestern University Feinberg School of Medicine, 240 East Huron Street, McGaw M300, Chicago, IL 60611, USA

[b] Medical Intensive Care Unit, Northwestern Memorial Hospital, Division of Pulmonary and Critical Care Medicine, Northwestern University School of Medicine, 675 North Saint Clair Street, Chicago, IL 60611, USA

* Corresponding author.

E-mail address: k-radigan@northwestern.edu

Clin Chest Med 32 (2011) 451–467

doi:10.1016/j.ccm.2011.05.010

Viral infection of the lower respiratory tract can produce severe disease through triggering an inflammatory and cytokine response sufficient to cause acute lung injury, eventually developing into diffuse alveolar damage or acute respiratory distress syndrome (ARDS). Mouse models suggest that the lethal effect of viral pneumonia is more likely secondary to the host response than to a direct cytopathic result of viral replication.[9] Although not as common, viral invasion and replication can directly cause a necrotizing bronchopneumonia with inflammatory and exudative reactions.

Immunosuppression and Viral Infections

In the past few decades, the number of patients who are immunosuppressed has increased dramatically. This growth is largely secondary to the global epidemic of HIV, the development of more aggressive and successful chemotherapy regimens, and the progress of solid organ transplantation (SOT) and hematopoietic stem cell transplantation (HSCT).[10] Despite advances in treating infections and significant progress with new preventative techniques,[11] infection continues to be the leading cause of death in these populations. Patients who are immunocompromised have long been recognized as higher risk for viral pneumonia, including herpes simplex virus (HSV), varicella-zoster virus (VZV), cytomegalovirus, and measles. Over the past few decades, RSV, influenza, parainfluenza (PIV), adenovirus, picornavirus, and human metapneumovirus (hMPV) have also been recognized as causes of pneumonia in the immunocompromised population. In a study of viral infections in patient who had undergone HSCT, the incidence of influenza ranged from 14% to 52%, RSV from 14% to 48%, adenovirus from 2% to 21%, and PIV from 11% to 49% of all viral isolates.[12] The incidence and outcome of these viral pneumonias can vary significantly based on the intensity and duration of T-cell–mediated immune suppression.[11,13] Other factors in the pathogenesis of viral infections include stem cell product, donor–recipient matching and appropriate screening in both, composition of the conditioning regimen, and graft-versus-host disease.

Bacterial Superinfection

Although influenza and other viral pneumonias can themselves be fatal, a substantial number of viral pneumonia deaths result from secondary bacterial pneumonia.[7,14] The most common culprit is *Streptococcus pneumoniae*, followed by *Staphylococcus aureus* and *Hemophilus influenzae*.[14,15]

This lethal combination may be partially from the viral effects on the host, such as epithelial damage within the respiratory tract and changes in airway function. Influenza A infection, the most commonly studied virus in this area of research, can also alter the inflammatory and immune response. Both influenza and bacterial infections use similar pathways, cofactors, and intermediates, and the overlap in the inflammatory mediators produced may create an interference with or augmentation of the host immune response.[16] This alteration of the immune response contributes to the severity of the resulting infection either through diminishing the ability of the host to clear the bacteria or through amplification of the inflammatory cascade. The overwhelming inflammatory cascade is usually the culprit in rapidly progressive lower respiratory tract disease resulting in ARDS.[17,18]

CLINICAL MANIFESTATIONS

The presentation of viral pneumonia varies widely. Unfortunately, no clinical predictors reliably distinguish between viral and bacterial pneumonia.[4] Many patients with viral pneumonia present with dyspnea, cough, sputum production, and pleuritic chest pain. Other patients, especially those who are over age of 65 years old, lack any of the above symptoms and instead present with altered mental status or falls. In studies of patients who are elderly and frail, those with viral pneumonia more often present with cardiac disease, lower white blood cell and neutrophil counts, and less frequent chest pain and rigors.[19]

RADIOLOGIC FINDINGS

Viral pneumonia has a variety of radiographic presentations. Again, no findings reliably predict a specific pathogen or differentiate between viral and bacterial pneumonia. Despite this, two different pathologic processes are reflected in two common radiographic patterns: a slowly progressive, insidious course of pneumonia and a rapidly progressive or virulent pneumonia.[20] The insidious form is characterized by lymphatic infiltrates in the alveolar septa, which may extend to the areas adjacent to the terminal and respiratory bronchioles. On CT scan, well-defined nodules and patchy areas of peribronchial ground-glass opacity and air-space consolidation are seen. Because the viruses are intracellular, most of the pathologic changes tend to occur in the epithelium and adjacent interstitial tissue. In the rapidly progressive form, the underlying disease process is often diffuse alveolar hemorrhage and the infiltrate often extends to the interstitium and alveolar space. The chest radiograph often shows a rapid presentation of patchy unilateral or bilateral consolidations and ground-glass opacities. Poorly defined centrilobular nodules may also be present.

SPECIFIC VIRUSES
Influenza

Pathogenesis
Influenza viruses are the only paramyxoviruses capable of causing disease in humans. Influenza A, the most virulent subtype, possesses eight negative-sense RNA segments that encode 11 known proteins. Of these proteins, two large viral surface glycoproteins on the outside of the viral particles, hemagglutinin (HA) and neuraminidase (NA), form the basis of multiple serologically distinct subtypes. To initiate infection, HA binds to sialic acid residues on the respiratory epithelial cell surface glycoproteins.[21] Protease-mediated cleavage of HA results in its endocytosis, where the low pH of the endosome promotes uncoating of the virion and viral replication, eventually leading to the death of the epithelial cell.[22] Once viral replication occurs, progeny virions are bound to the host cell. NA cleaves the links between the virions and host cell.[23] Recently, 16 HA and 9 NA subtypes have been identified in wild water birds, the natural host for all influenza A viruses.[24]

Epidemiology
Influenza viruses have distinct outbreaks every year. Although both influenza A and influenza B cause infection, influenza A virus has a remarkable ability to undergo periodic changes in the antigenic characteristics of NA and HA. Influenza A viruses that infect humans are from three major subtypes of HA (H1, H2, H3) and two subtypes of NA (N1 and N2). When NA or HA undergo stepwise point mutations in the RNA gene segments as the virus replicates, antigenic drift occurs.[25] When two different viruses coinfect a single host, this host can act as a "mixing vessel" and a new virus is created by reassortment of the genomic segments.[26] Major changes such as these antigenic shifts can cause epidemics and pandemics.

Although infection can occur all year round in tropical regions, outbreaks of influenza in the northern and southern hemisphere are almost exclusively in the winter months. People at higher risk for influenza include those with known pulmonary or cardiovascular disease, diabetes, or renal disease; immunosuppressed individuals; nursing home or chronic care facility residents; or healthy individuals older than 50 years.[27]

Recent H1N1 outbreak
In late March 2009, an outbreak of a novel H1N1 influenza A virus was detected in Mexico.[28] This outbreak represented a rare quadruple reassortment of two swine strains, one human strain, and one avian strain of influenza.[29] As a result of airline travel, the pandemic spread rapidly. Using a modeling study, the Centers for Disease Control and Prevention (CDC) estimated 61 million cases, 274,000 hospitalizations, and 12,470 deaths occurred in the United States from April 2009 to April 2010.[30] Even though deaths during the pandemic were fewer than the number of influenza deaths during nonpandemic years, mortality disproportionately affected younger individuals.[31] A similar outbreak in 1957 may have provided preexisting immunity to protect the elderly people. Of those hospitalized, 70% had a known underlying high-risk condition,[32] including chronic lung disease (37%), immunosuppressive conditions (17%), pregnancy (17%), cardiac disease (17%), obesity (13%), and diabetes (13%).[27] Asthma was also prevalent among children and adults who were hospitalized.[33]

The 2009 novel H1N1 pandemic gave several important insights into influenza pneumonia. Previously, antiviral therapy was only recommended for patients with a recent onset of symptoms. Because most studies showed a significant survival benefit for early antiviral treatment,[32,34] antivirals were also recommended for those with suspected or confirmed H1N1 influenza A infection who were severely ill or had risk factors for a complicated course. The U.S. Food and Drug Administration (FDA) authorized emergency use of a new intravenous neuraminidase inhibitor, peramivir,[35] for patients unable to take inhaled or oral neuraminidase inhibitors, and possibly for those who experienced no response to other neuraminidase inhibitors. Now that the outbreak has ended, peramivir is no longer approved for use in patients with influenza. Because of the H1N1 epidemic, vaccination is now recommended for all individuals older than 6 months.

Corticosteroids were also studied during the recent pandemic. Two of the most recently published studies showed that corticosteroids were associated with higher mortality, especially when given early.[36,37] These patients tended to have longer duration of mechanical ventilation in addition to higher incidences of acquired pneumonia, including both secondary bacterial pneumonia and invasive fungal infection. These findings are consistent with the results of steroid treatment in severe acute respiratory syndrome (SARS) and avian influenza, suggesting that steroid treatment of acute lung injury caused by viral pneumonia may be contraindicated.

Clinical findings

After an incubation period of 1 or 2 days, influenza usually presents acutely with fever, headache, malaise, and myalgias along with cough and sore throat.[38] Pneumonia is the most common complication of influenza, but other complications include central nervous involvement, myocarditis, myositis, and rhabdomyolysis. Primary influenza pneumonia presents with dyspnea, persistent high fever, and significant hypoxia. Secondary bacterial pneumonia is a common complication of influenza and is responsible for 25% of all influenza deaths.[39] These patients usually present with recurrence of fever and new respiratory symptoms after the initial viral syndrome has begun to abate. Increasingly, concomitant influenza and bacterial pneumonia is being recognized, with a significantly higher mortality, especially with S aureus. S aureus can express cytotoxins, such as Panton-Valentin leukocidin, that have the ability to cause severe necrotizing pneumonia both directly through direct toxic activity and indirectly through the upregulation of surface proteins.[40] The mortality associated from the Panton-Valentin leukocidin–associated staphylococcal infection ranges from 56% to 61%. Myositis and rhabdomyolysis often present with significant tenderness of the muscles along with elevated creatine phosphokinase levels, myoglobinuria, and renal failure.[41] Central nervous involvement may include transverse myelitis,[41] Guillain-Barré syndrome,[41] aseptic meningitis,[41] and encephalitis.[41]

Diagnosis

In many circumstances, influenza can be diagnosed clinically, and diagnostic testing is unnecessary. Reverse transcriptase-polymerase chain reaction (RT-PCR) is the preferred method of diagnosis.[41] RT-PCR can also distinguish between different subtypes of influenza infection, which is important when different strains with different antiviral resistance patterns are both circulating. RT-PCR only takes 4 to 6 hours to run but may be delayed if not performed in-house. Although rapid antigen and immunofluorescence assays are useful if positive, the limited sensitivity of presently available tests does not warrant their use. Cultures are less sensitive and clearly delayed compared with RT-PCR.

Prevention

Vaccination is a major method of disease control during influenza season. The CDC regularly tracks influenza viral isolates throughout the world to monitor disease activity and predict components for the annual influenza vaccine that best match the circulating viruses for the next season.[42] As seen in the recent H1N1 pandemic, vaccine strains are chosen according to previous viral strains. Consequently, anticipating pandemics or epidemics created by large antigenic shifts can be difficult.

In 2010, new recommendations from the Advisory Committee on Immunization Practices (ACIP) included vaccination for all individuals older than 6 months,[43] expanding the previous recommendation of only individuals at high risk for influenza complications and people in close contact with those individuals.

The influenza vaccines licensed for use in the United States are the intramuscular trivalent inactivated influenza vaccine and an intranasal trivalent live, attenuated, cold-adapted influenza vaccine. The inactivated vaccine includes inactivated preparations of the whole virus or subvirion components (also called the "split product"). Only split product vaccines are available in the United States and are preferred for use of children younger than 12 years.[44] The live, attenuated intranasal vaccine should not be administered to patients who are immunosuppressed or pregnant; have a history of Guillain-Barré syndrome; or have cardiovascular, pulmonary, or metabolic disease[43]; or to household members or health care professionals in close contact with patients who are immunocompromised.[45] Neither vaccine should be given to individuals with history of anaphylaxis caused by eggs or other components of vaccine.[43]

In general, vaccine and placebo recipients report similar rates of fever, myalgias, fatigue, malaise, and headaches. Concern over an association between Guillain-Barré syndrome and influenza vaccine was highlighted with the A/New Jersey (swine) influenza vaccine administered in 1976.[46] Subsequent studies show a significant decline in the association between influenza inoculation and Guillain-Barré syndrome.[47]

Treatment

All patients with severe disease or high-risk status (**Box 1**) should be treated with antiviral therapy.[41,48] People with severe disease include those with evidence of LRTI or who are hospitalized.[49] Adults younger than 65 years without chronic medical conditions and only mild illness do not require testing, but treatment within 48 hours of their illness onset may reduce duration of symptoms.

Adamantanes

The adamantanes, amantadine and rimantadine, prevent viral replication through blocking the viral

---

Box 1
High-risk individuals with influenza infection

Age older than 65 years

Pregnant

Resident in a chronic care facility

Chronic medical conditions (renal failure, liver failure, cardiac disease, pulmonary disease, diabetes mellitus, malignancy, hemoglobinopathies)

Chronic immunosuppression

Neurologic disease (difficulty handling respiratory secretions)

M2 protein ion channel, preventing fusion of virus and host cell membranes.[50] The ACIP recommended against the routine use of adamantanes for influenza infection in 2008.[48] Amantadines are now recommended only for patients at risk of oseltamivir-resistant influenza and who have a contraindication to zanamivir therapy. Although side effects are not common for rimantadine, amantadine has significant central nervous system side effects (eg, nervousness, anxiety, insomnia, difficulty concentrating, lightheadedness).[51]

Neuraminidase inhibitors
The neuraminidase inhibitors, zanamivir and oseltamivir, selectively inhibit the neuraminidase of both influenza A and B viruses.[21] Neuraminidase inhibitors block the active sites of NA and leave uncleaved sialic acid residues on the surfaces of host cells and influenza viral envelopes. As a result, viral HA binding to the uncleaved sialic acid residues leads to viral aggregation at the host cell surface and a reduced release of virus.[52]

When administered within 24 to 48 hours, antivirals can reduce the duration of symptoms from 1 to 3 days.[53,54] In addition to shortening the duration of symptoms, early initiation of oseltamivir decreases overall mortality[32,55] and length of hospitalization in cases of severe influenza.[56] Zanamivir is available for oral inhalation, but intravenous administration is still being evaluated in clinical trials.[57] Because zanamivir induced bronchospasm and decreased lung function in some patients, it is contraindicated in patients with underlying asthma or other chronic respiratory conditions. Before 2007, resistance to oseltamivir occurred in 1% to 5% of patients.[58,59] Since 2007, several different outbreaks of oseltamivir-resistant influenza have occurred.[60,61] Patients who are immunocompromised seem to have a higher incidence of resistance, which is thought to result from prolonged viral shedding.[62]

PIV

PIVs are important respiratory viral pathogens with presentations ranging from mild upper respiratory tract infections in adults who are immunocompetent to life-threatening LRTIs in those who are immunocompromised. PIV-3, representing 52% of all PIV infections, and is endemic year-round.[63] PIV-1 and PIV-2 (representing 26% and 12% of all the PIV infections) tend to peak during the fall months. Although pneumonia is rare, infection usually recurs throughout adulthood and accounts for 1% to 15% of acute febrile respiratory illnesses. In a prospective study of the role of viruses in CAP since the advent of nucleic amplification tests, 3 of 75 (4%) of patients who had a pathogen identified were found to have PIV.[19] Despite the low incidence of pneumonia in the general adult population, PIV pneumonia commonly afflicts elderly people, especially nursing home residents.[64]

Among patients who are immunocompromised, PIV infection is known to cause significant morbidity and mortality.[65] For example, in a study of more than 1000 patients who underwent bone marrow transplants, although only 5.2% tested positive for PIV, 44% of these developed pneumonia, with a mortality of 37% (10 of 27 patients).[66] Glucocorticoids were associated with an increased risk of progression from upper to lower tract disease and mortality in patients who had undergone HSCT.[67] Lung transplant recipients are also prone to PIV infection, with an estimated incidence of 5.3 per every 100 patients,[68] with LRTIs in 10% to 66% of cases. Patients who have undergone lung transplants and acquire PIV have worse short- and long-term pulmonary dysfunction, along with more acute rejection episodes[68] and bronchiolitis obliterans.[69]

Because most of these studies involve inpatients, the incidence of PIV infection may be underestimated and severity may therefore be overestimated. However, outbreaks have been discovered among HSCT units, and asymptomatic shedding of HSCT recipients is common.[70,71] Therefore, nosocomial acquisition is a major concern.

Polymerase chain reaction (PCR), specifically multiplex PCR, is now the preferred method of testing, especially in the immunocompromised population. Compared with culture, RT-PCR enzyme hybridization assay shows 100% sensitivity (95% CI, 0.66–1.00) and 95% specificity (95% CI, 0.88–0.99).[72–74]

No treatment has proven efficacy for PIV infection. In patients who are immunosuppressed, the most common treatment is reduction of immunosuppression.[65] Aerosolized ribavirin with or without intravenous immunoglobulin in HSCT recipients did not change mortality or viral shedding from the nasopharynx with either treatment group.[67] An inhibitor of HA and NA and a recombinant sialidase fusion protein with potent in vitro and in vivo activity against PIV are being studied.[75,76]

RSV

Epidemiology

Although widely known to be the leading cause of LRTI among infants and children, RSV also causes significant LRTI among older children and adults, especially people who are elderly and immunocompromised.[61,77] Although mortality from RSV in children has declined, the number of hospitalizations climbs yearly; recent estimates are approximately 120,000 hospitalizations each year.[78] RSV infections are responsible for approximately 2700 deaths in adults and children every year.[77]

Direct contact is the most common form of transmission, but RSV can also be transmitted through large aerosol droplets.[79] In temperate climates, RSV typically peaks in winter months, whereas in tropical and semitropical climates, the outbreaks usually occur throughout the rainy season. Patients at risk for more severe infections include infants, children with comorbid conditions, institutionalized adults, and people who are immunosuppressed.[80–82]

Clinical findings

The clinical presentation of RSV infection varies significantly. Typically, younger children and infants with RSV infection develop LRTI symptoms, including pneumonia, bronchiolitis, or severe respiratory failure. Although LRTI is common with an individual's first RSV infection, it decreases with subsequent infections.[83] RSV infection can also alter the sensitivity of the laryngeal chemoreceptors and cause apnea in infants.[84] Almost 20% of infants who present with apnea are found to have RSV infection.[85] Upper respiratory tract infections are also common in children and adults,[86] with wheezing the most common presenting symptom.[61] Adults who are immunocompetent rarely develop pneumonia with RSV infection. Patients who are immunocompromised often present with pneumonia that may progress to respiratory failure. Although RSV infection can cause substantial mortality in patients who have undergone a bone marrow transplant, no long-term sequelae to RSV infection are found and pulmonary function returns to normal.[87]

Radiographic findings

In children, the radiographic appearance of RSV infection also varies. Controlling for several factors, including bacterial superinfection and age of child, the most common findings on chest radiograph are normal (30%), central pneumonia (32%), or peribronchitis (26%).[88] Less common findings are emphysema (11%), pleural effusion (6%), lobar- or broncho-pneumonia (each 6%), atelectasis (5%), or pneumothorax. In immuno-compromised patients, radiographic findings vary from ground-glass attenuation to tree-in-bud opacities to consolidation.

Diagnosis

In mild cases of RSV infection, the diagnosis can be made clinically. If hospitalization and treatment are necessary, diagnosis should be confirmed. In children, nasopharyngeal wash is preferred, although nasopharyngeal swab or throat culture is often adequate.[89] In patients who are intubated or immunocompromised, bronchoalveolar lavage provides the highest diagnostic yield.[90] Because the definitive diagnosis through isolation of the virus in HEp-2 cells can take weeks, multiplex PCR assay is preferred, especially in the immuno-compromised population.[91]

Treatment

The primary management of significant RSV infection is supportive care. If lower airway obstruction is present, a trial of β-agonist or aerosolized racemic epinephrine is recommended but should not be continued if no significant clinical improvement results. Although racemic epinephrine did not shorten hospital stay nor improve other comorbid conditions associated with bronchiolitis after hospital discharge, the medication improved respiratory distress.[92] Despite the potential benefit of decreased bronchiolar swelling and airway obstruction, corticosteroids have not been shown to benefit patients with bronchiolitis and are not recommended for infants with RSV bronchiolitis or pneumonia.[93,94] If RSV causes an asthma exacerbation in older children or adults, corticosteroid treatment is reasonable.

The FDA has approved ribavirin, a synthetic nucleoside analog administered through continuous aerosol, for the treatment of RSV infection. Although FDA-approved, routine use of nebulized ribavirin in infants and children with RSV is not recommended by the American Academy of Pediatrics (AAP). A beneficial effect of this therapy has not been proven and several studies show conflicting results.[95–97] Concerns for toxicity limit use, and ribavirin should never be administered to pregnant patients, and supportive staff working with the patient should not be pregnant. Intravenous immunoglobulin with high neutralizing activity against RSV or monoclonal antibody for infants or young children has no proven benefit with RSV infection.[74] Ribavirin and immunotherapy also have shown no substantial benefit in patients who are immunocompromised and severely ill with RSV infection.[84,98,99] Ribavirin may have the greatest potential benefit in preventing the progression of upper respiratory tract infection to LRTI.

Prevention

Intravenous immunoglobulin has been shown to be safe and effective in decreasing the severity of RSV infections.[100,101] The AAP now recommends that palivizumab, a humanized monoclonal antibody against the RSV F glycoprotein, be considered for infants and children at risk for severe RSV infection, including those with bronchopulmonary dysplasia, prematurity, and hemodynamically significant congenital heart disease.[102] Multiple factors have limited the development of more effective live, attenuated RSV vaccines, including potentiation of disease in people who have been vaccinated and subsequently become infected with wild-type virus.[103]

Adenovirus

Epidemiology

Adenovirus is the most common cause of pharyngitis and coryza in young children,[104] and causes 5% to 10% of all febrile illnesses in infants and young children.[105] Of all young children who contract adenovirus, 10% will develop pneumonia, most commonly with serotype 14.[106] Although most infections are self-limiting and mild, adenovirus also causes potentially fatal pneumonia in patients who are immunocompromised.[107] In a study of more than 200 of bone marrow transplant recipients, 20.9% had evidence of adenovirus infection and 6.2% developed invasive disease. The high incidence of adenovirus infection in this particular study may be secondary to more intensive immunosuppressive regimens.[108] Nonpneumonic disease, such as colitis, hepatitis, hemorrhagic cystitis, tubulointerstitial nephritis, encephalitis, or disseminated disease, can also be seen in patients who have undergone HSCT.[109,110] For patients who have undergone solid organ transplants, the most common presenting symptom for adenovirus infection is strongly associated with the transplanted organ (eg, liver transplant recipients present with hepatitis, lung transplant recipients with pneumonia).[111]

In the early 1950s to 1960s, almost 10% of all military recruits were infected with adenovirus, representing 90% of the pneumonia hospitalizations in that population.[112] As a result, all military recruits received oral, live enteric-coated vaccines starting in 1971. In 1996, the manufacturer of the vaccine ceased production and outbreaks of adenoviral respiratory illness reemerged, with approximately 10% of all recruits again ill with adenovirus infection. Efforts to contain the virus have not been successful.[112,113] Therefore, interest in vaccination has again increased. A double-blind placebo-controlled study of new live, oral, type 4 and type 7 adenovirus vaccines in adult military recruits found the vaccines to be safe and to induce an appropriate immune response. Further trials are in progress.[114]

Once again, PCR has become the diagnostic method of choice, replacing viral culture of a nasopharyngeal aspirate or swab, throat swab, or sputum.[115] Since adenoviral infection is usually self-limited, treatment is mostly supportive. Antiviral treatments are usually reserved for immunocompromised patients and those individuals with severe disease. Cidofovir, an acyclic nucleoside phosphonate with broad-spectrum activity against a wide variety of DNA viruses, has been tried.[116] Small studies have shown mixed results,[99,117] particularly with adenoviral pneumonia.[118] Combination with pooled intravenous immunoglobulin (IVIg) may be more effective.[119] Mortality was only 19% in patients who are severely immunocompromised with adenovirus infection treated with cidofovir and IVIg,[119] compared with the historical control mortality of 26% overall, with 73% mortality in patients with pneumonia.[120]

Rhinovirus

Rhinovirus is responsible for 30% of all upper respiratory tract infections, including a third to half of all colds in adults.[121,122] Rhinovirus is responsible for one to three respiratory illnesses per year in adults and four to eight per year in healthy children.[121] Although most often self-limited, rhinovirus can cause LRTIs, particularly in patients who are immunocompromised,[123] and can trigger asthma exacerbations.[124] Although aerosol transmission is possible, the most common mode of transmission is self-inoculation through the nose or conjunctival surfaces.[125]

Rhinovirus usually presents as the common cold, including cough, nasal discharge, and nasal obstruction.[126] In contrast to adults, children may have fever early in the illness. Symptoms in adults usually resolve within a week, whereas children often continue to report symptoms for at least 7 to 10 days.[127] Rhinovirus may significantly contribute to asthma exacerbations and wheezing in both children and young adults.[124] The virus is responsible for 15% of pneumonias within the first month of life[128] and is also very common in patients who are immunosuppressed.[123,129] Mortality as high as 32% has been reported in bone marrow transplant recipients.

In most cases, diagnosis is not necessary and patients are given supportive care. If diagnosis is necessary, PCR is the gold standard.[130] Viral culture is time-consuming and has poor sensitivity and specificity. Because of the multiplicity of serotypes, rapid antigen detection and serologic tests do not exist for rhinovirus infections.[131]

Treatment

Rhinovirus is usually self-limited and the mainstay of therapy usually includes rest, hydration, and nasal decongestants. In a double-blind, randomized, placebo-controlled trial of oral pleconaril for treatment of colds caused by picornaviruses in adults,[132] median time to alleviation of symptoms was found to be 1 day shorter compared with placebo. Prednisolone was also found to be promising for the treatment of rhinovirus infection. During a 2-month period after the first episodes of wheezing, prednisolone was found to reduce rhinovirus relapses.[133] A randomized double-blind study of a recombinant soluble intercellular adhesion molecule-1 (ICAM-1) administered intranasally sex times per day, beginning either 7 hours before or 12 hours after rhinovirus challenge,[134] showed no effect on the incidence of infection, although clinical colds, total symptoms score, and nasal secretion weight decreased. A virally encoded enzyme, 3C protease, which cleaves viral proteins from precursor polyproteins essential for the viral replication and virion assembly, is currently in phase II trials.[135] Although some of these treatments show promise, more studies must be completed, and standard treatment for rhinovirus remains supportive care.

hMPV

Although in retrospect hMPV has caused infection for the past 50 years, it was only recently discovered after successful isolation from symptomatic children in the Netherlands.[136] Because hMPV is only newly recognized, detailed data are limited. Although hMPV can cause upper respiratory tract infection and LRTIs in all age groups, symptomatic infection is most common in young children and older adults. In individuals with LRTIs, bronchiolitis (59%), croup (18%), asthma exacerbation (14%), and pneumonia (8%) are the most common presentations.[137,138] For adults, the most common presentations include cough (100%), nasal congestion (85%), rhinorrhea (75%), dyspnea (69%),

hoarseness (67%), and wheezing (62%). Despite usually being self-limiting, hMPV infection may account for the hospitalization of a significant portion of persons with respiratory infections.

Similar to the other viral infections, hMPV has more severe consequences in the immunocompromised population. In a prospective study of 251 patients with hematologic malignancies presenting with upper respiratory tract infections and LRTIs, 9% of the infections were associated with hMPV.[139] Of these, 16 of 22 occurred in patients who underwent HSCT. Only 9 of 251 (3.6%) had hMPV pneumonia but 3 died. Another retrospective study of HSCT patients found hMPV in the bronchoalveolar lavage of 5 of 163 patients (3%), and 4 of 5 patients died from overwhelming respiratory failure and shock. This study emphasized the importance of waiting for mild upper respiratory tract infections to clear before transplantation.[140]

hMPV can be isolated from viral culture but grows slowly and inefficiently. RT-PCR is the most sensitive method for diagnosing hMPV infection. Serology is another method of detection.[141]

Treatment of hMPV is supportive. Ribavirin has been shown to be active against hMPV in vitro[142] and in animal studies,[143] but efficacy in human subjects is unknown.

SARS Coronavirus

Epidemiology

The SARS coronavirus was discovered during the near-pandemic that infected 8096 individuals with 774 confirmed deaths between November 2002 and July 2003.[144] SARS is a highly contagious, severe, atypical pneumonia first noted in Guangdong Providence in Southern China. The index case for the epidemic was a physician who traveled to Hong Kong 5 days after the onset of his symptoms.[145] The virus spread rapidly from southern China and Hong Kong to Vietnam, Thailand, and Singapore, eventually spreading to Europe, Canada, and the United States. The virus was not identified as a new viral strain from the coronavirus family until February/March 2003.[146] After extraordinary efforts at containment, no new cases were identified after July 2003. Most of the patients were adults; health care workers accounted for nearly 23% of these cases, testifying to the high infectivity.[147] Since then, smaller outbreaks have occurred because of laboratory transmission and contact with animal sources.[148,149]

This SARS epidemic case-fatality rate was 9.6%.[144] Mortality was strongly associated with age: the estimated case fatality rate was 13.2% for patients younger than 60 years and 43.3% for patients aged 60 years or older.[150] Younger children (<12 years) had milder disease with no mortality.[151]

Because of the rapid and extensive spread of SARS, multiple modes of transmission, including droplet, airborne, and close contact, were suspected.[152] Environmental sampling showed that both air samples and swab samples from surfaces of a room containing a patient with SARS were PCR-positive.[153] Even the medication refrigerator door in the nursing station was PCR-positive. These findings stressed the need for adequate respiratory protection along with strict surface hygiene practices.

Clinical presentation

SARS is a respiratory viral disease with an atypical prolonged prodrome, most commonly presenting with fever, cough, chills, rigors, myalgias, dyspnea, and headache.[145,154] As the disease progresses, respiratory symptoms become more severe, often necessitating admission to the intensive care unit (ICU) and mechanical ventilation (approximately 26% of patients).[155] Death is most commonly attributable to ARDS and multiorgan failure.[145,156] Laboratory findings include lymphopenia, thrombocytopenia, elevated alanine aminotransferase, elevated C-reactive protein, and elevated lactate dehydrogenase.[147,154] Elevated lactate dehydrogenase is associated with poor outcome. Although chest radiographs often vary in appearance, the most common presentation is focal peripheral air-space disease with gradual resolution.[157] Even when initial chest radiographs are normal, CT scan usually shows parenchymal abnormalities.[158]

Diagnosis

Because of both limited sensitivity and specificity, positive RT-PCR from two separate samples (either two different sites or the same site on two different occasions) is recommended for diagnosis. The alternative is culture of the virus from any clinical specimen or detection of antibody by enzyme-linked immunosorbent assay or immunofluorescent assay. When SARS is suspected, initially negative RT-PCR should be repeated, because the sensitivity can be poor in the early stages of disease.[159] Although serologic testing is the most sensitive test available, several weeks are required before antibodies develop: the mean time to seroconversion is 19 to 20 days.[156,160] Because these tests can cross-react with other human coronaviruses, false-positive results are also seen.[161]

Treatment

Although several different treatments were tried during the recent epidemic, none were proven to have beneficial effect, including high-dose glucocorticoids and ribavirin.[162] Since the outbreak, lopinavir-ritonavir, interferon-α, and convalescent plasma have been tried in a smaller number of patients or in animal models without proven clinical efficacy.[163–165] Aggressive infection control standards were the key to control of the most recent epidemic. Vaccination and monoclonal antibodies are currently not ready for human subjects.[166–169] Concern that subsequent exposure to the SARS coronavirus after vaccination could lead to paradoxically severe disease may limit vaccination trials.

Varicella Pneumonia

Epidemiology

Varicella pneumonia is a rare complication in immunocompetent children. In adults, the reported incidence of varicella pneumonia is approximately 1 in every 400 cases.[170] Although the incidence of varicella pneumonia has decreased significantly since the introduction of the vaccine, most morbidity and mortality seen from varicella infection in adults are from pneumonia. The decrease in adult pneumonia is likely secondary to herd immunity from child immunization rather than adult immunization.[171] Despite the lower incidence, mortality from varicella pneumonia in immunocompetent individuals is staggering (up to 25%).[172] Risk factors for the development of varicella pneumonia include cigarette smoking, immunocompromised state, and pregnancy.[173–175] Overall, the severity of varicella pneumonia is highest in immunosuppressed individuals (mortality, 15%–18%) and in pregnant women in the second and third trimesters (mortality, 41%). Although only 0.1% of varicella infections develop in patients who are immunosuppressed, they accounted for approximately 25% of varicella-related deaths before the development of the vaccine.[176] The incidence and complication rates have decreased because of early initiation of acyclovir for high-risk individuals and vaccination of those in close contact with people who are immunosuppressed and were not candidates for varicella vaccination.[177]

Pathogenesis

VZV is a human herpesvirus that infects nearly all humans and causes chickenpox (varicella). Once a patient contracts chickenpox, VZV becomes latent in cranial nerve, dorsal root, and autonomic nervous system ganglia. Reactivation of the virus can produce shingles (herpes zoster), which is characterized by pain and rash.[178]

Clinical presentation

The varicella rash usually starts with fever along with a pruritic, vesicular rash commonly involving the mucosa.[179] Typically, varicella pneumonia develops 1 to 6 days after the appearance of the rash. Symptoms include progressive tachypnea, dry cough, and dyspnea. Patients often have progressive hypoxia with diffuse bilateral infiltrates.[180] In one of the rare times that radiographic pattern is diagnostic of the cause of pneumonia, nodular infiltrates can become calcified, especially in the early stages of disease.[181]

Although not more frequent, varicella pneumonia in pregnancy is considerably more severe than in nonpregnant women. Varicella in people who are immunocompromised is also similar to that in people who are immunocompetent, except in the severity of the infection. These patients are at increased risk for dissemination throughout their organs, disseminated intravascular coagulation, persistent development of new skin lesions for weeks, more severe vesicles becoming large and hemorrhagic, and, of course, increased risk of pneumonia.[182]

Diagnosis

Most cases of varicella infection (chicken pox and varicella zoster) are diagnosed clinically through the appearance of the typical vesicular rash at different stages. For varicella zoster, a painful, unilateral vesicular eruption usually occurs in a restricted dermatomal distribution. Further diagnostic testing is needed for an atypical rash or concern for disseminated disease in an immunocompromised host without typical cutaneous lesions. In these cases, PCR provides rapid and sensitive confirmation of VZV from clinical specimens obtained from skin lesions and body fluids, such as bronchoalveolar lavage.[183] The bronchoalveolar lavage may be most helpful in patients with pneumonia-like symptoms in whom the diagnosis of varicella has not been confirmed. Performing direct immunofluorescent test on the scrapings from active vesicular lesions is also a rapid helpful test to diagnose varicella.[184] Viral culture and serologic testing have not been found to be very helpful for diagnosis.

Treatment

Immediate treatment with intravenous acyclovir has been associated with improved outcomes.[180,185] Steroids have also been used for treatment but are controversial. In an uncontrolled study of patients in the ICU already on antiviral and antibiotic therapy,[186] those given steroids had shorter hospitalization (median difference, 10 days) and shorter ICU stay (median difference, 8 days) than historical controls.

Cytomegalovirus

Cytomegalovirus pneumonia is the most common viral pathogen in transplant recipients, acquired through either transfer of virus with the allograft or reactivation of the latent virus in the recipient, typically 1 to 3 months after transplantation. Incidence ranges from 1% to 9% of autologous HSCT recipients, 10% to 30% of allogeneic HSCT recipients,[187] and 15% to 55% of lung transplant recipients. Mortality is high, at 31% to 100% in HSCT recipients and 54% to 100% in solid organ transplant recipients. Patients who have undergone HSCT usually present after engraftment but can also present much later in disease. In patients who have undergone lung transplant, cytomegalovirus pneumonia develops 15 to 60 days posttransplant. In cases of cytomegalovirus donor-positive/recipient-negative patients, the progression of the infection is rapid.

Cytomegalovirus is also among the most frequent viruses detected among patients in the ICU who are not immunosuppressed. This occurrence was first documented in 1996 when autopsies and lung biopsies performed on patients with acute respiratory failure and possible ventilator-associated pneumonia showed that 25 of 86 of patients who were not immunocompromised had histologic findings compatible with cytomegalovirus lung disease.[188] Of course, viral detection does not necessarily correlate with viral disease, and this topic is still under much scrutiny.[189] Regardless, subsequent studies have shown enough evidence that an interventional randomized trial using anticytomegalovirus drugs would be warranted.

Although patients can be asymptomatic, common presenting symptoms usually include fever, dyspnea, nonproductive cough, and hypoxia. The most common chest CT scan findings of cytomegalovirus pneumonia are multiple, small centrilobular nodules, patchy ground-glass opacities, and small bilateral/asymmetric foci of consolidation.[190]

Cytomegalovirus pneumonia is established through the presence of viral inclusions on a cytologic or histologic specimen. Because the yield of these findings can be low, bronchoalveolar lavage fluid is often sent for rapid shell vial culture.

The primary treatment for acute cytomegalovirus pneumonia is ganciclovir (5 mg/kg intravenously every 12 hours for 14 to 21 days) followed by valganciclovir, 900 mg, orally daily for suppression.[191] An alternative agent is foscarnet.

Although evidence is lacking, high-dose intravenous immunoglobulin has been used successfully in conjunction with ganciclovir to treat cytomegalovirus pneumonia.[192]

Bocavirus

Bocavirus, a linear nonenveloped DNA virus, was newly discovered by Swedish scientists in 2005. Although the pathogenesis of the virus is unknown, bocavirus has been implicated in respiratory tract infections in adults, along with acute gastroenteritis in children and adults. Human bocavirus was detected through PCR in 4 of 273 respiratory samples of hospitalized adults.[193] Another study performed in children showed that 36 of 1539 respiratory specimens were positive for bocavirus. Although described in immunocompromised individuals, the incidence is not known.[194] In children, symptoms of bocavirus include cough, dyspnea, wheezing, rhinitis, fever, and diarrhea.[195] In adults, symptoms are similar to atypical pneumonia or acute bronchitis. Although limited by availability, most diagnoses are PCR-based.[196] Treatment is supportive care.

SUMMARY

Viruses cause a high percentage of community-acquired pneumonias. The advent of PCR and other molecular techniques has been associated with the detection of a higher prevalence of common respiratory viruses than previously suspected. Better diagnostics have shown new viral pathogens regularly in epidemics, immunocompromised patients, and occasionally children. Despite better diagnostics, treatment for all but influenza is still very limited.

REFERENCES

1. Heikkinen T, Jarvinen A. The common cold. Lancet 2003;361(9351):51–9.
2. Eccles R. Understanding the symptoms of the common cold and influenza. Lancet Infect Dis 2005;5(11):718–25.
3. Jennings GH. The clinical features of the pneumonias undergoing virus tests. Br Med J 1952;1(4750):123–9.
4. Jennings LC, Anderson TP, Beynon KA, et al. Incidence and characteristics of viral community-acquired pneumonia in adults. Thorax 2008;63(1):42–8.
5. de Roux A, Marcos MA, Garcia E, et al. Viral community-acquired pneumonia in nonimmunocompromised adults. Chest 2004;125(4):1343–51.
6. Niederman MS. Community-acquired pneumonia: the U.S. perspective. Semin Respir Crit Care Med 2009;30(2):179–88.
7. Irwin RS, Rippe JM. Irwin and Rippe's intensive care medicine. 6th edition. Philadelphia: Wolters Kluwer Health/Lippincott Williams & Wilkins; 2008.
8. Zhang Y, Hinojosa ME, Yoo N, et al. Viral and host strategies to take advantage of the innate immune response. Am J Respir Cell Mol Biol 2010;43(5):507–10.
9. Akaike T. Role of free radicals in viral pathogenesis and mutation. Rev Med Virol 2001;11(2):87–101.
10. Ison MG, Hayden FG. Viral infections in immunocompromised patients: what's new with respiratory viruses? Curr Opin Infect Dis 2002;15(4):355–67.
11. Fishman JA. Medical progress: infection in solid-organ transplant recipients. N Engl J Med 2007;357(25):2601–14.
12. Barton TD, Blumberg EA. Viral pneumonias other than cytomegalovirus in transplant recipients. Clin Chest Med 2005;26(4):707–20.
13. Dykewicz CA, Jaffe HW, Kaplan JE, et al. Guidelines for preventing opportunistic infections among hematopoietic stem cell transplant recipients: recommendations of CDC, the Infectious Diseases Society of America, and the American Society of Blood and Marrow Transplantation. Biol Blood Marrow Transplant 2000;6(6A):659–64.
14. McCullers JA. Insights into the interaction between influenza virus and pneumococcus. Clin Microbiol Rev 2006;19(3):571–82.
15. Sethi S. Bacterial pneumonia. Managing a deadly complication of influenza in older adults with co-morbid disease. Geriatrics 2002;57(3):56–61.
16. Shahangian A, Chow EK, Tian XL, et al. Type I IFNs mediate development of postinfluenza bacterial pneumonia in mice. J Clin Invest 2009;119(7):1910–20.
17. Bauer TT, Ewig S, Rodloff AC, et al. Acute respiratory distress syndrome and pneumonia: a comprehensive review of clinical data. Clin Infect Dis 2006;43(6):748–56.
18. Hagau N, Slavcovici A, Gonganau DN, et al. Clinical aspects and cytokine response in severe H1N1 influenza A virus infection. Crit Care 2010;14(6):R203.
19. Johnstone J, Majumdar SR, Fox JD, et al. Viral infection in adults hospitalized with community-acquired pneumonia: prevalence, pathogens, and presentation. Chest 2008;134(6):1141–8.
20. Kim EA, Lee KS, Primack SL, et al. Viral pneumonias in adults: radiologic and pathologic findings. Radiographics 2002;(Spec No)22:S137–49.
21. Moscona A. Neuraminidase inhibitors for influenza. N Engl J Med 2005;353(13):1363–73.
22. Steinhauer DA. Role of hemagglutinin cleavage for the pathogenicity of influenza virus. Virology 1999;258(1):1–20.

23. Gubareva LV, Kaiser L, Hayden FG. Influenza virus neuraminidase inhibitors. Lancet 2000;355(9206): 827–35.

24. Gorbach SL, Bartlett JG, Blacklow NR. Infectious diseases. 3rd edition. Philadelphia: Lippincott Williams & Wilkins; 2004.

25. Webster RG, Kendal AP, Gerhard W. Analysis of antigenic drift in recently isolated influenza A (H1N1) viruses using monoclonal antibody preparations. Virology 1979;96(1):258–64.

26. Webster RG, Wright SM, Castrucci MR, et al. Influenza—a model of an emerging virus disease. Intervirology 1993;35(1–4):16–25.

27. Centers for Disease Control and Prevention (CDC). Hospitalized patients with novel influenza A (H1N1) virus infection—California, April–May, 2009. MMWR Morb Mortal Wkly Rep 2009;58(19): 536–41.

28. Centers for Disease Control and Prevention (CDC). Outbreak of swine-origin influenza A (H1N1) virus infection—Mexico, March–April 2009. MMWR Morb Mortal Wkly Rep 2009;58(17):467–70.

29. Khanna M, Kumar B, Gupta N, et al. Pandemic swine influenza virus (H1N1): a threatening evolution. Indian J Microbiol 2009;49(4):365–9.

30. Shrestha SS, Swerdlow DL, Borse RH, et al. Estimating the burden of 2009 pandemic influenza A (H1N1) in the United States (April 2009–April 2010). Clin Infect Dis 2011;52(Suppl 1):S75–82.

31. Viboud C, Miller M, Olson D, et al. Preliminary Estimates of Mortality and Years of Life Lost Associated with the 2009 A/H1N1 Pandemic in the US and Comparison with Past Influenza Seasons. Version 59. PLoS Currents: Influenza. 2010.

32. Jain S, Kamimoto L, Bramley AM, et al. Hospitalized patients with 2009 H1N1 influenza in the United States, April–June 2009. N Engl J Med 2009;361(20):1935–44.

33. Centers for Disease Control and Prevention (CDC). Patients hospitalized with 2009 pandemic influenza A (H1N1)—New York City, May 2009. MMWR Morb Mortal Wkly Rep 2010;58(51):1436–40.

34. Siston AM, Rasmussen SA, Honein MA, et al. Pandemic 2009 influenza A(H1N1) virus illness among pregnant women in the United States. JAMA 2010;303(15):1517–25.

35. Mancuso CE, Gabay MP, Steinke LM, et al. Peramivir: an intravenous neuraminidase inhibitor for the treatment of 2009 H1N1 influenza. Ann Pharmacother 2010;44(7–8):1240–9.

36. Kim SH, Hong SB, Yun SC, et al. Corticosteroid treatment in critically Ill patients with pandemic influenza A/H1N1 2009 infection: analytic strategy using propensity scores. Am J Respir Crit Care Med 2011;183(9):1207–14.

37. Brun-Buisson C, Richard JC, Mercat A, et al. Early corticosteroids in severe influenza A/H1N1 pneumonia and acute respiratory distress syndrome. Am J Respir Crit Care Med 2011;183(9): 1200–6.

38. Zuckerman AJ. Principles and practice of clinical virology. 6th edition. Chichester (United Kingdom): John Wiley & Sons; 2009.

39. Simonsen L. The global impact of influenza on morbidity and mortality. Vaccine 1999;17(Suppl 1): S3–10.

40. Gillet Y, Vanhems P, Lina G, et al. Factors predicting mortality in necrotizing community-acquired pneumonia caused by Staphylococcus aureus containing Panton-Valentine leukocidin. Clin Infect Dis 2007;45(3):315–21.

41. Harper SA, Bradley JS, Englund JA, et al. Seasonal influenza in adults and children–diagnosis, treatment, chemoprophylaxis, and institutional outbreak management: clinical practice guidelines of the Infectious Diseases Society of America. Clin Infect Dis 2009;48(8):1003–32.

42. Glezen WP. Clinical practice. Prevention and treatment of seasonal influenza. N Engl J Med 2008; 359(24):2579–85.

43. Fiore AE, Uyeki TM, Broder K, et al. Prevention and control of influenza with vaccines: recommendations of the Advisory Committee on Immunization Practices (ACIP), 2010. MMWR Recomm Rep 2010;59(RR-8):1–62.

44. Belshe RB, Edwards KM, Vesikari T, et al. Live attenuated versus inactivated influenza vaccine in infants and young children. N Engl J Med 2007; 356(7):685–96.

45. Kamboj M, Sepkowitz KA. Risk of transmission associated with live attenuated vaccines given to healthy persons caring for or residing with an immunocompromised patient. Infect Control Hosp Epidemiol 2007;28(6):702–7.

46. Lehmann HC, Hartung HP, Kieseier BC, et al. Guillain-Barré syndrome after exposure to influenza virus. Lancet Infect Dis 2010;10(9):643–51.

47. Haber P, DeStefano F, Angulo FJ, et al. Guillain-Barré syndrome following influenza vaccination. JAMA 2004;292(20):2478–81.

48. Fiore AE, Shay DK, Broder K, et al. Prevention and control of influenza: recommendations of the Advisory Committee on Immunization Practices (ACIP), 2008. MMWR Recomm Rep 2008;57(RR-7):1–60.

49. Updated interim recommendations for the use of antiviral medications in the treatment and prevention of influenza for the 2009–2010 season. Centers for Disease Control and Prevention Web site. Available at: http://www.cdc.gov/h1n1flu/recommendations. htm. Accessed January 15, 2011.

50. Weinstock DM, Zuccotti G. Adamantane resistance in influenza A. JAMA 2006;295(8):934–6.

51. Dolin R, Reichman RC, Madore HP, et al. A controlled trial of amantadine and rimantadine

in the prophylaxis of influenza A infection. N Engl J Med 1982;307(10):580–4.

52. Palese P, Compans RW. Inhibition of influenza virus replication in tissue culture by 2-deoxy-2,3-dehydro-N-trifluoroacetylneuraminic acid (FANA): mechanism of action. J Gen Virol 1976;33(1):159–63.

53. Hayden FG, Osterhaus AD, Treanor JJ, et al. Efficacy and safety of the neuraminidase inhibitor zanamivir in the treatment of influenzavirus infections. GG167 Influenza Study Group. N Engl J Med 1997;337(13):874–80.

54. Jefferson T, Jones M, Doshi P, et al. Neuraminidase inhibitors for preventing and treating influenza in healthy adults: systematic review and meta-analysis. BMJ 2009;339:b5106.

55. McGeer A, Green KA, Plevneshi A, et al. Antiviral therapy and outcomes of influenza requiring hospitalization in Ontario, Canada. Clin Infect Dis 2007; 45(12):1568–75.

56. Lee N, Chan PK, Choi KW, et al. Factors associated with early hospital discharge of adult influenza patients. Antivir Ther 2007;12(4):501–8.

57. Calfee DP, Peng AW, Cass LM, et al. Safety and efficacy of intravenous zanamivir in preventing experimental human influenza A virus infection. Antimicrob Agents Chemother 1999;43(7):1616–20.

58. Hayden FG, Pavia AT. Antiviral management of seasonal and pandemic influenza. J Infect Dis 2006;194(Suppl 2):S119–26.

59. Kiso M, Mitamura K, Sakai-Tagawa Y, et al. Resistant influenza A viruses in children treated with oseltamivir: descriptive study. Lancet 2004; 364(9436):759–65.

60. Influenza A (H1N1) virus resistance to oseltamivir. World Health Organization Web site. Available at: http://www.who.int/csr/disease/influenza/h1n1_table/en/index.html. Accessed January 15, 2011.

61. Falsey AR, Walsh EE. Respiratory syncytial virus infection in adults. Clin Microbiol Rev 2000;13(3): 371–84.

62. Ison MG, Gubareva LV, Atmar RL, et al. Recovery of drug-resistant influenza virus from immunocompromised patients: a case series. J Infect Dis 2006;193(6):760–4.

63. Hall CB. Respiratory syncytial virus and parainfluenza virus. N Engl J Med 2001;344(25):1917–28.

64. Parainfluenza infections in the elderly 1976–82. Br Med J (Clin Res Ed) 1983;287(6405):1619.

65. Ison MG. Respiratory viral infections in transplant recipients. Antivir Ther 2007;12(4 Pt B):627–38.

66. Lewis VA, Champlin R, Englund J, et al. Respiratory disease due to parainfluenza virus in adult bone marrow transplant recipients. Clin Infect Dis 1996; 23(5):1033–7.

67. Nichols WG, Corey L, Gooley T, et al. Parainfluenza virus infections after hematopoietic stem cell transplantation: risk factors, response to antiviral therapy, and effect on transplant outcome. Blood 2001;98(3):573–8.

68. Vilchez RA, Dauber J, McCurry K, et al. Parainfluenza virus infection in adult lung transplant recipients: an emergent clinical syndrome with implications on allograft function. Am J Transplant 2003;3(2):116–20.

69. Billings JL, Hertz MI, Savik K, et al. Respiratory viruses and chronic rejection in lung transplant recipients. J Heart Lung Transplant 2002;21(5): 559–66.

70. Nichols WG, Erdman DD, Han A, et al. Prolonged outbreak of human parainfluenza virus 3 infection in a stem cell transplant outpatient department: insights from molecular epidemiologic analysis. Biol Blood Marrow Transplant 2004;10(1):58–64.

71. Zambon M, Bull T, Sadler CJ, et al. Molecular epidemiology of two consecutive outbreaks of parainfluenza 3 in a bone marrow transplant unit. J Clin Microbiol 1998;36(8):2289–93.

72. Fan J, Henrickson KJ. Rapid diagnosis of human parainfluenza virus type 1 infection by quantitative reverse transcription-PCR-enzyme hybridization assay. J Clin Microbiol 1996;34(8):1914–7.

73. Fan J, Henrickson KJ, Savatski LL. Rapid simultaneous diagnosis of infections with respiratory syncytial viruses A and B, influenza viruses A and B, and human parainfluenza virus types 1, 2, and 3 by multiplex quantitative reverse transcription-polymerase chain reaction-enzyme hybridization assay (Hexaplex). Clin Infect Dis 1998;26(6):1397–402.

74. Fuller H, Del Mar C. Immunoglobulin treatment for respiratory syncytial virus infection. Cochrane Database Syst Rev 2006;4:CD004883.

75. Alymova IV, Taylor G, Takimoto T, et al. Efficacy of novel hemagglutinin-neuraminidase inhibitors BCX 2798 and BCX 2855 against human parainfluenza viruses in vitro and in vivo. Antimicrob Agents Chemother 2004;48(5):1495–502.

76. Moscona A, Porotto M, Palmer S, et al. A recombinant sialidase fusion protein effectively inhibits human parainfluenza viral infection in vitro and in vivo. J Infect Dis 2010;202(2):234–41.

77. Thompson WW, Shay DK, Weintraub E, et al. Mortality associated with influenza and respiratory syncytial virus in the United States. JAMA 2003; 289(2):179–86.

78. Shay DK, Holman RC, Roosevelt GE, et al. Bronchiolitis-associated mortality and estimates of respiratory syncytial virus-associated deaths among US children, 1979–1997. J Infect Dis 2001;183(1): 16–22.

79. Hall CB, Douglas RG Jr, Geiman JM. Quantitative shedding patterns of respiratory syncytial virus in infants. J Infect Dis 1975;132(2):151–6.

80. Whimbey E, Couch RB, Englund JA, et al. Respiratory syncytial virus pneumonia in hospitalized adult

patients with leukemia. Clin Infect Dis 1995;21(2): 376–9.

81. Wald TG, Miller BA, Shult P, et al. Can respiratory syncytial virus and influenza A be distinguished clinically in institutionalized older persons? J Am Geriatr Soc 1995;43(2):170–4.

82. McCarthy AJ, Kingman HM, Kelly C, et al. The outcome of 26 patients with respiratory syncytial virus infection following allogeneic stem cell transplantation. Bone Marrow Transplant 1999;24(12): 1315–22.

83. Glezen WP, Taber LH, Frank AL, et al. Risk of primary infection and reinfection with respiratory syncytial virus. Am J Dis Child 1986;140(6):543–6.

84. Glanville AR, Scott AI, Morton JM, et al. Intravenous ribavirin is a safe and cost-effective treatment for respiratory syncytial virus infection after lung transplantation. J Heart Lung Transplant 2005;24(12): 2114–9.

85. Bruhn FW, Mokrohisky ST, McIntosh K. Apnea associated with respiratory syncytial virus infection in young infants. J Pediatr 1977;90(3):382–6.

86. Hall CB, Long CE, Schnabel KC. Respiratory syncytial virus infections in previously healthy working adults. Clin Infect Dis 2001;33(6):792–6.

87. Wendt CH, Fox JM, Hertz MI. Paramyxovirus infection in lung transplant recipients. J Heart Lung Transplant 1995;14(3):479–85.

88. Kern S, Uhl M, Berner R, et al. Respiratory syncytial virus infection of the lower respiratory tract: radiological findings in 108 children. Eur Radiol 2001; 11(12):2581–4.

89. Ahluwalia G, Embree J, McNicol P, et al. Comparison of nasopharyngeal aspirate and nasopharyngeal swab specimens for respiratory syncytial virus diagnosis by cell culture, indirect immunofluorescence assay, and enzyme-linked immunosorbent assay. J Clin Microbiol 1987; 25(5):763–7.

90. Englund JA, Piedra PA, Jewell A, et al. Rapid diagnosis of respiratory syncytial virus infections in immunocompromised adults. J Clin Microbiol 1996;34(7):1649–53.

91. Puppe W, Weigl JA, Aron G, et al. Evaluation of a multiplex reverse transcriptase PCR ELISA for the detection of nine respiratory tract pathogens. J Clin Virol 2004;30(2):165–74.

92. Langley JM, Smith MB, LeBlanc JC, et al. Racemic epinephrine compared to salbutamol in hospitalized young children with bronchiolitis; a randomized controlled clinical trial [ISRCTN46561076]. BMC Pediatr 2005;5(1):7.

93. Patel H, Platt R, Lozano JM, et al. Glucocorticoids for acute viral bronchiolitis in infants and young children. Cochrane Database Syst Rev 2004;3:CD004878.

94. King VJ, Viswanathan M, Bordley WC, et al. Pharmacologic treatment of bronchiolitis in infants and children: a systematic review. Arch Pediatr Adolesc Med 2004;158(2):127–37.

95. Meert KL, Sarnaik AP, Gelmini MJ, et al. Aerosolized ribavirin in mechanically ventilated children with respiratory syncytial virus lower respiratory tract disease: a prospective, double-blind, randomized trial. Crit Care Med 1994;22(4):566–72.

96. Guerguerian AM, Gauthier M, Lebel MH, et al. Ribavirin in ventilated respiratory syncytial virus bronchiolitis. A randomized, placebo-controlled trial. Am J Respir Crit Care Med 1999;160(3):829–34.

97. Smith DW, Frankel LR, Mathers LH, et al. A controlled trial of aerosolized ribavirin in infants receiving mechanical ventilation for severe respiratory syncytial virus infection. N Engl J Med 1991; 325(1):24–9.

98. Ghosh S, Champlin RE, Englund J, et al. Respiratory syncytial virus upper respiratory tract illnesses in adult blood and marrow transplant recipients: combination therapy with aerosolized ribavirin and intravenous immunoglobulin. Bone Marrow Transplant 2000;25(7):751–5.

99. Ljungman P, Ribaud P, Eyrich M, et al. Cidofovir for adenovirus infections after allogeneic hematopoietic stem cell transplantation: a survey by the Infectious Diseases Working Party of the European Group for Blood and Marrow Transplantation. Bone Marrow Transplant 2003;31(6):481–6.

100. Meissner HC, Fulton DR, Groothuis JR, et al. Controlled trial to evaluate protection of high-risk infants against respiratory syncytial virus disease by using standard intravenous immune globulin. Antimicrob Agents Chemother 1993;37(8):1655–8.

101. Groothuis JR, Levin MJ, Rodriguez W, et al. Use of intravenous gamma-globulin to passively immunize high-risk children against respiratory syncytial virus: safety and pharmacokinetics. Antimicrob Agents Chemother 1991;35(7):1469–73.

102. Committee on Infectious Diseases. From the American Academy of Pediatrics: policy statements—modified recommendations for use of palivizumab for prevention of respiratory syncytial virus infections. Pediatrics 2009;124(6):1694–701.

103. Polack FP, Teng MN, Collins PL, et al. A role for immune complexes in enhanced respiratory syncytial virus disease. J Exp Med 2002;196(6): 859–65.

104. Pacini DL, Collier AM, Henderson FW. Adenovirus infections and respiratory illnesses in children in group day care. J Infect Dis 1987;156(6):920–7.

105. Fox JP, Hall CE, Cooney MK. The Seattle Virus Watch. VII. Observations of adenovirus infections. Am J Epidemiol 1977;105(4):362–86.

106. Wen CC, Kuo YH, Jan JT, et al. Specific plant terpenoids and lignoids possess potent antiviral activities against severe acute respiratory syndrome coronavirus. J Med Chem 2007;50(17):4087–95.

107. Kojaoghlanian T, Flomenberg P, Horwitz MS. The impact of adenovirus infection on the immunocompromised host. Rev Med Virol 2003;13(3):155–71.

108. Flomenberg P, Babbitt J, Drobyski WR, et al. Increasing incidence of adenovirus disease in bone marrow transplant recipients. J Infect Dis 1994;169(4):775–81.

109. Ison MG. Adenovirus infections in transplant recipients. Clin Infect Dis 2006;43(3):331–9.

110. Shields AF, Hackman RC, Fife KH, et al. Adenovirus infections in patients undergoing bone-marrow transplantation. N Engl J Med 1985; 312(9):529–33.

111. Ohori NP, Michaels MG, Jaffe R, et al. Adenovirus pneumonia in lung transplant recipients. Hum Pathol 1995;26(10):1073–9.

112. Centers for Disease Control and Prevention. Two fatal cases of adenovirus-related illness in previously healthy young adults—Illinois, 2000. MMWR Morb Mortal Wkly Rep 2001;50(26):553–5.

113. Trei JS, Johns NM, Garner JL, et al. Spread of adenovirus to geographically dispersed military installations, 2007. Emerg Infect Dis 2010;16(5): 769–75.

114. Lyons A, Longfield J, Kuschner R, et al. A double-blind, placebo-controlled study of the safety and immunogenicity of live, oral type 4 and type 7 adenovirus vaccines in adults. Vaccine 2008; 26(23):2890–8.

115. Heim A, Ebnet C, Harste G, et al. Rapid and quantitative detection of human adenovirus DNA by real-time PCR. J Med Virol 2003;70(2):228–39.

116. De Clercq E. Therapeutic potential of Cidofovir (HPMPC, Vistide) for the treatment of DNA virus (i.e. herpes-, papova-, pox- and adenovirus) infections. Verh K Acad Geneeskd Belg 1996;58(1): 19–47.

117. Doan ML, Mallory GB, Kaplan SL, et al. Treatment of adenovirus pneumonia with cidofovir in pediatric lung transplant recipients. J Heart Lung Transplant 2007;26(9):883–9.

118. Symeonidis N, Jakubowski A, Pierre-Louis S, et al. Invasive adenoviral infections in T-cell-depleted allogeneic hematopoietic stem cell transplantation: high mortality in the era of cidofovir. Transpl Infect Dis 2007;9(2):108–13.

119. Neofytos D, Ojha A, Mookerjee B, et al. Treatment of adenovirus disease in stem cell transplant recipients with cidofovir. Biol Blood Marrow Transplant 2007;13(1):74–81.

120. La Rosa AM, Champlin RE, Mirza N, et al. Adenovirus infections in adult recipients of blood and marrow transplants. Clin Infect Dis 2001;32(6): 871–6.

121. Monto AS, Ullman BM. Acute respiratory illness in an American community. The Tecumseh study. JAMA 1974;227(2):164–9.

122. Hendley JO. The host response, not the virus, causes the symptoms of the common cold. Clin Infect Dis 1998;26(4):847–8.

123. Ghosh S, Champlin R, Couch R, et al. Rhinovirus infections in myelosuppressed adult blood and marrow transplant recipients. Clin Infect Dis 1999; 29(3):528–32.

124. Heymann PW, Platts-Mills TA, Johnston SL. Role of viral infections, atopy and antiviral immunity in the etiology of wheezing exacerbations among children and young adults. Pediatr Infect Dis J 2005; 24(Suppl 11):S217–22 [discussion: S220–1].

125. Hendley JO. Clinical virology of rhinoviruses. Adv Virus Res 1999;54:453–66.

126. Pappas DE, Hendley JO, Hayden FG, et al. Symptom profile of common colds in school-aged children. Pediatr Infect Dis J 2008;27(1):8–11.

127. Gwaltney JM Jr, Hendley JO, Simon G, et al. Rhinovirus infections in an industrial population. II. Characteristics of illness and antibody response. JAMA 1967;202(6):494–500.

128. Abzug MJ, Beam AC, Gyorkos EA, et al. Viral pneumonia in the first month of life. Pediatr Infect Dis J 1990;9(12):881–5.

129. Malcolm E, Arruda E, Hayden FG, et al. Clinical features of patients with acute respiratory illness and rhinovirus in their bronchoalveolar lavages. J Clin Virol 2001;21(1):9–16.

130. Gambarino S, Costa C, Elia M, et al. Development of a RT real-time PCR for the detection and quantification of human rhinoviruses. Mol Biotechnol 2009;42(3):350–7.

131. Makela MJ, Puhakka T, Ruuskanen O, et al. Viruses and bacteria in the etiology of the common cold. J Clin Microbiol 1998;36(2):539–42.

132. Hayden FG, Herrington DT, Coats TL, et al. Efficacy and safety of oral pleconaril for treatment of colds due to picornaviruses in adults: results of 2 double-blind, randomized, placebo-controlled trials. Clin Infect Dis 2003;36(12):1523–32.

133. Jartti T, Lehtinen P, Vanto T, et al. Evaluation of the efficacy of prednisolone in early wheezing induced by rhinovirus or respiratory syncytial virus. Pediatr Infect Dis J 2006;25(6):482–8.

134. Turner RB, Wecker MT, Pohl G, et al. Efficacy of tremacamra, a soluble intercellular adhesion molecule 1, for experimental rhinovirus infection: a randomized clinical trial. JAMA 1999;281(19):1797–804.

135. McKinlay MA. Recent advances in the treatment of rhinovirus infections. Curr Opin Pharmacol 2001; 1(5):477–81.

136. van den Hoogen BG, de Jong JC, Groen J, et al. A newly discovered human pneumovirus isolated from young children with respiratory tract disease. Nat Med 2001;7(6):719–24.

137. Esper F, Martinello RA, Boucher D, et al. A 1-year experience with human metapneumovirus in

children aged <5 years. J Infect Dis 2004;189(8): 1388–96.

138. Williams JV, Harris PA, Tollefson SJ, et al. Human metapneumovirus and lower respiratory tract disease in otherwise healthy infants and children. N Engl J Med 2004;350(5):443–50.

139. Williams JV, Martino R, Rabella N, et al. A prospective study comparing human metapneumovirus with other respiratory viruses in adults with hematologic malignancies and respiratory tract infections. J Infect Dis 2005;192(6):1061–5.

140. Englund JA, Boeckh M, Kuypers J, et al. Brief communication: fatal human metapneumovirus infection in stem-cell transplant recipients. Ann Intern Med 2006;144(5):344–9.

141. Falsey AR, Erdman D, Anderson LJ, et al. Human metapneumovirus infections in young and elderly adults. J Infect Dis 2003;187(5):785–90.

142. Wyde PR, Chetty SN, Jewell AM, et al. Comparison of the inhibition of human metapneumovirus and respiratory syncytial virus by ribavirin and immune serum globulin in vitro. Antiviral Res 2003;60(1):51–9.

143. Hamelin ME, Prince GA, Boivin G. Effect of ribavirin and glucocorticoid treatment in a mouse model of human metapneumovirus infection. Antimicrob Agents Chemother 2006;50(2):774–7.

144. World Health Organization. Summary of probable SARS cases with onset of illness from 1 November 2002 to 31 July 2003 (based on data as of the 31 December 2003). World Health Organization Web site. Available at: http://www.who.int/csr/sars/country/table2004_04_21/en/index.html. Accessed January 15, 2011.

145. Tsang KW, Ho PL, Ooi GC, et al. A cluster of cases of severe acute respiratory syndrome in Hong Kong. N Engl J Med 2003;348(20):1977–85.

146. Ksiazek TG, Erdman D, Goldsmith CS, et al. A novel coronavirus associated with severe acute respiratory syndrome. N Engl J Med 2003; 348(20):1953–66.

147. Leung GM, Hedley AJ, Ho LM, et al. The epidemiology of severe acute respiratory syndrome in the 2003 Hong Kong epidemic: an analysis of all 1755 patients. Ann Intern Med 2004;141(9):662–73.

148. Liang G, Chen Q, Xu J, et al. Laboratory diagnosis of four recent sporadic cases of community-acquired SARS, Guangdong Province, China. Emerg Infect Dis 2004;10(10):1774–81.

149. Wang M, Yan M, Xu H, et al. SARS-CoV infection in a restaurant from palm civet. Emerg Infect Dis 2005;11(12):1860–5.

150. Donnelly CA, Ghani AC, Leung GM, et al. Epidemiological determinants of spread of causal agent of severe acute respiratory syndrome in Hong Kong. Lancet 2003;361(9371):1761–6.

151. Snider MT, Campbell DB, Kofke WA, et al. Venovenous perfusion of adults and children with severe acute respiratory distress syndrome. The Pennsylvania State University experience from 1982–1987. ASAIO Trans 1988;34(4):1014–20.

152. Poutanen SM, Low DE, Henry B, et al. Identification of severe acute respiratory syndrome in Canada. N Engl J Med 2003;348(20):1995–2005.

153. Booth TF, Kournikakis B, Bastien N, et al. Detection of airborne severe acute respiratory syndrome (SARS) coronavirus and environmental contamination in SARS outbreak units. J Infect Dis 2005; 191(9):1472–7.

154. Christian MD, Poutanen SM, Loutfy MR, et al. Severe acute respiratory syndrome. Clin Infect Dis 2004;38(10):1420–7.

155. Chan JW, Ng CK, Chan YH, et al. Short term outcome and risk factors for adverse clinical outcomes in adults with severe acute respiratory syndrome (SARS). Thorax 2003;58(8):686–9.

156. Peiris JS, Chu CM, Cheng VC, et al. Clinical progression and viral load in a community outbreak of coronavirus-associated SARS pneumonia: a prospective study. Lancet 2003;361(9371):1767–72.

157. Bitar R, Weiser WJ, Avendano M, et al. Chest radiographic manifestations of severe acute respiratory syndrome in health care workers: the Toronto experience. AJR Am J Roentgenol 2004;182(1):45–8.

158. Muller NL, Ooi GC, Khong PL, et al. Severe acute respiratory syndrome: radiographic and CT findings. AJR Am J Roentgenol 2003;181(1):3–8.

159. Tang P, Louie M, Richardson SE, et al. Interpretation of diagnostic laboratory tests for severe acute respiratory syndrome: the Toronto experience. CMAJ 2004;170(1):47–54.

160. Chen X, Zhou B, Li M, et al. Serology of severe acute respiratory syndrome: implications for surveillance and outcome. J Infect Dis 2004;189(7): 1158–63.

161. Chan KH, Cheng VC, Woo PC, et al. Serological responses in patients with severe acute respiratory syndrome coronavirus infection and cross-reactivity with human coronaviruses 229E, OC43, and NL63. Clin Diagn Lab Immunol 2005;12(11):1317–21.

162. Stockman LJ, Bellamy R, Garner P. SARS: systematic review of treatment effects. PLoS Med 2006; 3(9):1525–31.

163. Groneberg DA, Poutanen SM, Low DE, et al. Treatment and vaccines for severe acute respiratory syndrome. Lancet Infect Dis 2005;5(3):147–55.

164. Loutfy MR, Blatt LM, Siminovitch KA, et al. Interferon alfacon-1 plus corticosteroids in severe acute respiratory syndrome: a preliminary study. JAMA 2003;290(24):3222–8.

165. Wong VW, Dai D, Wu AK, et al. Treatment of severe acute respiratory syndrome with convalescent plasma. Hong Kong Med J 2003;9(3):199–201.

166. Enjuanes L, Dediego ML, Alvarez E, et al. Vaccines to prevent severe acute respiratory syndrome

coronavirus-induced disease. Virus Res 2008; 133(1):45–62.

167. Sui J, Li W, Murakami A, et al. Potent neutralization of severe acute respiratory syndrome (SARS) coronavirus by a human mAb to S1 protein that blocks receptor association. Proc Natl Acad Sci U S A 2004;101(8):2536–41.

168. Bian C, Zhang X, Cai X, et al. Conserved amino acids W423 and N424 in receptor-binding domain of SARS-CoV are potential targets for therapeutic monoclonal antibody. Virology 2009;383(1):39–46.

169. Yasui F, Kai C, Kitabatake M, et al. Prior immunization with severe acute respiratory syndrome (SARS)-associated coronavirus (SARS-CoV) nucleocapsid protein causes severe pneumonia in mice infected with SARS-CoV. J Immunol 2008;181(9): 6337–48.

170. Guess HA, Broughton DD, Melton LJ 3rd, et al. Population-based studies of varicella complications. Pediatrics 1986;78(4 Pt 2):723–7.

171. Marin M, Watson TL, Chaves SS, et al. Varicella among adults: data from an active surveillance project, 1995–2005. J Infect Dis 2008;197:S94–100.

172. Feldman S. Varicella-zoster virus pneumonitis. Chest 1994;106(1):S22–7.

173. Knyvett AF. Is smoking a risk factor for pneumonia in adults with chickenpox. Br Med J (Clin Res Ed) 1987;295(6590):122.

174. Mohsen AH, McKendrick M. Varicella pneumonia in adults. Eur Respir J 2003;21(5):886–91.

175. Esmonde TF, Herdman G, Anderson G. Chickenpox pneumonia: an association with pregnancy. Thorax 1989;44(10):812–5.

176. Straus SE, Ostrove JM, Inchauspe G, et al. Varicella-zoster virus-infections - biology, natural-history, treatment, and prevention. Ann Intern Med 1988;108(2):221–37.

177. Nguyen HQ, Jumaan AO, Seward JF. Decline in mortality due to varicella after implementation of varicella vaccination in the United States. N Engl J Med 2005;352(5):450–8.

178. Gilden DH, Cohrs RJ, Mahalingam R. Clinical and molecular pathogenesis of varicella virus infection. Viral Immunol 2003;16(3):243–58.

179. Heininger U, Seward JF. Varicella. Lancet 2006; 368(9544):1365–76.

180. Schlossberg D, Littman M. Varicella pneumonia. Arch Intern Med 1988;148(7):1630–2.

181. Floudas CS, Kanakis MA, Andreopoulos A, et al. Nodular lung calcifications following varicella zoster virus pneumonia. QJM 2008;101(2):159.

182. Balfour HH. Varicella zoster virus infections in immunocompromised hosts. A review of the natural history and management. Am J Med 1988;85(2A): 68–73.

183. Schmutzhard J, Riedel HM, Wirgart BZ, et al. Detection of herpes simplex virus type 1, herpes simplex virus type 2 and varicella-zoster virus in skin lesions. Comparison of real-time PCR, nested PCR and virus isolation. J Clin Virol 2004;29(2): 120–6.

184. Dahl H, Marcoccia J, Linde A. Antigen detection: the method of choice in comparison with virus isolation and serology for laboratory diagnosis of herpes zoster in human immunodeficiency virus-infected patients. J Clin Microbiol 1997;35(2): 347–9.

185. Haake DA, Zakowski PC, Haake DL, et al. Early treatment with acyclovir for varicella pneumonia in otherwise healthy-adults - retrospective controlled-study and review. Rev Infect Dis 1990;12(5): 788–98.

186. Mer M, Richards GA. Corticosteroids in life-threatening varicella pneumonia. Chest 1998; 114(2):426–31.

187. Ison MG, Fishman JA. Cytomegalovirus pneumonia in transplant recipients. Clin Chest Med 2005; 26(4):691–705.

188. Papazian L, Fraisse A, Garbe L, et al. Cytomegalovirus. An unexpected cause of ventilator-associated pneumonia. Anesthesiology 1996;84(2):280–7.

189. Chiche L, Forel JM, Papazian L. The role of viruses in nosocomial pneumonia. Curr Opin Infect Dis 2011;24(2):152–6.

190. Kotloff RM, Ahya VN, Crawford SW. Pulmonary complications of solid organ and hematopoietic stem cell transplantation. Am J Respir Crit Care Med 2004;170(1):22–48.

191. Harbison MA, De Girolami PC, Jenkins RL, et al. Ganciclovir therapy of severe cytomegalovirus infections in solid-organ transplant recipients. Transplantation 1988;46(1):82–8.

192. D'Alessandro AM, Pirsch JD, Stratta RJ, et al. Successful treatment of severe cytomegalovirus infections with ganciclovir and CMV hyperimmune globulin in liver transplant recipients. Transplant Proc 1989;21(3):3560–1.

193. Chow BD, Huang YT, Esper FP. Evidence of human bocavirus circulating in children and adults, Cleveland, Ohio. J Clin Virol 2008;43(3):302–6.

194. Kupfer B, Vehreschild J, Cornely O, et al. Severe pneumonia and human bocavirus in adult. Emerg Infect Dis 2006;12(10):1614–6.

195. Dina J, Vabret A, Gouarin S, et al. Detection of human bocavirus in hospitalised children. J Paediatr Child Health 2009;45(3):149–53.

196. Choi JH, Chung YS, Kim KS, et al. Development of real-time PCR assays for detection and quantification of human bocavirus. J Clin Virol 2008;42(3): 249–53.

Defining Severe Pneumonia

Samuel M. Brown, MD, MS[a,b,]*, Nathan C. Dean, MD[a,b]

KEYWORDS
- Pneumonia • Severity assessment • Prognostic models

Community-acquired pneumonia (CAP) is an important public health problem. When combined with influenza, it is currently the eighth leading cause of death in the United States[1] and the most common infectious cause of death in the developed world.[2–4] Because the site of care is the major determinant of cost and appropriate site of care presumably improves outcome, the correct assessment of severity in CAP is understood to be crucial.[5,6] One persistent problem in studies of CAP is the difficulty in defining and predicting pneumonia severity, although however it is defined severe CAP (SCAP) is a significant clinical and public health problem.[7]

The Infectious Disease Society of America and the American Thoracic Society in 2007 issued consensus guidelines on CAP and SCAP (IDSA/ATS 2007),[5] as have the British Thoracic Society and other professional organizations.[8–10] Several investigators, including the authors' group, have published general reviews relative to CAP, SCAP, and severity assessment.[3,11–17] In this review, the authors consider the many approaches to defining pneumonia severity, their applications, implications, and limitations. The authors emphasize that definitions depend on goals. Different definitions may be required in different situations, and care should also be taken to distinguish descriptive from predictive applications of such definitions.

DEFINING SEVERE PNEUMONIA

Pneumonia severity is necessarily contextual; the question of whether a given case of CAP is severe depends on the question being asked. Different clinical or logistical questions may require different definitions. Several of the relevant questions include the possible microbial etiology, possibility of benefit from specific or supportive therapy, possible benefit from experimental therapies (ie, for enrollment in clinical trials), and probability of morbidity or mortality (eg, for prognostic discussions). Most commonly, the question of location of care, the major driver of the cost of treatment, has been the central problem of CAP severity. In many cases, the question of which antibiotic to prescribe may depend more on chronic airways disease and recent antibiotic exposures than acute physiology. On the other hand, the expected response to administration of activated protein C (APC) depends more on acute derangement of physiology and thrombotic imbalance in the microvascular circulation. A definition of severity that guides antibiotic therapy may fail to identify patients likely to benefit from specific adjunctive therapies and vice versa.

Definitions to Guide Choice of Anti-infective Agents

Both common sense physiologic reasoning and observational data have suggested that delay in treatment with appropriate antibiotics is associated with poor outcome in sepsis generally and CAP specifically.[18] SCAP could increase both the urgency of appropriate antibiotics and the risk that a particular pathogen may be present. Organisms that merit special attention include methicillin-resistant *Staphylococcus aureus* (MRSA), which

The authors' research is supported by the National Institute of General Medical Sciences (1K23GM094465 to SMB), the Easton Fund, and the Deseret Research Foundation. The authors have no conflicts of interest relevant to this article.

a Division of Pulmonary and Critical Care Medicine, Intermountain Medical Center, Salt Lake City, UT, USA
b Division of Pulmonary and Critical Care Medicine, University of Utah, Salt Lake City, UT, USA
* Corresponding author. Shock Trauma ICU, 5121 South Cottonwood Street, Murray, UT 84157.
E-mail address: Samuel.Brown@imail.org

chestmed.theclinics.com

is resistant to all β-lactam antibiotics, and the non–lactose-fermenting gram-negative bacilli (eg, *Pseudomonas aeruginosa*). By most definitions, SCAP varies in microbial etiologic predominance from CAP, with a higher representation of *Staphylococcus aureus* and gram-negative organisms.[5,19–21] However, the inciting organism can be independent of the physiologic severity of CAP, as with pneumococcus, which is heavily represented in both SCAP and non-SCAP. Acute physiology may represent host immune response or intercurrent disease more than the infecting microorganism. The independence of disease severity and microbial etiology has been demonstrated with regard to health care–associated pneumonia; a similar discordance has been suggested for CAP.[22] Predictive models for the presence of *Pseudomonas* have been developed but highlight chronic airways disease and recent antibiotic exposure rather than acute physiologic derangements.[23] Age is no longer considered a relevant predictor.[23–26] Nevertheless, pseudomonal pneumonia generally is associated with physiologic derangement,[23,27,28] and, in at least 1 study, 1 in 5 patients with pneumonia admitted to the intensive care unit (ICU) had *Pseudomonas* infection.[23] No study has specifically assessed the effect of withholding antipseudomonal therapy in ICU-admitted patients without risk factors for *Pseudomonas* colonization or infection, although in the age of multiple drug resistance, such a study could be clinically and ecologically important. Evolving clinical understanding of the role of community-acquired (CA) MRSA in CAP suggests a predominance of necrotizing infection, a higher rate of pleural and/or metastatic involvement, leukopenia, and an association with influenza infection.[29–31] No validated prediction rule exists for CA-MRSA. The close connection between CA-MRSA pneumonia and severity has recently been challenged, perhaps on the basis of improved therapy[30]; some studies suggesting high degrees of severity and/or mortality exhibit ascertainment bias, for example, by restricting the case definition to semi-invasively (bronchoscopically) obtained cultures.[32]

Definitions to Guide Choice of Supportive Therapy

Preliminary work has suggested tailoring nonantibiotic therapies on the basis of patient presentation and/or severity in CAP. To date, these therapies are limited to the administration of APC and corticosteroids. There is post hoc evidence that APC may benefit certain subgroups of patients with CAP complicated by severe sepsis.

In the main study of APC in undifferentiated severe sepsis (PROWESS [Recombinant Human Protein C Worldwide Evaluation in Severe Sepsis] trial), the benefit of therapy appeared limited to patients with severe rather than nonsevere disease, a finding that may be relevant in CAP as well.[33] The findings relative to APC in patients with SCAP are only post hoc and, even on subgroup analysis, may be limited to patients with inappropriate initial antibiotic therapy.[34,35] A randomized trial limited to SCAP has not been undertaken. The recently completed CAPTIVATE (Community-Acquired Pneumonia Tifacogin Intravenous Administration Trial for Efficacy) study of tifacogin in SCAP[36] showed negative results, as was observed in a randomized trial of surfactant protein C, although the latter study may have been affected by inadvertent inactivation of the study drug.[37]

Controversial data suggest that steroid therapy may be beneficial in SCAP,[38] a finding the same group has described in acute respiratory distress syndrome,[39] despite negative results from the much larger multicenter LaSRS (Late Steroid Rescue Study).[40] One systematic review, based largely on the single randomized trial, also concluded that steroids should be administered in SCAP.[41] However, the recently published CORTICUS (Corticosteroid Therapy of Septic Shock) trial showed no benefit of steroid therapy in an undifferentiated cohort of patients with septic shock in which the largest subgroup of patients had pneumonia.[42] There are inadequate data to support routine corticosteroid therapy in SCAP. Given the morbidity of steroid therapy, it is likely that SCAP rather than non-SCAP would be the target if sufficient evidence were to accrue in support of a therapeutic benefit.

Definitions to Guide Enrollment in Clinical Trials

The question of CAP severity for enrollment in clinical trials of novel therapies is important. If trials are powered for a primary outcome of mortality, mortality needs to be reasonably high in the study population. For such an application, a model of SCAP that emphasizes mortality may be more useful, although comorbid illnesses may be important to near- and intermediate-term mortality and could be less amenable to acute therapies. Other end points such as cost of care, duration of hospitalization, and ventilator-free or ICU-free days may be linked to other definitions of pneumonia severity. Biomarkers may be particularly helpful in the setting of targeted therapy, although this has not been reliably demonstrated.

Definitions to Guide Site-of-Care Decisions

Reliable prediction of mortality is important for a variety of reasons, including triage and accounting of health care resources and prognostic counseling for patients and families. Pneumonia-specific mortality may be the best measure, which is reasonably well represented by 30-day all-cause mortality.[43] However it is defined, SCAP has a higher mortality rate than non-SCAP.[44] However, the use of mortality as the definition of CAP severity is often clouded by questions of limitations of care in patients of advanced age or with significant comorbidities.

A composite definition of severity that meets all needs simultaneously may not be achievable. At present, the most commonly discussed goal of severity assessment serves the needs of health services research by predicting the patients who will require intensive therapies and/or ICU admission. The question of identifying the patients who should use scarce ICU beds should probably be driven by the likelihood of benefit from intensive therapy, although current definitions have not evolved to that level of sophistication. Patients with acute physiologic derangements may be more likely to respond to intensive therapy than those whose comorbidities make a relatively modest physiologic derangement life threatening, although this has not been demonstrated in the literature.

ICU admission is often used as a surrogate for SCAP, although it varies considerably based on local practice patterns.[45–48] Angus and coauthors[48] evaluated hospital costs, late convalescence, and the length of stay in the hospital and ICU as alternative outcomes of SCAP. The investigators compared these outcomes based on four different definitions of severity: ICU admission, receipt of mechanical ventilation, development of medical complications, and mortality. Leroy and colleagues[49] evaluated mechanical ventilation, shock, or medical complications to define SCAP, whereas Buising and colleagues[50] proposed mortality, ICU admission, mechanical ventilation, or inotrope/vasopressor therapy. Charles and colleagues[51] used mechanical ventilation (invasive or noninvasive) and vasopressors, regardless of site of care. The authors' group validated the IDSA/ATS 2007 guidelines against a reference definition of SCAP that incorporated both admission to the ICU and receipt of intensive therapy, overcoming many of the problems with other definitions of CAP severity relevant to the question of patient triage.[52]

A word of caution is advised with regard to the testing of predictive models. Some have used receipt of mechanical ventilation or vasopressors in the emergency department (ED) as predictors of ICU admission, but the requirement for preadmission intensive therapies of this sort is more a determination of the location of therapy than a prediction of severity because almost no health care environments would recommend the care of mechanically ventilated or vasopressor-dependent patients outside the ICU, as Charles[53] has correctly observed. The authors and others therefore focused on the IDSA/ATS 2007 minor criteria in validation studies.

CLINICAL PREDICTION RULES

Clinical judgment has often been proved inadequate to the task of assessing severity in CAP.[3,54–56] However, there is some evidence and good reason to believe that a combination of prediction models and clinical judgment is superior to either alone.[57] To standardize initial assessments of the anticipated course of CAP, two main predictive models have been proposed. These models, simplified regression equations used to generate scores that classify patients based on their predicted 30-day mortality, have proved useful at excluding the need for hospital admission but unsatisfactory in predicting the need for ICU admission or receipt of intensive therapies.[3]

The best known of the prediction models, the Pneumonia Severity Index (PSI)[58] and the British Thoracic Society simplified prediction model, the CURB-65 model in various versions,[59,60] have demonstrated utility in recommending outpatient therapy for low-risk patients.[46,47,61–63] The American Thoracic Society has also proposed severity models with multiple iterations[45,64] and validations.[46–48,57] The IDSA/ATS 2007[5] guidelines include new predictors that are in the process of validation with reasonable performance.[52,65–67]

Other models specific to SCAP have been developed, including a recent Australian model called SMART-COP,[51] a Spanish model called CURXO (although the investigators of this prediction model designate it SCAP, the authors find this usage confusing because the score is designed to predict SCAP but is one of several competing prediction models; the authors therefore refer to it as CURXO),[68–70] and a mixed French-American score called the REA-ICU index.[71] The SMART-COP, which predicts mechanical ventilation or vasopressors, has been externally validated in patients younger than 50 years.[72] The CURXO and the REA-ICU models predict ICU admission only and thus seem less well validated than the IDSA/ATS 2007 or the SMART-COP. **Table 1** presents the constituent elements of these severity models, underscoring the considerable overlap among the

Table 1
Elements of pneumonia severity models

Predictor	IDSA/ATS 2007	SMART-COP	CURXO	CURB-65
Confusion	X	X	X	X
Uremia	X	—	X	X
Tachypnea	X	X	X	X
Hypotension	X	X	X	X
Age	—	X	X	X
Tachycardia	—	X	—	—
Multilobar involvement	X	X	X	—
Leukopenia	X	—	—	—
Thrombocytopenia	X	—	—	—
Acidemia	—	X	X	—
Hypoxemia	X	X	X	—
Hypoalbuminemia	—	X	—	—
Hypothermia	X	—	—	—

various models. When compared within a cohort, the IDSA/ATS 2007 predictors outperformed (area under the receiver operating curve [AUC], 0.88) other prediction models, including SMART-COP, CURB-65, and CURXO (AUC, 0.76–0.83). **Table 2** displays the results of various comparative validations of severity prediction models.

Other investigators have proposed a method based on the PIRO (Predisposition, Insult, Response, Organ dysfunction) classification for sepsis generally, which remains largely a schema rather than a detailed prediction model.[73,74] Although conceptually satisfying, PIRO requires substantial further work to allow implementation in useful predictive models, particularly in light of

evidence that acute physiology has the greatest effect on near-term outcomes from CAP.[75] Others have argued that generic mortality models, such as the Acute Physiology and Chronic Health Evaluation (APACHE), would perform better, although these are mortality predictors for ICU-admitted patients rather than predictors of need for ICU admission or intensive therapy, and are more cumbersome to calculate than the simplified pneumonia models.

Competing prediction models have been compared in many different populations. A prospective follow-on study by the investigators of the PSI suggested slightly better prediction of 30-day mortality for this system than for the

Table 2
Comparative validations of severity models

	Phua[66]	Charles[51]	Yandiola[69]	Brown[52]
ATS2007 (AUC)	0.85	NA	NA	0.88
SMART-COP (AUC)	NA	0.87	NA	0.83
CURXO (AUC)	NA	NA	0.75	0.83
CURB-65 (AUC)	0.68	0.67	0.61	0.76
Primary outcome	ICU admission[a]	Intensive therapy[b]	ICU admission[a]	Intensive therapy[c] and ICU admission
Sample size (Total:SCAP)	1017:>91	882:91	671:57[d]	1540:298

Abbreviation: NA, not applicable.
   [a] Evaluated multiple outcomes; results generally consistent.
   [b] Mechanical ventilation or vasopressor therapy.
   [c] Mechanical ventilation, vasopressor therapy, emergent renal replacement, high-volume fluid resuscitation, inspired oxygen fraction greater than 60%.
   [d] External validation cohort.

CURB or CURB-65 models.[76] A variety of other studies have suggested that these scores are reasonably similar, although the PSI is more weighted toward age and comorbidity and the CURB-65 model is more weighted toward acute physiologic dysfunction.[77–79] Both these models do not perform well at predicting which patients require ICU admission or intensive therapy. These models tend to overestimate severity in patients with advanced age or chronic organ failure and underestimate severity in younger patients.[47,48,57,61,63] They also poorly discriminate among patients with a high risk of death.[80] One investigator has proposed using a combination of the CURB-65 model and the PSI scores in tandem evaluation of patients to consider both comorbidities and acute physiologic derangements, although the CURB-65 model is also limited in predictive utility for SCAP. This technique needs external validation and is encumbered by the complex statistical nature of this seemingly simple proposal.[81] The authors do not recommend the use of the CURB-65 model or the PSI in the validation of new models of SCAP. Rather, the new prediction models for SCAP should be compared against the IDSA/ATS 2007 definition.

Some investigators have begun to evaluate the utility of severity prediction models in other pneumonia populations, such as human immunodeficiency virus–infected patients presenting with CAP,[82] or resource-limited settings.[83,84] Much additional work is required in this area.

The authors stress that the most popular current method of evaluating the utility of a diagnostic test (such as a prediction model) is the AUC, equivalent to the C statistic. This statistic measures how often, in a pair of patients drawn at random from both populations, an affected patient has a higher score than an unaffected patient. Although a minimum AUC of 0.75 is proposed as statistically adequate, it is important to recognize that when the AUC is much less than 0.90, it is more useful as a measure of how populations differ than as a predictor of the fate of any individual patient. Even composite predictors can have frustratingly small effects on the risk prediction of an individual patient.[85] Predictive models with high AUC may highlight possible physiologic relationships but may not perform as well in the management of individual patients. Furthermore, most techniques of logistic regression, the most common method of building predictive models, are unstable in populations in which separation is near complete, such as would be seen with an AUC greater than 0.95. In addition, if there are substantially more unaffected patients than affected patients, even a very low false-negative rate yields a significant

proportion of affected patients with a low score. Most of the prediction rules have AUC in the 0.75 to 0.85 range, and non-SCAP is much more common than SCAP. As a result, as many as 30% of the patients admitted to the ICU will be in low-risk categories. The proportion of low-risk patients admitted to ICUs may depend as much on the prevalence of the high-risk phenotype as on the diagnostic utility of the test. Many statisticians prefer the positive and negative likelihood ratios, which do not depend on baseline prevalence. These specify, in the spirit of Bayesian statistics, the ratio of posttest to pretest probability. However, likelihood ratios require that the clinicians estimate the pretest probability, something few clinicians have been willing to do. Positive and negative predictive values seem more intuitive for clinicians. For a given baseline prevalence, these predictive values estimate the chance of SCAP among patients with a score above a given threshold. However, positive and negative predictive values are unreliable if the baseline prevalence changes significantly. Health services research focused on human factors in the interpretation and use of such prediction rules is clearly needed. Statistical rigor may be of little significance if real-world applications yield unintended or undesired outcomes.

BIOMARKERS OF PNEUMONIA SEVERITY

There is considerable clinical and research interest in the use of novel biomarkers to diagnose and classify CAP. The use of the term biomarker should not obscure the fact that a variety of biomarkers are already in routine clinical use, including serum creatinine or bilirubin, lactate, the ratio of arterial to inspired oxygen, hemoglobin concentrations, or platelet count. Simple measures of multiple organ dysfunction syndrome may be more useful than any of the newer assays, as suggested in the IDSA/ATS 2007 guidelines, which incorporate platelet count[86] and measures of renal function. The Sequential Organ Failure Assessment score[87] summarizes the dysfunction of multiple organ systems in critical illness and may prove useful as a biomarker summary in SCAP, although this has not been established. The 2 most lethal complications of CAP in the first 30 days are hypoxemic respiratory failure and the multiple organ dysfunction syndrome. Before making decisions about the utility of biomarkers, it should be borne in mind that after 30 days, comorbidities such as neurologic impairment, cancer, or atherosclerotic events or cardiac failure play a much larger role in mortality complicating CAP.[43] New biomarkers should prove their superiority over established scores and similar assays before they are widely implemented; none is yet ready for clinical use.[3]

Of the novel biomarkers, most attention has been focused on procalcitonin, the CALC-1 gene product and prohormone of calcitonin, probably involved in chemoattraction and nitric oxide production. Evolving data on procalcitonin suggest possible utility in deciding the duration of antibiotic therapy[88] and in identifying a bacterial cause of lower respiratory tract infection[89] (or severe sepsis generally[90]). However, procalcitonin has no established role in triage decisions or severity assessments.[91]

A variety of pulmonary-specific biomarkers have been evaluated with mixed results, including the receptor for advanced glycation end products,[92] high-mobility group box protein 1,[93] soluble triggering receptor expressed on myeloid cells 1,[94] pro–atrial natriuretic peptide and provasopressin,[95] and proadrenomedullin.[96] Although the concentrations of these biomarkers are generally higher in serum and bronchoalveolar lavage in patients with lung injury, their application in severity assessment should remain limited, awaiting further evaluation. Unfortunately, most biomarkers are useful primarily at extremely low or extremely high values. The more commonly encountered intermediate levels rarely discriminate well in individual patients. It seems likely that combinations of clinical scores and laboratory biomarkers perform better than either of these methods used alone, although this remains to be demonstrated.[97]

A report from the German CAPNETZ (Community-Acquired Pneumonia Competence Network) study group adding biomarkers to CURB-65 predictors for short- and long-term outcomes in CAP suggested that proadrenomedullin outperformed other biomarkers and improved the prediction of the CURB-65 model. Procalcitonin performed less well at mortality prediction than other biomarkers in this multicenter cohort, a result that was possibly confounded by the presence of viral pneumonias. This study had few patients with SCAP and also failed to clarify whether proadrenomedullin levels reflected pneumonia-related morbidity and mortality or comorbidity-related mortality.[98]

Another approach to biomarkers emphasizes the role of microbe-related factors. Although early in its validation, mounting data suggest that, for instance, the bacterial load in blood among patients with pneumococcal pneumonia may strongly affect outcome.[99,100] Such microbe-related biomarkers may have the added advantage of implications for the timing and nature of adjunctive and anti-infective therapy,[101] although the final endorsement of such techniques awaits the results of prospective controlled trials.

IMPLICATIONS OF SEVERITY ASSESSMENT

As with all procedures in medicine, the possible effects of severity assessment should be explicitly considered. The definition of SCAP can affect triage, therapy, and prognostic estimates. Application of definitions and predictive models may have real-world consequences. Clinicians and investigators should be thoughtful about the appropriate contexts in which to apply definitions of CAP severity.

That failure to triage a critically ill patient directly to the ICU could lead to worse outcomes drives much of the work on severity as a triage tool for the ICU.[102,103] One early study suggested that admission to the ICU did not improve patient outcomes. However, it had methodological limitations because patients were only admitted to the ICU late in the course of illness, perhaps too late for benefit from intensive therapy.[104] A recent study showed that patients with CAP requiring vasopressor therapy in the ED admitted to the ICU had a lower mortality than those admitted to the floor, although this finding likely reflected unstated or unrecorded requests to limit care because it seems unusual to admit a patient with vasopressor dependence to the hospital ward.[65] A study of a large British cohort suggested worse outcomes for late ICU admissions but did not control for disease severity.[103] A recent post hoc analysis of multicenter prospective observational studies,[105] two retrospective case series,[106,107] and the authors' preliminary data[108] suggest that initial ICU triage may be associated with better outcomes, although no analysis has yet controlled for the entity of progressive pneumonia, a crucial confounder of the proposed relationship between ICU triage and mortality.[109]

Designation as SCAP does not accurately predict microbial etiology, as noted earlier. Nevertheless, there are data, mostly observational, suggesting that particular antibiotic regimens may be superior to others in patients with SCAP. Several studies have suggested that dual antibiotic therapy is superior to monotherapy, perhaps reflecting the effect of macrolide therapy.[110–113]

There is little evidence that SCAP definitions are used for prognostic estimates. Whether they would be superior to traditional ICU prognostic models is an open question. The APACHE and Mortality Probability Model regression-based prediction equations perform reasonably well in prognostication in general ICU populations.[114,115] Little data exist to suggest that CAP-specific models would be superior (in an unpublished analysis of the authors' cohort of approximately 1500 hospitalized patients with CAP the Simplified Acute Physiology Score II[116] and the IDSA/ATS 2007 guidelines predicted 30-day mortality with similar AUC of approximately 0.83). Whether the absence of SCAP classification should restrict admission to the ICU is an open question, unlikely to be implemented without prospective validation.

Areas for future research include application of general prediction models to other pulmonary infections, such as health care–associated pneumonia, the possibility of incorporating biomarkers into prediction rules, phenotypic and genotypic models that might predict the likelihood of benefiting from intensive therapies, and the role of patient response or institutional characteristics (eg, presence of board-certified subspecialists, use of clinical protocols) in predicting and modifying outcomes from SCAP. Another area for research is the analysis of data-rich hemodynamic information derived from telemetry monitors in the ED or ICU. Preliminary studies in sepsis have suggested a role for the broader application of these techniques.[117]

SUMMARY

Attempts to define SCAP are not merely questions of semantics. Specific definitions may affect triage, therapy, and clinical outcome. In important respects, the definition of severity is contextual. Severity definitions and predictive models should be applied for the purposes for which they were formulated and validated. In coming years, laboratory biomarkers of pneumonia severity may improve our ability to estimate the benefit from intensive supportive therapies. With the advance of personalized medicine, severity assessments coupled with broader phenotypic assessments of patients will lead to more specific and effective therapy for patients with SCAP.

REFERENCES

1. Heron M, Hoyert DL, Murphy SL, et al. Deaths: final data for 2006. Natl Vital Stat Rep 2009;57(14): 1–134.

2. Armstrong GL, Conn LA, Pinner RW. Trends in infectious disease mortality in the United States during the 20th century. JAMA 1999;281(1): 61–6.

3. Singanayagam A, Chalmers JD, Hill AT. Severity assessment in community-acquired pneumonia: a review. QJM 2009;102(6):379–88.

4. Marston BJ, Plouffe JF, File TM Jr, et al. Incidence of community-acquired pneumonia requiring hospitalization. Results of a population-based active surveillance study in Ohio. The Community-Based Pneumonia Incidence Study Group. Arch Intern Med 1997;157(15):1709–18.

5. Mandell LA, Wunderink RG, Anzueto A, et al. Infectious Diseases Society of America/American Thoracic Society consensus guidelines on the management of community-acquired pneumonia in adults. Clin Infect Dis 2007;44(Suppl 2):S27–72.

6. Bartolome M, Almirall J, Morera J, et al. A population-based study of the costs of care for community-acquired pneumonia. Eur Respir J 2004;23(4):610–6.

7. The aetiology, management and outcome of severe community-acquired pneumonia on the intensive care unit. The British Thoracic Society Research Committee and The Public Health Laboratory Service. Respir Med 1992;86(1):7–13.

8. Guidelines for the management of community-acquired pneumonia in adults admitted to hospital. The British Thoracic Society. Br J Hosp Med 1993; 49(5):346–50.

9. Lim WS, Baudouin SV, George RC, et al. BTS guidelines for the management of community acquired pneumonia in adults: update 2009. Thorax 2009;64(Suppl 3):iii1–55.

10. Mandell LA, Marrie TJ, Grossman RF, et al. Summary of Canadian guidelines for the initial management of community-acquired pneumonia: an evidence-based update by the Canadian Infectious Disease Society and the Canadian Thoracic Society. Can J Infect Dis 2000;11(5):237–48.

11. Niederman MS. Recent advances in community-acquired pneumonia: inpatient and outpatient. Chest 2007;131(4):1205–15.

12. Laterre PF. Severe community acquired pneumonia update: mortality, mechanisms and medical intervention. Crit Care 2008;12(Suppl 6):S1.

13. Lim WS, Macfarlane JT. Importance of severity of illness assessment in management of lower respiratory infections. Curr Opin Infect Dis 2004;17(2): 121–5.

14. Ewig S, Schafer H, Torres A. Severity assessment in community-acquired pneumonia. Eur Respir J 2000;16(6):1193–201.

15. Niederman MS. Making sense of scoring systems in community acquired pneumonia. Respirology 2009;14(3):327–35.

16. Brown SM, Dean NC. Defining and predicting severe community-acquired pneumonia. Curr Opin Infect Dis 2010;23(2):158–64.

17. Chalmers JD, Singanayagam A, Akram AR, et al. Severity assessment tools for predicting mortality in hospitalised patients with community-acquired pneumonia. Systematic review and meta-analysis. Thorax 2010;65(10):878–83.

18. Ibrahim EH, Sherman G, Ward S, et al. The influence of inadequate antimicrobial treatment of bloodstream infections on patient outcomes in the ICU setting. Chest 2000;118(1):146–55.

19. Restrepo MI, Jorgensen JH, Mortensen EM, et al. Severe community-acquired pneumonia: current outcomes, epidemiology, etiology, and therapy. Curr Opin Infect Dis 2001;14(6):703–9.

20. Ruiz M, Ewig S, Torres A, et al. Severe community-acquired pneumonia. Risk factors and follow-up epidemiology. Am J Respir Crit Care Med 1999; 160(3):923–9.

21. Paganin F, Lilienthal F, Bourdin A, et al. Severe community-acquired pneumonia: assessment of microbial aetiology as mortality factor. Eur Respir J 2004;24(5):779–85.

22. Brito V, Niederman MS. Healthcare-associated pneumonia is a heterogeneous disease, and all patients do not need the same broad-spectrum antibiotic therapy as complex nosocomial pneumonia. Curr Opin Infect Dis 2009;22(3):316–25.

23. Arancibia F, Bauer TT, Ewig S, et al. Community-acquired pneumonia due to gram-negative bacteria and Pseudomonas aeruginosa: incidence, risk, and prognosis. Arch Intern Med 2002;162(16):1849–58.

24. Riquelme R, Torres A, El-Ebiary M, et al. Community-acquired pneumonia in the elderly: a multivariate analysis of risk and prognostic factors. Am J Respir Crit Care Med 1996;154(5):1450–5.

25. Venkatesan P, Gladman J, Macfarlane JT, et al. A hospital study of community acquired pneumonia in the elderly. Thorax 1990;45(4):254–8.

26. Marrie TJ, Durant H, Yates L. Community-acquired pneumonia requiring hospitalization: 5-year prospective study. Rev Infect Dis 1989;11(4):586–99.

27. Feldman C, Ross S, Mahomed AG, et al. The aetiology of severe community-acquired pneumonia and its impact on initial, empiric, antimicrobial chemotherapy. Respir Med 1995;89(3):187–92.

28. Torres A, Serra-Batlles J, Ferrer A, et al. Severe community-acquired pneumonia. Epidemiology and prognostic factors. Am Rev Respir Dis 1991; 144(2):312–8.

29. Gillet Y, Vanhems P, Lina G, et al. Factors predicting mortality in necrotizing community-acquired pneumonia caused by Staphylococcus aureus containing Panton-Valentine leukocidin. Clin Infect Dis 2007;45(3):315–21.

30. Lobo LJ, Reed KD, Wunderink RG. Expanded clinical presentation of community-acquired methicillin-resistant Staphylococcus aureus pneumonia. Chest 2010;138(1):130–6.

31. Rubinstein E, Kollef MH, Nathwani D. Pneumonia caused by methicillin-resistant Staphylococcus aureus. Clin Infect Dis 2008;46(Suppl 5):S378–85.

32. Kollef KE, Reichley RM, Micek ST, et al. The modified APACHE II score outperforms Curb65 pneumonia severity score as a predictor of 30-day mortality in patients with methicillin-resistant Staphylococcus aureus pneumonia. Chest 2008;133(2):363–9.

33. Bernard GR, Vincent JL, Laterre PF, et al. Efficacy and safety of recombinant human activated protein C for severe sepsis. N Engl J Med 2001;344(10): 699–709.

34. Laterre PF, Opal SM, Abraham E, et al. A clinical evaluation committee assessment of recombinant human tissue factor pathway inhibitor (tifacogin) in patients with severe community-acquired pneumonia. Crit Care 2009;13(2):R36.

35. Laterre PF, Garber G, Levy H, et al. Severe community-acquired pneumonia as a cause of severe sepsis: data from the PROWESS study. Crit Care Med 2005;33(5):952–61.

36. Wunderink RG, Laterre PF, Francois B, et al. Recombinant tissue factor pathway inhibitor in severe community-acquired pneumonia: a randomized trial. Am J Respir Crit Care Med 2011;183(11):1561–8.

37. Spragg RG, Taut FJ, Lewis JF, et al. Recombinant surfactant protein C based surfactant for patients with severe direct lung injury. Am J Respir Crit Care Med 2011;183(8):1055–61.

38. Confalonieri M, Urbino R, Potena A, et al. Hydrocortisone infusion for severe community-acquired pneumonia: a preliminary randomized study. Am J Respir Crit Care Med 2005;171(3):242–8.

39. Meduri GU, Golden E, Freire AX, et al. Methylprednisolone infusion in early severe ARDS: results of a randomized controlled trial. Chest 2007;131(4): 954–63.

40. Steinberg KP, Hudson LD, Goodman RB, et al. Efficacy and safety of corticosteroids for persistent acute respiratory distress syndrome. N Engl J Med 2006;354(16):1671–84.

41. Salluh JI, Povoa P, Soares M, et al. The role of corticosteroids in severe community-acquired pneumonia: a systematic review. Crit Care 2008;12(3): R76.

42. Sprung CL, Annane D, Keh D, et al. Hydrocortisone therapy for patients with septic shock. N Engl J Med 2008;358(2):111–24.

43. Mortensen EM, Coley CM, Singer DE, et al. Causes of death for patients with community-acquired pneumonia: results from the Pneumonia Patient Outcomes Research Team cohort study. Arch Intern Med 2002;162(9):1059–64.

44. Restrepo MI, Mortensen EM, Velez JA, et al. A comparative study of community-acquired pneumonia patients admitted to the ward and the ICU. Chest 2008;133(3):610–7.

45. Niederman MS, Bass JB Jr, Campbell GD, et al. Guidelines for the initial management of adults with community-acquired pneumonia: diagnosis, assessment of severity, and initial antimicrobial therapy. American Thoracic Society. Medical

Section of the American Lung Association. Am Rev Respir Dis 1993;148(5):1418–26.

46. Ewig S, Ruiz M, Mensa J, et al. Severe community-acquired pneumonia. Assessment of severity criteria. Am J Respir Crit Care Med 1998;158(4):1102–8.

47. Ewig S, de Roux A, Bauer T, et al. Validation of predictive rules and indices of severity for community acquired pneumonia. Thorax 2004;59(5):421–7.

48. Angus DC, Marrie TJ, Obrosky DS, et al. Severe community-acquired pneumonia: use of intensive care services and evaluation of American and British Thoracic Society Diagnostic criteria. Am J Respir Crit Care Med 2002;166(5):717–23.

49. Leroy O, Santre C, Beuscart C, et al. A five-year study of severe community-acquired pneumonia with emphasis on prognosis in patients admitted to an intensive care unit. Intensive Care Med 1995;21(1):24–31.

50. Buising KL, Thursky KA, Black JF, et al. A prospective comparison of severity scores for identifying patients with severe community acquired pneumonia: reconsidering what is meant by severe pneumonia. Thorax 2006;61(5):419–24.

51. Charles PG, Wolfe R, Whitby M, et al. SMART-COP: a tool for predicting the need for intensive respiratory or vasopressor support in community-acquired pneumonia. Clin Infect Dis 2008;47(3):375–84.

52. Brown SM, Jones BE, Jephson AR, et al. Validation of the Infectious Disease Society of America/American Thoracic Society 2007 guidelines for severe community-acquired pneumonia. Crit Care Med 2009;37(12):3010–6.

53. Charles PG. Predicting need for ICU in community-acquired pneumonia. Chest 2008;133(2):587 [author reply: 588].

54. Tang CM, Macfarlane JT. Early management of younger adults dying of community acquired pneumonia. Respir Med 1993;87(4):289–94.

55. Neill AM, Martin IR, Weir R, et al. Community acquired pneumonia: aetiology and usefulness of severity criteria on admission. Thorax 1996;51(10):1010–6.

56. McQuillan P, Pilkington S, Allan A, et al. Confidential inquiry into quality of care before admission to intensive care. BMJ 1998;316(7148):1853–8.

57. Riley PD, Aronsky D, Dean NC. Validation of the 2001 American Thoracic Society criteria for severe community-acquired pneumonia. Crit Care Med 2004;32(12):2398–402.

58. Fine MJ, Auble TE, Yealy DM, et al. A prediction rule to identify low-risk patients with community-acquired pneumonia. N Engl J Med 1997;336(4):243–50.

59. Community-acquired pneumonia in adults in British hospitals in 1982–1983: a survey of aetiology, mortality, prognostic factors and outcome. The British Thoracic Society and the Public Health Laboratory Service. Q J Med 1987;62(239):195–220.

60. Lim WS, van der Eerden MM, Laing R, et al. Defining community acquired pneumonia severity on presentation to hospital: an international derivation and validation study. Thorax 2003;58(5):377–82.

61. Kamath A, Pasteur MC, Slade MG, et al. Recognising severe pneumonia with simple clinical and biochemical measurements. Clin Med 2003;3(1):54–6.

62. Leroy O, Georges H, Beuscart C, et al. Severe community-acquired pneumonia in ICUs: prospective validation of a prognostic score. Intensive Care Med 1996;22(12):1307–14.

63. Lim WS, Lewis S, Macfarlane JT. Severity prediction rules in community acquired pneumonia: a validation study. Thorax 2000;55(3):219–23.

64. Niederman MS, Mandell LA, Anzueto A, et al. Guidelines for the management of adults with community-acquired pneumonia. Diagnosis, assessment of severity, antimicrobial therapy, and prevention. Am J Respir Crit Care Med 2001;163(7):1730–54.

65. Liapikou A, Ferrer M, Polverino E, et al. Severe community-acquired pneumonia: validation of the Infectious Diseases Society of America/American Thoracic Society guidelines to predict an intensive care unit admission. Clin Infect Dis 2009;48(4):377–85.

66. Phua J, See KC, Chan YH, et al. Validation and clinical implications of the IDSA/ATS minor criteria for severe community-acquired pneumonia. Thorax 2009;64(7):598–603.

67. Kontou P, Kuti JL, Nicolau DP. Validation of the Infectious Diseases Society of America/American Thoracic Society criteria to predict severe community-acquired pneumonia caused by Streptococcus pneumoniae. Am J Emerg Med 2009;27(8):968–74.

68. Espana PP, Capelastegui A, Gorordo I, et al. Development and validation of a clinical prediction rule for severe community-acquired pneumonia. Am J Respir Crit Care Med 2006;174(11):1249–56.

69. Yandiola PP, Capelastegui A, Quintana J, et al. Prospective comparison of severity scores for predicting clinically relevant outcomes for patients hospitalized with community-acquired pneumonia. Chest 2009;135(6):1572–9.

70. Espana PP, Capelastegui A, Quintana JM, et al. Validation and comparison of SCAP as a predictive score for identifying low-risk patients in community-acquired pneumonia. J Infect 2010;60(2):106–13.

71. Renaud B, Labarere J, Coma E, et al. Risk stratification of early admission to the intensive care unit of patients with no major criteria of severe

community-acquired pneumonia: development of an international prediction rule. Crit Care 2009; 13(2):R54.

72. Chalmers JD, Singanayagam A, Hill AT. Predicting the need for mechanical ventilation and/or inotropic support for young adults admitted to the hospital with community-acquired pneumonia. Clin Infect Dis 2008;47(12):1571–4.

73. Rello J, Rodriguez A, Lisboa T, et al. PIRO score for community-acquired pneumonia: a new prediction rule for assessment of severity in intensive care unit patients with community-acquired pneumonia. Crit Care Med 2009;37(2):456–62.

74. Rello J. Demographics, guidelines, and clinical experience in severe community-acquired pneumonia. Crit Care 2008;12(Suppl 6):S2.

75. Valencia M, Badia JR, Cavalcanti M, et al. Pneumonia Severity Index class V patients with community-acquired pneumonia: characteristics, outcomes, and value of severity scores. Chest 2007;132(2):515–22.

76. Aujesky D, Auble TE, Yealy DM, et al. Prospective comparison of three validated prediction rules for prognosis in community-acquired pneumonia. Am J Med 2005;118(4):384–92.

77. Man SY, Lee N, Ip M, et al. Prospective comparison of three predictive rules for assessing severity of community-acquired pneumonia in Hong Kong. Thorax 2007;62(4):348–53.

78. Ananda-Rajah MR, Charles PG, Melvani S, et al. Comparing the pneumonia severity index with CURB-65 in patients admitted with community acquired pneumonia. Scand J Infect Dis 2008; 40(4):293–300.

79. Capelastegui A, Espana PP, Quintana JM, et al. Validation of a predictive rule for the management of community-acquired pneumonia. Eur Respir J 2006;27(1):151–7.

80. Loke YK, Kwok CS, Niruban A, et al. Value of severity scales in predicting mortality from community-acquired pneumonia: systematic review and meta-analysis. Thorax 2010;65(10):884–90.

81. Niederman MS, Feldman C, Richards GA. Combining information from prognostic scoring tools for CAP: an American view on how to get the best of all worlds. Eur Respir J 2006;27(1):9–11.

82. Cordero E, Pachon J, Rivero A, et al. Community-acquired bacterial pneumonia in human immunodeficiency virus-infected patients: validation of severity criteria. The Grupo Andaluz para el Estudio de las Enfermedades Infecciosas. Am J Respir Crit Care Med 2000;162(6):2063–8.

83. Shah BA, Ahmed W, Dhobi GN, et al. Validity of pneumonia severity index and CURB-65 severity scoring systems in community acquired pneumonia in an Indian setting. Indian J Chest Dis Allied Sci 2010;52(1):9–17.

84. Aydogdu M, Ozyilmaz E, Aksoy H, et al. Mortality prediction in community-acquired pneumonia requiring mechanical ventilation; values of pneumonia and intensive care unit severity scores. Tuberk Toraks 2010;58(1):25–34.

85. Ware JH. The limitations of risk factors as prognostic tools. N Engl J Med 2006;355(25):2615–7.

86. Mirsaeidi M, Peyrani P, Aliberti S, et al. Thrombocytopenia and thrombocytosis at time of hospitalization predict mortality in patients with community-acquired pneumonia. Chest 2010;137(2):416–20.

87. Vincent JL, Moreno R, Takala J, et al. The SOFA (Sepsis-related Organ Failure Assessment) score to describe organ dysfunction/failure. On behalf of the Working Group on Sepsis-Related Problems of the European Society of Intensive Care Medicine. Intensive Care Med 1996;22(7):707–10.

88. Christ-Crain M, Stolz D, Bingisser R, et al. Procalcitonin guidance of antibiotic therapy in community-acquired pneumonia: a randomized trial. Am J Respir Crit Care Med 2006;174(1):84–93.

89. Muller B, Harbarth S, Stolz D, et al. Diagnostic and prognostic accuracy of clinical and laboratory parameters in community-acquired pneumonia. BMC Infect Dis 2007;7:10.

90. Uzzan B, Cohen R, Nicolas P, et al. Procalcitonin as a diagnostic test for sepsis in critically ill adults and after surgery or trauma: a systematic review and meta-analysis. Crit Care Med 2006;34(7):1996–2003.

91. Kruger S, Ewig S, Marre R, et al. Procalcitonin predicts patients at low risk of death from community-acquired pneumonia across all CRB-65 classes. Eur Respir J 2008;31(2):349–55.

92. Uchida T, Shirasawa M, Ware LB, et al. Receptor for advanced glycation end-products is a marker of type I cell injury in acute lung injury. Am J Respir Crit Care Med 2006;173(9):1008–15.

93. Angus DC, Yang L, Kong L, et al. Circulating high-mobility group box 1 (HMGB1) concentrations are elevated in both uncomplicated pneumonia and pneumonia with severe sepsis. Crit Care Med 2007;35(4):1061–7.

94. Gibot S, Cravoisy A, Levy B, et al. Soluble triggering receptor expressed on myeloid cells and the diagnosis of pneumonia. N Engl J Med 2004; 350(5):451–8.

95. Kruger S, Papassotiriou J, Marre R, et al. Pro-atrial natriuretic peptide and pro-vasopressin to predict severity and prognosis in community-acquired pneumonia: results from the German competence network CAPNETZ. Intensive Care Med 2007; 33(12):2069–78.

96. Christ-Crain M, Morgenthaler NG, Stolz D, et al. Pro-adrenomedullin to predict severity and outcome in community-acquired pneumonia [ISRCTN04176397]. Crit Care 2006;10(3):R96.

97. Menendez R, Martinez R, Reyes S, et al. Biomarkers improve mortality prediction by prognostic scales in community-acquired pneumonia. Thorax 2009;64(7):587–91.

98. Kruger S, Ewig S, Giersdorf S, et al. Cardiovascular and inflammatory biomarkers to predict short- and long-term survival in community-acquired pneumonia: results from the German Competence Network, CAPNETZ. Am J Respir Crit Care Med 2010;182(11):1426–34.

99. Rello J, Lisboa T, Lujan M, et al. Severity of pneumococcal pneumonia associated with genomic bacterial load. Chest 2009;136(3):832–40.

100. Peters RP, de Boer RF, Schuurman T, et al. Streptococcus pneumoniae DNA load in blood as a marker of infection in patients with community-acquired pneumonia. J Clin Microbiol 2009;47(10):3308–12.

101. Waterer G, Rello J. Why should we measure bacterial load when treating community-acquired pneumonia? Curr Opin Infect Dis 2011;24(2):137–41.

102. Ewig S, Bauer T, Hasper E, et al. Prognostic analysis and predictive rule for outcome of hospital-treated community-acquired pneumonia. Eur Respir J 1995;8(3):392–7.

103. Woodhead M, Welch CA, Harrison DA, et al. Community-acquired pneumonia on the intensive care unit: secondary analysis of 17,869 cases in the ICNARC Case Mix Programme Database. Crit Care 2006;10(Suppl 2):S1.

104. Hook EW 3rd, Horton CA, Schaberg DR. Failure of intensive care unit support to influence mortality from pneumococcal bacteremia. JAMA 1983; 249(8):1055–7.

105. Renaud B, Santin A, Coma E, et al. Association between timing of intensive care unit admission and outcomes for emergency department patients with community-acquired pneumonia. Crit Care Med 2009;37(11):2867–74.

106. Phua J, Ngerng WJ, Lim TK. The impact of a delay in intensive care unit admission for community-acquired pneumonia. Eur Respir J 2010;36(4): 826–33.

107. Restrepo MI, Mortensen EM, Rello J, et al. Late admission to the ICU in patients with community-acquired pneumonia is associated with higher mortality. Chest 2010;137(3):552–7.

108. Brown SM, Jephson AR, Jones BE, et al. Effect of delayed ICU admission on patients with severe community-acquired pneumonia [abstract]. Am J Respir Crit Care Med 2009;179:A6111.

109. Lisboa T, Blot S, Waterer GW, et al. Radiologic progression of pulmonary infiltrates predicts a worse prognosis in severe community-acquired pneumonia than bacteremia. Chest 2009;135(1): 165–72.

110. Metersky ML, Ma A, Houck PM, et al. Antibiotics for bacteremic pneumonia: improved outcomes with macrolides but not fluoroquinolones. Chest 2007; 131(2):466–73.

111. Baddour LM, Yu VL, Klugman KP, et al. Combination antibiotic therapy lowers mortality among severely ill patients with pneumococcal bacteremia. Am J Respir Crit Care Med 2004;170(4): 440–4.

112. Leroy O, Saux P, Bedos JP, et al. Comparison of levofloxacin and cefotaxime combined with ofloxacin for ICU patients with community-acquired pneumonia who do not require vasopressors. Chest 2005;128(1):172–83.

113. Restrepo MI, Mortensen EM, Waterer GW, et al. Impact of macrolide therapy on mortality for patients with severe sepsis due to pneumonia. Eur Respir J 2009;33(1):153–9.

114. Higgins TL, Teres D, Nathanson B. Outcome prediction in critical care: the mortality probability models. Curr Opin Crit Care 2008;14(5): 498–505.

115. Knaus WA, Draper EA, Wagner DP, et al. APACHE II: a severity of disease classification system. Crit Care Med 1985;13(10):818–29.

116. Le Gall JR, Lemeshow S, Saulnier F. A new Simplified Acute Physiology Score (SAPS II) based on a European/North American multicenter study. JAMA 1993;270(24):2957–63.

117. Chen WL, Kuo CD. Characteristics of heart rate variability can predict impending septic shock in emergency department patients with sepsis. Acad Emerg Med 2007;14(5):392–7.

The Use of Large Databases to Study Pneumonia: What is Their Value?

Timothy Wiemken, PhD, MPH, CIC, Paula Peyrani, MD,
Forest W. Arnold, DO, Julio Ramirez, MD*

KEYWORDS

- Pneumonia • Database • Community-acquired pneumonia
- Hospital-acquired pneumonia
- Ventilator-associated pneumonia
- Health care–associated pneumonia

The generation of new knowledge to improve the management of pneumonia primarily originates through clinical studies. Clinical studies in pneumonia published during the 1990s were frequently from single centers and included limited numbers of patients. As the management of pneumonia became more complex and investigators were interested in testing hypotheses with less frequent predictor or outcome variables, the need emerged to generate large databases to study pneumonia. A large database can be defined as one containing more than 1000 patients. **Fig. 1** depicts the number of publications in the field of community-acquired pneumonia (CAP) that were based on large databases. The increasing trend in the number of publications using large databases is likely to continue as the need to analyze large numbers of patients increases.

The primary objective of this article is to describe the value of large databases to study pneumonia. The authors review elements including how to develop a large pneumonia database, examples of large databases in pneumonia, the strengths and weaknesses in the analysis of large databases, research opportunities using large databases, and the challenge of merging large databases to generate new knowledge using a very large database to study pneumonia.

The Community-Acquired Pneumonia Organization (CAPO) database is one of several large databases to study pneumonia.[1] In this review, data from the CAPO project are emphasized because the authors are members of the CAPO Data and Statistical Coordinating Center.

DEVELOPING A LARGE PNEUMONIA DATABASE

The development of a database that incorporates data on more than 1000 patients with pneumonia requires the collaboration of a network of clinical investigators. Selection of investigators that will participate in the network is an important first step in the development of a large database.

There are two potential models for the development of large databases for clinical research. The traditional model begins with a hypothesis and a prespecified sample size to be entered into the database. Data collection ceases when the sample size or a prespecified period of time is reached. This database can be considered as "bound" by the sample size or begin and end dates. The analysis of the primary hypothesis as well as secondary analyses of the database can be performed. The second, less traditional model, also begins with a hypothesis, but investigators

The authors have no conflicts of interest to disclose.
Division of Infectious Diseases, University of Louisville, 501 East Broadway #380, Louisville, KY 40202, USA
* Corresponding author.
E-mail address: j.ramirez@louisville.edu

Clin Chest Med 32 (2011) 481–489
doi:10.1016/j.ccm.2011.05.007
0272-5231/11/$ – see front matter © 2011 Elsevier Inc. All rights reserved.

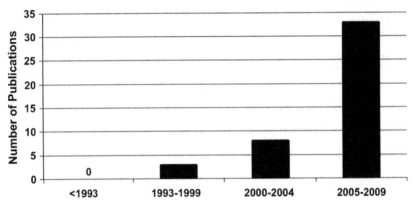

Fig. 1. Peer-reviewed pneumonia publications using large databases, 1993 to 2009.

are committed to continue data collection with the goal of generating a large database. This model can be seen as an "unbound" one for the development of a large database. There is a specific start-point, but no predefined end point for data collection (**Fig. 2**). The analysis of the primary hypothesis is performed when a particular number of patients is reached. This second model facilitates secondary analyses as well as ancillary studies.

The CAPO database is an example of an unbound model. Modifications of the data collection form and the study database allows for a multiplicity of ancillary studies. For example, in March 2009 when the pandemic of H1N1 influenza A began, the CAPO data collection form and study database was modified to include influenza-specific CAP data. Data from this ancillary study generated two peer-reviewed publications.[2,3]

Large databases can be generated with national or international models for research collaboration. Development of international collaborations has been greatly facilitated with the increased global access to electronic forms of communication. The Internet can be used to perform data collection, data transfer, and data quality. Free electronic video communication through the Internet

(eg, Skype) has made it possible for investigators to freely interact in all aspects of clinical research.

The CAPO study is an example of a database developed at the international level. To evaluate the management of CAP worldwide, the participating centers are grouped into 4 international regions (**Fig. 3**). The CAPO study uses a secure, Internet-based data collection through the study Web site (www.caposite.com).

There are several elements that are critical to ensure the development of a high-quality database. Because these projects are almost always multicenter, the development and implementation of a data-coordinating center is imperative. The data-coordinating center should minimally be responsible for maintaining administrative aspects of the project. The data-coordinating center can also coordinate other aspects of the project, such as development and maintenance of all study Web sites, as well as database administration. Database administration can include such things as data backup, timely updating of the database as the case report form changes, and data validation. The database administration duties must include data quality control to ensure the data is of the highest quality before analysis takes place. A more robust model is the creation of a center

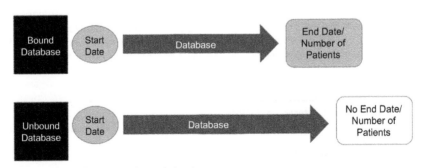

Fig. 2. An overview of bound versus unbound databases.

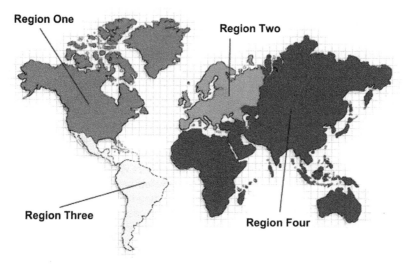

Fig. 3. The 4 international regions of the Community-Acquired Pneumonia Organization.

to provide data management and statistical support. These models are defined as Data and Statistical Coordinating Centers (DSCC).

The CAPO database is managed by the CAPO DSCC, located at the Division of Infectious Diseases of the University of Louisville. At present, the DSCC coordinates the administrative aspects of the project, conducts database administration, and acts as the project statistical-coordinating center. A director, a project manager, and 8 other positions responsible for statistical support, database development, and Web site development, as well as grant, manuscript, and administrative support make up the organization of the CAPO DSCC. The CAPO DSCC supports and manages the ongoing core CAPO study as well as other CAPO-sponsored clinical research projects.

For the CAPO project, the DSCC trains all clinical site staff for various tasks such as data collection, data system access, and data entry into the study database. When a local study site submits a case, the DSCC performs quality control of the data by viewing all entries and ensuring the data are entered per protocol. If an error is found, a query is sent to the local site. After all queries are addressed, the case is entered into the CAPO database for analysis.

The current activities of the CAPO DSCC include:

- Develops the study database and Web site
- Maintains administrative and institutional review board documents
- Coordinates research
- Provides data quality control
- Provides data management
- Performs secondary data analysis

- Coordinates ancillary studies
- Supports the preparation of abstracts for presentation and manuscripts for publication
- Organizes meetings for the steering committee and organizes the annual meeting of international CAPO investigators.

Another important element in the development of a large database is to have a clear publication policy. One of the primary goals for investigators to participate in the creation of a large database is to facilitate the generation of manuscripts and publications. A publication committee clarifies the order and role of each author. Some investigators provide a focused contribution such as analyzing and interpreting data or drafting part of the manuscript. Others may provide a supervisory role, helping with the concept and design or critically revising the manuscript.

As an example, the CAPO database publication guidelines were developed with the goal of maintaining a fair authorship distribution. The investigator with an original idea to perform an evaluation of the database and who is willing to oversee the study will be the leading author on the manuscript. Other investigators will be invited to work on the project in various roles and thus will constitute the coauthors. The selection of investigators invited to participate in a particular project is based on the number of cases collected and entered into the CAPO database during the prior year of the study. Investigators are encouraged to include, at the end of the list of authors, "and the CAPO investigators." At the end of the manuscript, an appendix is included with the list of all participating CAPO investigators. This mechanism allows all participating investigators to obtain fair credit for their work according with their contributions to the database.

EXAMPLES OF LARGE DATABASES

Much of the current literature in pneumonia originates from analysis of large databases. The authors have performed a survey of investigators with recent publications in the field of pneumonia, in an attempt to exemplify the structure of current databases in the study of pneumonia. **Table 1** describes the names of the databases, the type of study, the current number of patients, whether the database is national or international, and whether the database is bound or unbound. All of the described databases are available for analysis. **Table 1** also identifies the contact person who can explain the requirements of database use.

Other large databases that have been used for pneumonia research include those generated by insurance companies. For example, the United States government-run Medicare insurance program grants insurance to patients aged 65 years and older, under age 65 with certain disabilities, and those with end-stage renal disease. This very large database has been used by multiple investigators to generate new knowledge in the study of pneumonia.

STRENGTHS AND WEAKNESSES IN THE ANALYSIS OF LARGE DATABASES

There are many strengths and weaknesses to studying large numbers of patients. Some of the strengths include (1) reduced error and selection bias, (2) ability to examine rare predictors, (3) ability to control for multiple confounding variables, (4) increased statistical power, and (5) increased generalizability. Weaknesses of using large databases include (1) sampling error, (2) dealing with missing data, and (3) potential "overpowering."

Strengths

Including large numbers of patients, especially from multiple study sites, can reduce sampling error and selection bias.[4] As the size of the sample grows, it becomes more representative of the population. Furthermore, by including patients from different study sites, errors in the selection of patients and data collection may become less harmful to the results.

A major issue in clinical research is often the ability to study rare predictor variables. For example, if one were to examine the association between an infrequently used antibiotic and the

likelihood of CAP-related outcome, the sample size must be very large to attain an adequate number of patients with the predictor variable. Statistical analysis of databases is also controlled to some extent by the sample size of the study. To control for confounding variables, a common rule of thumb is to use no more than 1 confounding variable for every 10 cases of the outcome. For example, if one were to examine the likelihood of all-cause mortality in CAP patients with statin therapy versus those without statin therapy, clearly there would be many confounding variables associated with mortality and statin therapy that would need to be controlled: cholesterol levels, blood pressure, age, gender, prior history of myocardial infarction, and so forth. To be able to adjust for these confounding variables and examine their effects on the outcome, one would need 10 cases of mortality for every single confounder to be controlled. As confounding variables are identified, clearly the sample size necessary to control for them increases substantially. Recent advances in the use of the propensity score methodology can help reduce reliance on this rule, though it is not without its limitations.[5]

Statistical power is often cited as a reason for not identifying statistical significance in a study. Statistical power is reached when a sufficient sample size is reached to identify, with a prespecified level of confidence, a difference between the outcomes in one study group versus another.

The goal of every study is to be able to generalize the results back to the population in order to increase the quality of patient care. Through reducing bias (selection, confounding, and so forth) and studying a sample that is closer to the size of the actual population, the likelihood of concluding that the results of a study can be generalized to the population of patients under care is increased.

Weaknesses

A major weakness of every database is sampling error. If the sample for the database is not adequate, the results of any study, regardless of the size of the database, will also not be adequate. For example, imagine a large database was produced of nonconsecutive CAP patients from 8 different study sites. In each study site, if data not collected happen to relate to the most severe cases, due to lack of staffing or difficulty in identifying data elements from the medical record for these patients, it is clear that sampling error has occurred. Here the most severe patients will not be included in the study and therefore the results of the study will be missing key patients. As the

Table 1
A sample of pneumonia databases available for analysis

Study Name	Type of Study	No. of Patients	Member Network	Enrollment Dates	Contact Person
Community-Acquired Pneumonia Organization (CAPO)[1]	Retrospective cohort	5653	International	2001–present	Paula Peyrani, MD P0peyr01@louisville.edu
IMPACT-HAP[16]	Retrospective cohort	567	Multicenter (USA)	2006–present	Paula Peyrani, MD P0peyr01@louisville.edu
Atypical Pathogens Database[14]	Prospective clinical rial	4337	International	1996–2004	James Summersgill, PhD Jtsumm01@louisville.edu
Edinburgh Pneumonia Study[17]	Prospective cohort	1883	Multicenter (Scotland)	2005–present	James Chalmers, MD jamesdchalmers@googlemail.com
Australian CAP Study (ACAPS)[18]	Prospective cohort	885	Multicenter (Australia)	2004–2006	Patrick Charles, MD Patrick.charles@austin.org.au
Not titled[19]	Retrospective cohort	408	Single center (Australia)	2002	Patrick Charles, MD Patrick.charles@austin.org.au
CAPUCI[20]	Prospective cohort	529	Multicenter (Spain)	December 1, 2000–February 28, 2002	Jordi Rello, MD Jrello.aj23.ics@gencat.cat
CAPUCI2	Prospective cohort	150	Multicenter (Spain)	2009–present	Alejandro Rodriguez, MD ahr1161@yahoo.es
EUVAP/CAP[21]	Prospective cohort	2436 intubated patients, 465 VAP	Multicenter 27 ICUs, 9 European countries	Closed	Jordi Rello, MD Jrello.aj23.ics@gencat.cat
Latin-VAP/CAP	Prospective cohort	900 intubated patients	Multicenter	2009–June 2010	Jordi Rello, MD Jrello.aj23.ics@gencat.cat
CAPNETZ[22]	Prospective cohort	6209 inpatient CAP, 2679 outpatient CAP	Multicenter (Germany)	June 1, 2002–April 30, 2007	Tobias Welte, MD welte.tobias@mh-hannover.de
Not titled	Retrospective cohort	714	Single center (Milan, Italy)	2005–2006	Stefano Aliberti, MD Stefano.aliberti@unimib.it
FAILCAP	Prospective cohort	935	Single center (Milan, Italy)	2010–present	Stefano Aliberti, MD Stefano.aliberti@unimib.it
Universidad Católica de Chile[23]	Prospective cohort	463	Single center (Chile)	1999–2001	Fernando Saldías fsaldias@med.puc.cl
Universidad Católica de Chile[24]	Prospective cohort	176	Single center (Chile)	2003–2005	Fernando Saldías fsaldias@med.puc.cl

Abbreviations: CAP, community-acquired pneumonia; HAP, hospital-acquired pneumonia; ICU, intensive care unit; VAP, ventilator-associated pneumonia.

sample size approaches the size of the full population, this error is dramatically reduced.

With any database, some data elements may not be collected. The lack of collection of certain elements may be due to many reasons, such as lack of documentation in the medical record or simply that the element is not used in that particular facility. For example, if a large database of CAP patients was being created and one of the data elements was the C-reactive protein level, those facilities that do not regularly order this laboratory test would not have these data available to include in the database. Missing data can be very detrimental to a study, especially if systematically missing. Systematic missing data might occur if data are missing in a nonrandom manner. Analyzing a database with missing data can cause many issues, as cases may be dropped from analysis or nonrandom missing values may bias the results in a certain direction. If data cannot be collected, data management methods are available to impute these values. For example, imputation may replace a missing value with the value directly above it or below it. Higher-level statistical imputation methods are also available, such as using multivariate regression techniques.[6]

A particular weakness when using large databases generated by insurance companies is that the primary diagnosis is based on the clinical diagnosis by the primary physician as documented in the patient's medical record. From the perspective of coding for reimbursement purposes, the diagnosis documented in the medical record is valid. On the other hand, from the perspective of clinical research, the diagnosis of pneumonia is usually based on predefined criteria and not on the physician's diagnosis. To overcome this limitation, investigators can define the presence of pneumonia by reviewing imaging studies linked to the database.

With large databases, the appropriate statistical power may be reached easily. An issue arises when there are many more patients than needed for a specified power. Although "overpowering" a study is not an issue from a statistical point of view, interpretation of the study results must be done with caution. As the sample size increases, the chance of finding a statistically significant result also increases. The issue arises when a statistically significant result is not necessarily clinically significant.

RESEARCH OPPORTUNITIES USING LARGE DATABASES

An important value of large databases is that they provide several avenues to generate new knowledge. The most important research opportunities using large databases can be summarized as follows.

Analysis of the Database Core Study Question

The primary role of generating a database is to collect information on patients that will allow the investigator to answer the core study question or hypothesis. In the case of CAPO, the core study question is to define the current management of hospitalized patients with CAP, with the goal of evaluating compliance with national guidelines. This question can be answered at a global level, at a regional level, or at a national level. Another approach is to concentrate on the evaluation of a particular aspect of the management of patients with CAP. For example, articles have been published that evaluate the management of CAP at a global level.[7,8] Investigators in a particular country have also performed evaluation of the actual management of CAP. Under the leadership of Dr Carlos Luna, a CAPO network was developed in Argentina to evaluate quality of care in hospitalized patients in that country.[9] More recently, under the leadership of Dr Gur Levy, a network was developed in Venezuela. Some investigators have concentrated on certain aspects of the management of CAP. Recently, Aliberti and colleagues[10] evaluated the management of hospitalized patients with CAP regarding duration of antibiotic therapy.

Databases that are generated for clinical trials of pneumonia treatment have several exclusion criteria that limit the number of patients that can be enrolled into the trial. Database-generated observational studies have the advantage of not having extensive exclusion criteria, thus allowing these databases to contain data on patients with more complex medical problems. Patients are not excluded for participation if they are at high risk for poor outcomes. The CAPO database is an example of an observational cohort study with minimal exclusion criteria. These types of databases therefore more closely reflect the real-world experience of hospitalized patients with CAP.

Secondary Analyses of the Database

Investigators who are part of the network that developed the original database should always consider the possibility of developing new questions or hypotheses other than the core study hypothesis. Performing clinical research using existing data, defined as secondary data analysis, has the advantage of reducing the time and cost necessary to answer a research question. The original investigators can always perform secondary analysis. It is important to know if the database is available for investigators who are not part of the original network. All databases listed in **Table 1** are potentially available for secondary analysis to be performed by investigators who are not participants in the core study.

Several articles performing secondary analysis of the CAPO database have been recently published. In one of these the role of neutropenia in the outcomes of cancer patients with CAP was evaluated.[11] In another, the role of the pneumonia severity index as a predictor for time to clinical stability was examined.[12]

Expanding the Database with Ancillary Studies

Investigators can propose an expansion of the core database to collect new data with the goal of generating information to answer a new study question or hypothesis. These types of studies, defined as ancillary studies, have the advantage of being efficient and inexpensive. The original investigators may require approval of extensive modifications to the core study database.

The CAPO database, being an unbound database, is especially fit for the addition of ancillary studies. Several CAPO investigators have developed ancillary studies that significantly expanded the original CAPO database. For example, the original investigators agreed to add an ancillary

study to evaluate criteria for clinical failure and the etiology of clinical failure during the first 7 days of hospitalization.[13] Under the leadership of Dr Jose Bordon, the CAP human immunodeficiency (HIV) ancillary study evaluating the outcomes of HIV patients with CAP was recently completed.

Concurrently Analyzing Multiple Pneumonia Databases

Another research opportunity for investigators using pneumonia databases is to analyze data from more than one database that are then combined into a single report. There are two possibilities for concurrent analysis of multiple pneumonia databases. A single question can be asked of multiple databases to develop a stronger and more generalizable report. Another possibility is to ask specific questions of specific databases to generate a more robust report.

As an example, under the leadership of Dr Forest Arnold, a question regarding the incidence of atypical pathogens in different regions of the world was asked of the Atypical Pneumonia database. A different question regarding empiric therapy for atypical pathogens and patients' outcomes in different regions of the world was asked of the CAPO database. These two questions were merged into a single article entitled "A Worldwide Perspective on Atypical Pathogens."[14]

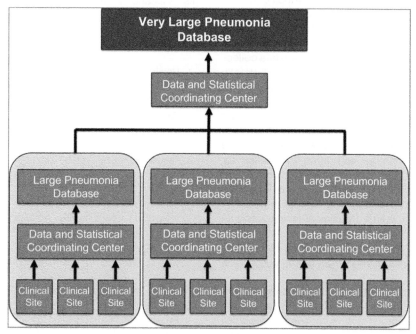

Fig. 4. A model for the development of a very large pneumonia database.

Future Directions: A Very Large Database to Study Pneumonia

In computer science, there is no official or standard definition for the terms "large database" or "very large database." In this article, from the perspective of clinical research in pneumonia, the authors have defined a large database as a database with more than 1000 cases of pneumonia. These types of databases are constructed by the collaboration of approximately 10 to 20 clinical sites. Very large databases can be defined as databases that combine several large databases. In terms of numbers, a very large pneumonia database may contain more than 50,000 cases of pneumonia that will be collected through a collaboration of at least 100 clinical sites. Computer technology that is able to merge large databases with the goal of generating a very large database is not yet available. In pneumonia research, we have reached a level of collaboration among clinical investigators that has allowed the generation of large databases to study pneumonia. The next step is to develop a level of collaboration among the software and database development teams from different centers with the goal of merging databases of pneumonia, and to create a very large global database of pneumonia (**Fig. 4**).

After the creation of a very large database of pneumonia, any investigator with a new question or hypothesis will first evaluate the data available to decide whether the question can be answered by performing a secondary data analysis. If not, the investigator would suggest a modification of the current data collection to expand the database and perform an ancillary study. The presence of an established, very large pneumonia database with standardized software, Internet-based data collection, and a solid data quality program will greatly simplify the development and implementation of new clinical research programs in pneumonia.

Researchers in computer science and computer engineering have been working on the challenges of how to merge large databases and how to develop and manage very large databases for several years. The first international convention fully dedicated to the topic of very large databases took place in Framingham, Massachusetts in 1975.[15] It is now time for clinical investigators in pneumonia to collaborate with colleagues in computer science and computer engineering with the goal of generating a very large, global pneumonia database.

The first step in accomplishing the development of a very large pneumonia database is for current clinical investigators in pneumonia to recognize that the possibility exists to merge large databases and thus generate a pneumonia database clearinghouse. The current DSCCs, located in different regions, will begin to work together to generate international harmonization of pneumonia variables. The very large database can incorporate information on all forms of pneumonia, CAP, health care–associated pneumonia, hospital-acquired pneumonia, and ventilator-associated pneumonia. A project of this magnitude will require funding that can be obtained from funding agencies with an international perspective.

SUMMARY

An important value of large databases is their capability to offer several opportunities for clinical research. Beyond analysis of the database core study question, large databases facilitate secondary analysis, expansion with ancillary studies, and concurrent analysis with other databases. Future collaboration among clinical investigators, software developers, and computer engineers will allow the generation of a global, very large pneumonia database, moving clinical research in pneumonia to a higher level.

ACKNOWLEDGMENTS

The authors would like to thank Dr Robert Kelley, Postdoctoral Associate in the University of Louisville Department of Computer Engineering and Computer Science Mobile Information Networks and Distributed Systems Laboratory, for his assistance in the section describing very large databases.

REFERENCES

1. Ramirez JA. Fostering international multicenter collaborative research: the CAPO Project. Int J Tuberc Lung Dis 2007;11(10):1062–5.
2. Riquelme R, Riquelme M, Rioseco ML, et al. Characteristics of hospitalized patients with 2009 H1N1 influenza in Chile. Eur Respir J 2010;36(4):864–9.
3. Riquelme R; CAPO H1N1 Study Group. Predicting mortality in hospitalized patients with 2009 H1N1 influenza pneumonia. Int J Tuberc Lung Dis 2011; 15(4):542–6.
4. Nguyen LL, Barshes NR. Analysis of large databases in vascular surgery. J Vasc Surg 2010;52(3): 768–74.
5. Imai K, van Dyk DA. Causal inference with general treatment regimes: generalizing the propensity score. J Am Stat Assoc 2004;99(467):854–86.
6. Donders AR, van der Heijden GJ, Stijnen T, et al. Review: a gentle introduction to imputation of missing values. J Clin Epidemiol 2006;59(10):1087–91.

7. Ramirez JA. Worldwide perspective of the quality of care provided to hospitalized patients with community-acquired pneumonia: results from the CAPO international cohort study. Semin Respir Crit Care Med 2005;26(6):543–52.

8. Arnold FW, LaJoie AS, Brock GN, et al. Improving outcomes in elderly patients with community-acquired pneumonia by adhering to national guidelines: Community-Acquired Pneumonia Organization International cohort study results. Arch Intern Med 2009;169(16):1515–24.

9. Christensen D, Luna CM, Martinez J, et al. Adherence with national guidelines in hospitalized patients with community-acquired pneumonia. Results of CAPO study in Argentina. Medicina (B Aires) 2007; 67(6 Pt 2):709–13.

10. Aliberti S, Blasi F, Zanaboni AM, et al. Duration of antibiotic therapy in hospitalised patients with community-acquired pneumonia. Eur Respir J 2010;36(1):128–34.

11. Aliberti S, Myers JA, Peyrani P, et al. The role of neutropenia on outcomes of cancer patients with community-acquired pneumonia. Eur Respir J 2009;33(1):142–7.

12. Arnold FW, Brock GN, Peyrani P, et al. Predictive accuracy of the pneumonia severity index vs CRB-65 for time to clinical stability: results from the Community-Acquired Pneumonia Organization (CAPO) International Cohort Study. Respir Med 2010;104(11):1736–43.

13. Aliberti S, Amir A, Peyrani P, et al. Incidence, etiology, timing, and risk factors for clinical failure in hospitalized patients with community-acquired pneumonia. Chest 2008;134(5):955–62.

14. Arnold FW, Summersgill JT, Lajoie AS, et al. A worldwide perspective of atypical pathogens in community-acquired pneumonia. Am J Respir Crit Care Med 2007;175(10):1086–93.

15. Kerr D. Proceedings of the international conference on very large databases. The Association for Computing Machinery (ACM). Framingham (MA), September 22–24, 1975.

16. Mirsaeidi M, Peyrani P, Ramirez JA. Predicting mortality in patients with ventilator-associated pneumonia: The APACHE II score versus the new IBMP-10 score. Clin Infect Dis 2009;49(1):72–7.

17. Chalmers JD, Singanayagam A, Murray MP, et al. Prior statin use is associated with improved outcomes in community-acquired pneumonia. Am J Med 2008;121(11):1002–7 e1001.

18. Charles PG, Whitby M, Fuller AJ, et al. The etiology of community-acquired pneumonia in Australia: why penicillin plus doxycycline or a macrolide is the most appropriate therapy. Clin Infect Dis 2008; 46(10):1513–21.

19. Ananda-Rajah MR, Charles PG, Melvani S, et al. Comparing the pneumonia severity index with CURB-65 in patients admitted with community acquired pneumonia. Scand J Infect Dis 2008; 40(4):293–300.

20. Rodriguez A, Lisboa T, Blot S, et al. Mortality in ICU patients with bacterial community-acquired pneumonia: when antibiotics are not enough. Intensive Care Med 2009;35(3):430–8.

21. Magret M, Amaya-Villar R, Garnacho J, et al. Ventilator-associated pneumonia in trauma patients is associated with lower mortality: results from EU-VAP study. J Trauma 2010;69(4):849–54.

22. Welte T, Kohnlein T. Global and local epidemiology of community-acquired pneumonia: the experience of the CAPNETZ Network. Semin Respir Crit Care Med 2009;30(2):127–35.

23. Saldias Penafiel F, O'Brien Solar A, Gederlini Gollerino A, et al. Community-acquired pneumonia requiring hospitalization in immunocompetent elderly patients: clinical features, prognostic factors and treatment. Arch Bronconeumol 2003;39(8):333–40 [in Spanish].

24. Diaz A, Barria P, Niederman M, et al. Etiology of community-acquired pneumonia in hospitalized patients in Chile: the increasing prevalence of respiratory viruses among classic pathogens. Chest 2007;131(3):779–87.

The Impact of Guidelines on the Outcomes of Community-acquired and Ventilator-associated Pneumonia

Miquel Ferrer, MD, PhD[a,b], Rosario Menendez, MD, PhD[b,c],
Rosanel Amaro, MD[a], Antoni Torres, MD, PhD[a,b],*

KEYWORDS

- Community-acquired pneumonia
- Ventilator-associated pneumonia • Guidelines
- Empiric antibiotic treatment

COMMUNITY-ACQUIRED PNEUMONIA

Respiratory tract infections constitute one of the most important causes of morbidity and mortality throughout the world, and, among them, pneumonia is the infection that most frequently causes death.[1,2] Although the greatest incidence of community-acquired pneumonia (CAP) occurs in the outpatient environment, where the mortality is lower, in hospitalized patients it varies between 5% and 15%, and is even higher than 25% when admittance to the intensive care unit (ICU) is required. The estimated incidence of CAP varies between 2 and 12 cases per 1000 inhabitants per year, and is more frequent in the extreme stages of life: children younger than 5 years and the elderly.

The evaluation of severity of CAP, the decision about the antibiotic treatment, and the overall management until complete resolution all play key roles in the prognosis of the disease. Furthermore, the recommendations of recently published guidelines have gradually broadened their function, and currently reflect aspects that include the empirical antibiotic treatment, risk factors for resistances, recommendations for hospitalization on the ward or in the ICU and subsequent discharge, definitions for nonresponding pneumonia, and recommendations for prevention.[3–5]

An appropriate way to evaluate the effect of guidelines for the management of pneumonias to analyze their impact on prognosis, because any deviation from the guidelines must be judged by its effect on patient outcome. In the past few years, there has been an increase in publications that have analyzed the independent effect of guideline compliance and its impact on prognosis.

Prediction of Causal Microorganisms According to Stratification of Patients

CAP is caused by a great variety of microorganisms. The classic approach, taking into account

This work was supported by 2009SGR911, Ciberes (CB06/06/0028)-ISCiii-MCI, Spain, and IDIBAPS.
The authors have nothing to disclose.
[a] Servei de Pneumologia, Institut del Torax, Hospital Clinic, IDIBAPS, Universitat de Barcelona, Villarroel 170, 08036 Barcelona, Spain
[b] Centro de Investigación Biomedica En Red-Enfermedades Respiratorias (CibeRes, CB06/06/0028), Barcelona, Spain
[c] Servicio de Neumologia, ISS Hospital Universitario La Fe, Avda de Campanar 21, 46009 Valencia, Spain
* Corresponding author. UVIR, Servei de Pneumologia, Hospital Clínic, Villarroel 170, 08036 Barcelona, Spain.
E-mail address: atorres@ub.edu

Clin Chest Med 32 (2011) 491–505
doi:10.1016/j.ccm.2011.06.002

symptoms, blood analyses, and radiographic results, is inefficient at identifying the causal microorganism. The cause in CAP mainly depends on the setting: outpatient, ward, or ICU admission. Therefore, empirical antibiotics recommended by guidelines are related to the site of care of patients. The Infectious Disease Society of America (IDSA)/ American Thoracic Society (ATS) recommendations stratifying patients into different groups for initial treatment according to the severity of illness.[4] Predicting microorganisms according to prognostic scales and how cause is associated with severity is important in selecting an empirical antibiotic regimen.

In patients with CAP, Carratala and colleagues[6] found a similar proportion of the most frequent causative microorganisms (*Streptococcus pneumoniae*, *Legionella pneumophila*, and *Hemophilus influenzae*) in patients with Pneumonia Severity Index (PSI) risk scale[7] II to III, irrespective of whether patients were hospitalized or not. Roson and colleagues[8] in 533 patients showed a correlation between cause of CAP and severity measured by the PSI. *S pneumoniae* was the most frequent microorganism in all risk classes, although it was more frequent in higher risk classes. Although reported in all risk classes, *Legionella* spp and *H influenzae* were also more frequent in higher risk classes. Atypical microorganisms were predominant in lower risk classes, whereas gram-negative bacilli were more common in higher risk classes. In that study, mixed infections were not associated with mortality. Mortality was higher with gram-negative bacilli, in aspiration pneumonia, and with *S pneumoniae*, and lower with atypical or viral causes.

Dambrava and colleagues[9] validated the recommendations in the 2001 ATS guidelines concerning stratification of groups for selecting initial antibiotics.[10] The groups were group I, outpatients with no cardiopulmonary disease or modifying factors; group II, outpatients with cardiopulmonary disease or modifying factors; group III-a, hospitalized patients without modifying factors; group III-b, hospitalized patients with modifying factors; group IV-a, patients in an ICU without risk factors for *Pseudomonas aeruginosa*; and group IV-b patients in an ICU with risk factors for *P aeruginosa*. After excluding nursing homes, they found a low proportion of *Pseudomonas* spp even in higher risk classes. *Legionella* spp were more frequent in patients in an ICU. In group I, atypical agents were a frequent cause, whereas *S pneumoniae* was the most common in all risk classes.

Cilloniz and colleagues[11] recently found an increasing frequency of *S pneumoniae* and mixed causes and decreasing frequency of atypical pathogens in hospitalized patients and patients in ICUs. Atypical bacteria are confidently recognized as low-risk conditions, whereas severity scores such as the PSI and CURB65 are more sensitive in identifying patients with Enterobacteriaceae and *P aeruginosa* as moderate-risk and high-risk causes.

Valencia and colleagues[12] reported a higher proportion of *P aeruginosa* in PSI risk class V patients, with similar proportions in those admitted to ICUs or wards (16% and 10%, respectively). In this ICU population, *P aeruginosa* was not related to nursing home residence. A German study on a large population found that independent risk factors for Enterobacteriaceae included cardiac and cerebrovascular disease, and, for *P aeruginosa*, chronic respiratory disease and enteral tube feeding.[13]

Swedish guidelines stratified cause depending on the prognostic scale CRB65. Stralin and colleagues[14] corroborated that *S pneumoniae* was the most frequent cause in low and high scores, whereas *Mycoplasma* sp was more frequent in low scores and *H influenzae* in the highest scores. Low frequencies of *Legionella* sp and other causes were reported (<3%).

Adequacy of Antibiotic Treatment Recommended by Guidelines and Outcome

Causal diagnosis is obtained in around 50% of cases, even when various microbiological studies are used, and it is sometimes obtained too late for selecting an initial antibiotic regimen. The choice of antibiotic treatment in CAP has prognostic implications, and an inappropriate initial treatment increases mortality.[15] In current practice, the decision to initiate antibiotic treatment is made at the time of the clinical diagnosis, without waiting for the microbiological results, except if urinary antigen data are available.

Debate exists about the importance of empirical versus targeted antibiotic treatment. Falguera and colleagues[16] designed a randomized study to initiate antibiotics, with 89 patients in the empirical treatment arm and 88 patients in the targeted treatment arm depending on urinary antigens findings. They found that antibiotic adherence to guidelines is better than adjusting treatment to urinary antigens, so they concluded that routine implementation of urine antigen does not carry substantial outcome-related or economic benefits to hospitalized patients with CAP. Narrowing the antibiotic treatment according to the urine antigen results may be associated with a higher risk of clinical relapse. However, van der Eerden and colleagues[17] did not find superiority of combined therapy versus pathogen-directed therapy, although the incidence of *Legionella* sp and the resistance of *S pneumoniae* to antibiotics are low in their geographic area.

Guidelines may help physicians to select the empirical antibiotic treatment in patients with CAP. Studies have addressed this issue in 3 different patient settings: outpatients, conventional hospitalization, and ICU admission.

Outpatient setting

There are few studies addressing antibiotic adherence and outcomes in the outpatient setting. In a Cochrane review using publications from a 12-year period, 6 studies with 1857 patients were selected.[18] No differences were found in the efficacy among antibiotics used in the outpatient setting. Gleason and colleagues[19] showed a good adherence to the ATS guidelines,[20] with differences in costs but not in outcomes. Suchyta and colleagues[21] found a decrease in admissions when there was higher adherence to a pneumonia guideline without reporting adverse effects.

Conventional hospitalization

Concerning hospitalized patients with CAP, there is more information about the impact of compliance with antibiotic treatment on outcomes (**Tables 1** and **2**). In a tertiary care hospital, Menendez and colleagues[22] compared the effect of adherence to 2 different guidelines: the Spanish (Spanish Society of Pulmonology and Thoracic Surgery [SEPAR]) and those of the ATS in hospitalized patients with CAP. This study found a lower mortality in the highest risk patients and the protective effect was more evident with the ATS guidelines and in PSI risk class

V patients. In a later multicenter study, the protective effect of the guideline-adherent treatment was confirmed, both on treatment failure and on mortality. Moreover, the hospital and the type of doctor prescribing the treatment were also associated with adherence and response to treatment.[23]

Dean and colleagues[24] analyzed the impact of the guidelines on 17,728 patients, including serious episodes with sepsis and/or respiratory failure, and adjusted for comorbidity. Key elements included in their health care pneumonia guidelines were the use of the CURB65 score for admission support, antibiotic prescription following guidelines, microbiological studies for inpatients, prophylaxis for deep venous thrombosis, and early ambulation, among others. These investigators showed a reduction in mortality in the adherent hospitals (odds ratio [OR] 0.89). The conclusion drawn from the findings was that, with this protocol, 20 lives could be saved yearly. The readmission rate was also lower.

Most of the previous studies analyzed mortality after 30 days. However, Mortensen and colleagues[25] showed in a retrospective study that the use of guideline-concordant antimicrobial therapy was significantly associated with decreased mortality (OR 0.37) at 48 hours after admission, after adjusting for confounders. One of the greatest limitations of the study is that, in the first 48 hours, only 2.5% of patients died, so these data should be confirmed with broader prospective studies.

More recently, Arnold and colleagues,[26] using a worldwide database, found that the patients with coverage against atypical organisms reached earlier clinical stability and had shorter hospital stays than those without this therapy. Menendez

Table 1
Impact of adherence to antibiotics recommended in the guidelines on selected outcomes

	Mortality	Treatment Failure	Time to Clinical Stability	Length of Stay	Readmission
Non-ICU					
Menendez et al[22]	↓	↓		=	
Blasi et al[52]	↓	↓			
Frei et al[55]	↓		↓	↓	
Mortensen et al[25]	↓				
Dean et al[24]	↓				↓
Capelastegui et al[51]	↓		↓	↓	
Dambrava et al[9]	↓			↓	
Arnold et al[28]	↓		↓	↓	
ICU					
Bodi et al[34]	↓				↓
Frei et al[36]	↓		=	=	

Table 2
Impact of adherence to guidelines and antibiotic regimens on length of stay

	N	Guidelines (% Adherence)	Median Length of Stay (d)		P
			Adherence	No Adherence	
Arnold et al[28,a]	4337	—	6.1	7.1	<0.001
Battleman et al[44]	609	IDSA (56)	OR 0.55	—	—
Stahl et al[32,b]	76	—	2.75	5.3	0.01
Dudas et al[33,c]	2963	ATS (81)	—	Higher	0.01
Meehan et al[54,d]	2388	—	5	7	<0.001
Shorr et al[37,e]	199	IDSA (56.8)	—	OR 1.40	—
Capelastegui et al[51,f]	1915	IDSA/ATS	7.3	5.7	<0.001

Abbreviation: OR, odds ratio.
  [a] Antibiotic regime with coverage for atypicals (77%) versus noncoverage for atypicals.
  [b] Treatment with macrolides within the first 24 hours or not.
  [c] Results from multivariate statistical analysis.
  [d] Connecticut Thoracic Society guideline. Number of patients: baseline period (1242 patients)/follow-up period (1146 patients).
  [e] Nonadherence increased the likelihood of longer mechanical ventilation.
  [f] Total patients 1915: 1 interventional hospital versus 4 control hospitals.

and colleagues[27] found that clinical stability was achieved 1 day earlier in patients treated according to the Spanish (SEPAR) or the ATS guidelines, after adjusting for severity and comorbidities. Dambrava and colleagues[9] reported shorter length of stay in patients receiving regimens that adhered to the 2001 ATS guidelines (7.6 vs 10.4 days); this result was confirmed after adjusting for confounders.

In elderly patients, adherence to the IDSA/ATS guidelines[4] at the local hospital level improved not only mortality and length of stay but also time to clinical stability, even when including patients who were residents of a nursing home.[28] In hospitalized patients with CAP, Orrick and colleagues[29] found that treatment according to the IDSA guidelines may result in cost savings to institutions (mean in the group treated with selected antibiotics $3009 vs $4992), although in this study there was no allowance for the initial severity, which is an important determinant of length of stay.

Cost-effectiveness analysis is a useful tool when evaluating costs and outcomes with different treatment modalities. This analysis, directed toward the initial empirical antibiotic treatment and adherence to the guidelines, has been rarely used in CAP.[30] Among the results, the mortality and readmission rates were 10% and 2.1% for adherent treatment versus 13.6% and 6.2% for nonadherent treatment. The incremental cost-effectiveness ratio showed that adherence to treatment guidelines saved 1121 Euros per patient cured, compared with nonadherence. Another study on the cost of the management and treatment of pneumonia showed that the therapeutic option with the best cost-effectiveness relationship was the one that followed the IDSA guidelines and was integrated into a pneumonia management plan.[31] Other studies have addressed the impact of guideline adherence on length of stay.[32,33]

ICU admission

In a multicenter prospective study in 23 hospitals, Bodi and colleagues[34] investigated the prognostic factors related to outcome in patients with CAP admitted to the ICU. This study, which included only severe CAP with a high mortality, analyzed adherence to the IDSA guidelines and confirmed the lower mortality in the adherent group of patients (24% vs 33%). Moreover, this finding was consistent after adjusting, in a multivariate analysis, for other confounders or risk factors, such as the APACHE-II score, age, and immune-compromised status. In addition, inadequate or insufficient initial treatment was most commonly found when P aeruginosa or methicillin-resistant Staphylococcus aureus (MRSA) were the causative microorganisms, even if patients were treated according to guidelines. The investigators reported that chronic obstructive pulmonary disease, malignancy, and prior antibiotic treatments were the most frequent risk factors for P aeruginosa. Dambrava and colleagues[9] also reported lower adherence to guidelines in patients in ICUs, and specifically in those at risk for Pseudomonas sp.

Martin-Loeches and colleagues[35] found that adherence to 2007 IDSA/ATS guidelines[4] in patients in ICUs with severe sepsis and septic shock was associated with lower mortality if treatment included a combination with macrolides (HR 0.44). In a retrospective study, Frei and colleagues[36] found a significantly lower mortality (25% vs 12%) in those patients treated with concordant antibiotic therapy.

Shorr and colleagues[37] analyzed the impact of antibiotic guideline compliance on the duration of mechanical ventilation (MV) in critically ill patients with CAP. They found that noncompliance with antibiotic recommendations for the treatment of CAP may increase the need for continuing MV. The investigators hypothesized that guideline compliance could represent a surrogate marker for other aspects of clinical care. However, the conclusion was that, given the costs associated with MV, guideline compliance may improve outcomes and enhance resource use.

Antibiotics Timing and Outcome

The timing of the initiation of the antibiotic treatment is one of the processes of care and a quality indicator that has aroused great interest in the past few years. Before the publication of the latest IDSA/ATS guidelines,[4] studies had already shown that adherence to guidelines and quality indicators were useful measures for improving the quality of care and prognosis. Nevertheless, the time elapsed until the initiation of the antibiotic treatment has produced a lot of controversy, because it is an indicator that can be modified by many factors, and because it can increase the number of unnecessary antibiotics used.[38] The detractors stated that timing has been adopted as a measure of quality of care in CAP based on 2 retrospective studies of large Medicare databases. In a prospective study, Waterer and colleagues[38] investigated, in 451 patients, the time (>4 hours) until the first antibiotic dose and the associated mortality. They found that altered mental state, absence of fever, absence of hypoxia, and increasing age were significant predictors of a delay in giving the first antibiotic dose. Moreover, in a multivariate analysis, they did not find an independent association between timing and mortality. Factors related to a delay in administering antibiotics in patients with CAP were an altered mental state or minimal signs of sepsis. The investigators stated that delayed antibiotic treatment was likely to be a marker of comorbidities driving both an atypical presentation and mortality, rather than directly contributing to outcome.

In a systematic review, Yu and Wyer[39] analyzed the results of 13 different retrospective and prospective observational studies that examined timing and evaluated whether the investigators controlled for severity. They failed to confirm decreased mortality with early administration of antibiotics in stable patients with CAP, and concluded that, although timely administration of antibiotics to patients with confirmed CAP should be encouraged, an inflated sense of the importance of the 4-hour time frame was not justified by the evidence. Nevertheless, there was inconsistency and no homogeneity of the results, because, in the studies analyzed, clinicians were more aware of severity and were prescribing antibiotics faster in those with recognized severity signs than those without. Cheng and Buising[40] reported no positive association between time to first antibiotic dose and mortality or prolonged length of stay, likely because patients at highest risk of death received antibiotics earlier than those less severely ill.

Furthermore, the implementation of any process of care might be accompanied by higher costs. In an intervention study, Barlow and colleagues[41] found that the increase in the proportion of patients who received an appropriate antibiotic treatment in the first 4 hours was accompanied by a significant increase in cost. Other recommendations, such as the usefulness of prognostic scales for the hospital admission decision, and the impact of the collection of blood cultures on mortality, have also created controversy.

The current perception is that timing is important in the most severely ill patients and that implementation of this recommendation should be specifically directed to them. In patients with septic shock, time to starting antibiotics is important, as indicated by a study of 14 ICUs in Canada and the United States.[42] The assessment of the medical records of 2731 adult patients with septic shock revealed a strong relationship between any delay in effective antimicrobial initiation and in-hospital mortality. Administration of an antimicrobial effective for isolated or suspected pathogens within the first hour of documented hypotension was associated with a survival rate of 80%, whereas each hour of delay in the next 6 hours was associated with an average decrease in survival of 7.6%.

Ferrer and colleagues[43] analyzed the effectiveness of treatments recommended in the sepsis guidelines. The early administration of broad-spectrum antibiotics in all patients and administration of drotrecogin-α (activated) in the most severe patients with sepsis reduced mortality. Battleman and colleagues[44] found that rapid antibiotic initiation and appropriate antibiotic selection in the emergency department reduced the hospital stay in CAP.

Barriers to the rapid administration of appropriate antibiotics in CAP are related to reasons such as knowledge and education, attitudes to CAP by doctors, work intensity and lack of senior support, and difficulty in using guidelines.[45] Some of the identified barriers could be overcome by undergraduate and postgraduate education, but organizational barriers can only be overcome by system redesign.

Rationale for Implementing Guidelines

The goals of the scientific guidelines are to improve management and outcome without increasing costs or reducing patient safety. There are many reasons for the lack of compliance[46–48]: (1) insufficient up-to-date training; (2) disagreement with the interpretation of the studies on which the treatments are based and/or the indications made by the guidelines[49]; and (3) external barriers or other circumstances.[46] In some specific circumstances, deviation from the guidelines may be appropriate if physicians recognize a clinical situation that is not appropriately addressed by the guidelines, such as an unusual causative microorganism or an underlying risk factor. Although it is not possible to routinely predict the causal microorganism, it is possible to identify risk factors for an unusual microorganism.

Several types of studies of guideline implementation have been conducted to evaluate their impact on outcomes. Randomized studies are not available because they are unethical. The most accessible studies are those with a before-after time series design. These studies compare the results in hospitals after the guideline implementation, either with their previous results or with hospitals that use the usual care (treatment according to guidelines vs usual care control). These studies also have limitations, such as the existence of other differences in the process of care, representing distinct study populations, or even different epidemiology across different geographic areas. Thus, Dean and colleagues,[50] in a multicenter study that included more than 28,000 cases of pneumonia in hospitals and outpatients, compared the effect of the implementation of the 1993 ATS guidelines[20] in some hospitals and centers with other hospitals that continued their usual care. Their results showed a decrease in the inpatient mortality after 30 days in the elderly admitted to those hospitals where the guidelines were in place. Furthermore, with the proposed admission criteria, they achieved a decrease in the hospitalization rate with no adverse effect on survival.

Capelastegui and colleagues[51] designed a before-after study in a hospital with guideline implementation compared with 4 control hospitals. Longitudinal measurement of outcomes before and after an intervention in one hospital was compared with the outcomes in 4 other hospitals. The measures implemented in the hospital were patient admission criteria, initiation of antibiotic, adherence to guidelines, antimicrobial coverage for atypical pathogens, and length of intravenous treatment. The study showed that the mortality, length of stay, and percentage of admissions in the control hospitals were similar in the 2 time periods of the study. In contrast, in the hospital with guideline implementation, the percentage of appropriate treatment increased, and the mortality and length of hospital stay were reduced.

Implementing guidelines is difficult. Blasi and colleagues[52] performed a before-after design in a population of almost 3000 patients. After a guideline implementation phase, although compliance with guidelines increased, the degree was low (44%), indicating the need for more aggressive and proactive approaches in future. This study highlighted that the risk of failure at the end of the first-line therapy, particularly in PSI risk class V patients, and the outcome in the overall population improved in compliant therapies. With regard to the type of antibiotic used, they pointed out that the use of levofloxacin alone and the combination of cephalosporin and macrolide resulted in higher success rates and in a significantly lower mortality.

The implementation of norms and clinical protocols to increase adherence to the guidelines has also shown a reduced hospitalization of patients with pneumonia.[51,53] In a multicenter study in 31 hospitals, Meehan and colleagues[54] achieved a reduction in the hospital stay from an average of 7 days to 5 days. In a retrospective study in 5 hospitals, Frei and colleagues[55] reported both a significant decrease in time to switch therapy and, consequently, length of hospital stay, in patients with guideline-compliant antibiotic therapy.

In summary, it seems that the stratification of CAP according to severity predicts fairly well the different causes of pneumonia, and this is the first step in selecting the different types of empirical antibiotic treatment. In addition, specific risk factors for particular microorganisms have to be taken into account. Compliance with the initial antibiotic guideline recommendations seems to favor a better outcome, although the different components of these recommendations (early antibiotic treatment, adherence and adequacy of recommendations, different combinations of antibiotics) have been studied separately and it is difficult to know the specific weight of each of these components.

HOSPITAL-ACQUIRED AND VENTILATOR-ACQUIRED PNEUMONIA

Hospital-acquired pneumonia (HAP) is the second most common nosocomial infection and accounts for approximately one-fourth of all infections in the ICU. When HAP occurs in mechanically ventilated patients, this is called ventilator-associated pneumonia (VAP).[56] The incidence of VAP ranges between 10% and 30% in patients who require MV for more than 48 hours. This incidence depends on the type of population studied, the presence or absence of risk factors, and the type and intensity of preventive measures implemented. Although mortality varies from one study to another, and the prognostic impact of nosocomial pneumonia is debated, it is recognized that one-third to one-half of all HAP deaths are directly attributable to the pneumonia itself.[57]

During the last decade, several risk factors associated with mortality have been detected. The most consistent and evident prognostic factor throughout the literature is the accuracy of initial empirical antibiotic treatment.[57] In a large series of patients with HAP, Alvarez Lerma[58] showed that patients with adequate antibiotic treatment had lower mortality than those with inadequate therapy (16% vs 25%). In addition, in that study, the number of complications and the presence of shock and of gastrointestinal hemorrhage were also lower in the group of patients receiving initial adequate antibiotic treatment. The percentage of inadequate treatment has varied in the literature between 22% and 73%.[57] In addition, the microorganisms not covered by the initial treatment in these studies were most often multidrug-resistant microorganisms such as *P aeruginosa*, *Acinetobacter* spp and MRSA.[57,58] For all the reasons mentioned earlier, it is important to set up antibiotic treatment protocols that potentially cover most of the microorganisms causing HAP or VAP.

The ATS released in 1996,[59] and later in 2005 jointly with the IDSA,[60] guidelines for the management of adults with HAP. The most recent guidelines, from 2005, included patients with VAP and patients with health care–associated pneumonia (HCAP). The stratification into different groups for initial treatment varied when comparing the 1996 (**Fig. 1**) and 2005 (**Fig. 2**) recommendations. In 1996, the guidelines recommended stratifying patients according to severity of illness (mild to moderate or severe), presence of risk factors, and the time of onset of pneumonia (early and late onset).[59] This algorithm was simplified in 2005 using only the time of onset and the presence of risk factor for multidrug-resistant microorganisms.[60]

In **Box 1** and **Table 3** the potential microorganisms in the different stratification groups from both the 1996 and 2005 guidelines are listed. An additional classification for mechanically ventilated patients was proposed by Trouillet and colleagues.[61] They classified patients in 4 categories according to the presence or absence of previous antimicrobial therapy and more or less than 7 days of MV (MV<7 days with no antibiotics, MV<7 days with antibiotics, MV>7 days with no antibiotics, and MV>7 days with antibiotics). The distribution of microorganisms in relation to these variables is shown in **Table 4**.

Prediction of Microorganisms According to Stratification Groups

Few studies have validated the accuracy of the prediction schemes for specific microorganisms. Leroy and colleagues[62] studied 124 patients with HAP-confirmed bacteriology and they assessed

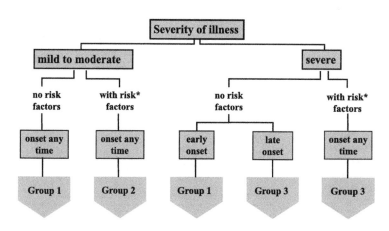

Fig. 1. Algorithm for classifying patients with HAP according to the Consensus Statement of the American Thoracic Society. Asterisk (*) indicates that risk factors for specific pathogens were specified in the guidelines. These included risk factors for anaerobes, *S aureus*, *Legionella* spp, and *P aeruginosa*. (*Adapted from* American Thoracic Society. Hospital-acquired pneumonia in adults: diagnosis, assessment of severity, initial antimicrobial therapy, and preventative strategies. A consensus statement. Am J Respir Crit Care Med 1996;153:1713; with permission.)

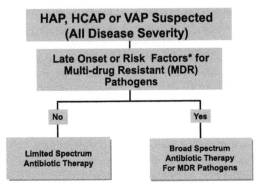

Fig. 2. Algorithm for initiating empirical antibiotic therapy for HAP, ventilator-associated pneumonia (VAP), and health care–associated pneumonia (HCAP), according to the 2005 American Thoracic Society/Infectious Disease Society of America. Asterisk (*) indicates prior antimicrobial therapy (90 days); hospitalization greater than or equal to 5 days; high frequency of antibiotic resistance in the community or the hospital unit; immunosuppressive disease or therapy. (*Adapted from* American Thoracic Society, Infectious Diseases Society of America. Guidelines for the Management of Adults with Hospital-acquired, Ventilator-associated, and Healthcare-associated Pneumonia. Am J Respir Crit Care Med 2005;171:401; with permission.)

the microbial prediction according to the 1996 ATS guidelines and to the Trouillet and colleagues[61] classification (see **Table 4**). In this study, the ATS classification was able to detect HAP episodes caused by resistant organisms with a negative predictive value of 100%, and was more specific than the Trouillet classification.

In another study with similar design, Ioanas and colleagues[63] also evaluated the 1996 ATS classification and Trouillet and colleagues'[61] criteria in 71 patients with ICU-acquired pneumonia. The ATS and Trouillet classifications showed an accuracy in predicting the causative microorganisms of 91% and 83%, respectively. The ATS approach failed to predict 2 microorganisms classified into ATS group 2 (*P aeruginosa* and MRSA) and 1 pathogen from a patient classified into group 3 (*Aspergillus* spp). The use of the Trouillet classification could properly predict the pathogen isolated in 15 of 18 (83%) patients, only failing to predict 3 pathogens: 1 MRSA in a Trouillet group 1, 1 MRSA in Trouillet group 2, and 1 *Aspergillus* spp in a Trouillet group 4 patients.

More recently, we evaluated a series of patients with HAP in the ICU and examined the prediction of microorganisms using both the 1996 ATS guidelines[59] and the 2005 ATS/IDSA recommendations.[60] We found that the 1996 guidelines better predicted the microorganisms causing HAP

Box 1
Potential microorganisms in each group according to the 1996 consensus statement of the ATS

Group 1: Core organisms

- Enteric gram-negative bacilli:
  - *Escherichia coli*
  - *Enterobacter* sp
  - *Klebsiella* sp
  - *Proteus* sp
  - *Serratia marcescens*
- *H influenzae*
- MS *S aureus*
- *S pneumoniae*

Group 2[a]: Core organisms plus

- Anaerobes
- *S aureus* (MS and MR)
- *Legionella* sp
- *P aeruginosa*

Group 3: Core organisms plus

- *P aeruginosa*
- *Acinetobacter* sp
- MR *S aureus*

Abbreviations: MS, methicillin sensitive; MR, methicillin resistant.
[a] Risk factors: abdominal surgery, witnessed aspiration, coma, head trauma, diabetes mellitus, renal failure, high-dose steroids, prolonged ICU stay, antibiotics, structural lung disease.
Data from American Thoracic Society. Hospital acquired pneumonia in adults: diagnosis, assessment of severity, initial antimicrobial therapy, and preventative strategies. A consensus statement. Am J Respir Crit Care Med 1996;153:1711–25.

---

or VAP in the ICU.[64] Specifically, 10 cases (26%) from group 1 of the 2005 classification[60] had potentially resistant bacteria despite the absence of risk factors for these microorganisms according to the guidelines. Reclassifying patients according to the 1996 guidelines, these microorganisms were correctly predicted in 9 (90%) of them. Further prospective studies in larger series are needed to confirm that the 1996 ATS guidelines were more accurate in predicting microorganisms compared with the 2005 ATS/IDSA recommendations.

Adequacy of Treatment and Outcome

Because adequacy of treatment is associated with lower mortality, the initial goal should be guideline

Table 3
Initial empirical antimicrobial treatment of patients with for hospital-acquired, ventilator-associated, and health care–associated pneumonia, according to the 2005 American Thoracic Society/Infectious Disease Society of America

No Risk Factors for MDR, Early Onset, and Any Disease Severity	Late-Onset Disease or Risk Factors for MDR Pathogens and all Disease Severity
Potential pathogens	Potential MDR pathogens
• S pneumoniae	P aeruginosa
• H influenzae	Klebsiella pneumoniae (ESBL)
• MS S aureus	Acinetobacter spp
• Antibiotic-sensitive enteric GNB:	L pneumophila
◦ E coli	MR S aureus
◦ K pneumoniae	
◦ Enterobacter sp	
◦ Proteus sp	
◦ S marcescens	
Recommended antibiotics	Recommended antibiotics
• Ceftriaxone, or	Combination antibiotic therapy:
• Levofloxacin, moxifloxacin, ciprofloxacin, or	Antipseudomonal cephalosporin (cefepime, ceftazidime), or
• Ampicillin/sulbactam, or	Antipseudomonal carbapenem (imipenem, meropenem), or
• Ertapenem	B-lactam, B-lactamase inhibitor (piperacillin/tazobactam) plus
	Antipseudomonal fluoroquinolone (ciprofloxacin, levofloxacin) plus
	Linezolid or vancomycin (if risk factors present)

Abbreviations: ESBL, extended-spectrum β-lactamase; GNB, gram-negative bacillus; MDR, multidrug resistant.
   Data from American Thoracic Society, Infectious Diseases Society of America. Guidelines for the Management of Adults with Hospital-acquired, Ventilator-associated, and Healthcare-associated Pneumonia. Am J Respir Crit Care Med 2005;171:388–416.

compliance. In a previous study, the adequacy of treatment according to the 1996 guidelines and Trouillet recommendations were 79% and 80%, respectively.[63] Microorganisms associated with inadequate treatment according to the ATS guidelines were P aeruginosa, Acinetobacter baumannii, Stenotrophomonas maltophilia, and MRSA, whereas P aeruginosa was associated with inadequate treatment according to the Trouillet classification.

Ibrahim and colleagues[65] implemented a treatment protocol based on accurate diagnosis definitions, microbiological confirmation of VAP, and the administration of imipenem plus ciprofloxacin as initial empirical antibiotic treatment. Fifty-two patients with VAP were evaluated before and after protocol implementation. The adequacy of initial treatment increased from 48% to 94%, comparing the preintervention and postintervention periods. The duration of antibiotic treatment was decreased from 15 to 9 days, and a second episode of VAP decreased from 24% to 8%. However, mortality was not changed.

To evaluate an antibiotic treatment protocol based on local microbiology data, Soo Hoo and colleagues[66] studied the treatment adequacy and outcome of 56 preguideline episodes and 61 guideline-treated episodes of severe HAP. They implemented an antibiotic protocol for HAP based on the 1996 ATS guidelines, adjusted according to local microbiological and resistance patterns. With the implementation of the local protocol, the adequacy of treatment increased from 46% to 81%. The 14-day mortality decreased from 27% to 8%. There were also differences in hospital and 30-day mortality in favor of the prospectively treated group, although differences were not significant.

Overall, there is not much evidence about the influence of guidelines on the outcome of patients with VAP, and this reflects the difficulties of these studies. A study validating the 2005 ATS/IDSA guidelines showed that adherence to the empirical treatment in the guidelines resulted in more treatment adequacy but did not influence major outcome variables such as hospital mortality.[64]

Table 4
Numbers and percentages of microorganisms responsible for 135 episodes of VAP classified according to the duration of MV and prior antibiotic therapy

	Group 1 (n = 22) MV<7 ATB = No	Group 2 (n = 12) MV<7 ATB = Yes	Group 3 (n = 17) MV>7 ATB = No	Group 4 (n = 84) MV>7 ATB = Yes
Total number of bacteria	41	20	32	152
Multiresistant bacteria (%)	0[a]	6 (30)	4 (13)[b]	89 (59)
P aeruginosa (%)	0	4 (20)	2 (6)	33 (22)
Acinetobacter baumannii (%)	0	1 (5)	1 (3)	20 (13)
Stenotrophomonas maltophilia (%)	0	0	0	6 (4)
MRSA (%)	0	1 (5)	1 (3)	30 (20)
Other bacteria (%)	41 (100)	14 (70)	28 (88)	63 (42)
Enterobacteriaceae (%)	10 (25)	4 (20)	7 (22)	23 (15)
Haemophilus spp (%)	8 (20)	2 (10)	1 (3)	4 (3)
MSSA (%)	6	0	7 (22)	7 (5)
S pneumoniae	3	0	0	0
Other streptococci (%)	7	5 (25)	7 (22)	14 (9)
Neisseria spp (%)	5	2 (10)	4 (13)	3 (2)
Other pathogens (%)	2	1 (5)	2 (6)	12 (8)

Abbreviation: ATB, antibiotics.
[a] P<.02 compared with groups 2, 3, and 4.
[b] P<.0001 compared with group 4.
Data from Trouillet JL, Chastre J, Vuagnat A, et al. Ventilator-associated pneumonia caused by potentially drug resistant bacteria. Am J Respir Crit Care Med 1998;157:531–9.

Additional concerns regarding the 2005 ATS/IDSA recommendations have recently been raised. In an observational study, patients in an ICU at risk for multidrug-resistant pneumonia who were treated according to these guidelines had higher mortality than those with nonadherent treatment.[67] The main reasons for noncompliance in this study were failure to use a second anti–gram-negative drug, or either a primary anti–gram-negative drug or anti-MRSA drug, resulting in more patients from the compliant group treated with triple antibiotic coverage. This study has several important limitations.[68] First, coverage of several multidrug-resistant bacteria was lower in patients with empirical treatment considered compliant with guidelines. Second, the timing of initiation of antimicrobial therapy, an important determination of outcome, particularly in patients with septic shock, was not assessed in this study. Third, excess mortality might be related to treatment toxicity of triple coverage, particularly renal failure, although no definitive data showed this to be the case.

The 2005 ATS/IDSA guidelines have several limitations in the definition of patients at risk for multidrug-resistant pneumonia and possibly promoting unnecessary use of empirical broad-spectrum combination antibiotics.[69] As mentioned earlier, more studies validating guidelines are needed to confirm the usefulness of these guidelines in clinical practice.

Elements to be Taken into Account to Validate Guidelines on HAP and VAP

Guideline implementation

One of the most difficult problems is to implement guidelines locally. A good example is the experience of Soo Hoo and colleagues.[66] In order to implement guidelines, they were first drafted and completed during several months. Then, a combined committee composed of members of the Pulmonary and Infectious Disease Services and the pharmacy met, and the guidelines were discussed and agreed on. The guidelines then underwent pilot testing for several months, and then they were posted and distributed to each group of house staff rotating through the medical ICU. Guidelines were distributed twice every 4 weeks. The guidelines were reviewed regularly by each group of stakeholders, and were also available on the Internet. The guidelines were also reviewed regularly by one of the staff physicians during daily rounds, or by one of the members of the pharmacy or Infectious Diseases Service. In the first few months after the introduction of the guidelines, regular conference sessions were held with house staff rotating through the medical ICU to reinforce the guidelines. In summary, implementation of local guidelines is a difficult task and a key element in performing studies with a before-and-after design.

Delay of initial antibiotic treatment

This variable may influence the results of any studies to validate guidelines. In retrospective studies it is difficult to know this information, but in prospective studies the time period from initial diagnosis to treatment needs to be standardized. For example, Iregui and colleagues[70] studied 107 patients and divided them in 2 groups according to whether or not the first dose of antibiotics was delayed for more than 24 hours. A delay of more than 24 hours was an independent risk factor of mortality (OR 7.68). The most common reason for delayed antibiotic administration was a delay in writing medical orders (78.5% of patients). The results of this study are a clear example of how outcomes of patients with VAP may be modified by other factors, in addition to adherence to guideline antibiotic recommendations.

Dosages of antibiotics

Dosages and intervals of administration of antibiotics may be associated with the outcomes for the patients, particularly with multidrug-resistant microorganisms. A classic manuscript from Paladino and colleagues[71] showed better survival in VAP caused by *P aeruginosa* when the area under the curve (AUC)/minimal inhibitory concentration (MIC) ratios for ciprofloxacin were optimized. The ATS/IDSA guidelines[60] recommend dosages and intervals of administration based on pharmacokinetic (PK)/pharmacodynamic (PD) information. When performing studies of validation, it is important to optimize dosages and avoid comparing patients with different dosages or intervals.

Local adaptation of guidelines

The patterns of microbial agents and their resistance vary from hospital to hospital and even in the same hospital from unit to unit. The variability of microorganisms and resistance to antibiotics was confirmed by Rello and colleagues[72] when comparing 4 different ICUs in Barcelona, Madrid, Seville, and Paris, finding a different incidence of multidrug-resistant pathogens in the 4 units.

Beardsley and colleagues[73] implemented nosocomial pneumonia guidelines and stratified the groups according to the onset period: early-late onset (<10 days) and late-late onset (>10 days). With this strategy, the initial treatment adequacy was greater than 90%. In addition, adding ciprofloxacin to β-lactams did not improve treatment adequacy, whereas adding a specific aminoglycoside (amikacin) did.

Hospital-acquired versus ICU-acquired pneumonia

Although nosocomial pneumonia acquired in the ward and ICU-acquired pneumonia are considered together in guideline recommendations, microorganisms and mortality are probably different. However, there are few studies on the epidemiology of nosocomial pneumonia outside the ICU. Sopena and Sabria[74] published a multicenter study in 165 patients with nosocomial pneumonia acquired in the ward. The overall mortality was 26%. *S pneumoniae* was one of the most frequent microorganisms and, in several cases, it was independent of the time of onset of nosocomial pneumonia. In our opinion, when validating guidelines, patients in ICUs and patients not in ICUs have to be investigated separately. This opinion is supported by a recent study in patients with nosocomial pneumonia in the ICU that compared VAP and pneumonia in nonventilated patients.[75] In this study, despite nonventilated patients having a lower proportion of pathogens compared with VAP, the type of isolates and outcomes were similar regardless of whether or not pneumonia was acquired during ventilation, indicating that outcomes may depend on patients' underlying disease severity rather than the presence of previous intubation.

Early microbiological diagnosis and resistance

Early microbiologic results may help to implement early antibiotic modifications. In addition, rapid tests to detect microbiologic resistance (eg, MRSA) may provide quick detection of drug-resistant organisms and consequently lead to changes in antibiotics. For example, Bouza and colleagues[76] randomized patients with VAP to the use in respiratory samples studied with a rapid E-test to detect microbiologic resistance. Although there were no differences in mortality, the median days of MV were lower in the group managed by the E- test. The findings of this study are important for the design of future validation studies.

In summary, the current evidence suggests that the stratification of HAP and VAP in 2 groups according the 2005 ATS/IDSA guidelines probably needs to be revisited to better define the risk factors for multidrug-resistant organisms in the group of early-onset pneumonia. The evidence available in a few studies also suggests that the implementation of guidelines for HAP and VAP is followed by a better outcome. New studies should take into account the different components of the recommendations, including time to the first dosage, initial adherence, adequacy of antibiotics, and the different combinations used.

SUMMARY

The crucial role of our decision-making process in pneumonia is made evident in the initial hours after diagnosis. The high degree of variability among professionals and hospitals in the management of CAP makes it clear that there is room for improvement. The implementation of updated guidelines is associated with less mortality, fewer days until clinical stability, and lower costs in patients with CAP.

Validation of guidelines in HAP is also important to confirm the reliability of these guidelines in clinical practice and their impact on outcome parameters. Overall, implementing guidelines is followed by an increase in initially adequate antibiotic treatment. In addition, only a few studies have shown that the prediction of microorganisms by HAP guidelines is reliable. Guideline validation studies are not easy and have to take into account different variables potentially related to the outcome of patients with HAP.

REFERENCES

1. Minino AM, Smith BL. Deaths: preliminary data for 2000. Natl Vital Stat Rep 2001;49:1–40.
2. Minino AM, Heron MP, Smith BL. Deaths: preliminary data for 2004. Natl Vital Stat Rep 2006;54:1–49.
3. Alfageme I, Aspa J, Bello S, et al. Guidelines for the diagnosis and management of community-acquired pneumonia. Spanish Society of Pulmonology and Thoracic Surgery (SEPAR). Arch Bronconeumol 2005;41:272–89 [in Spanish].
4. Mandell LA, Wunderink RG, Anzueto A, et al. Infectious Diseases Society of America/American Thoracic Society consensus guidelines on the management of community-acquired pneumonia in adults. Clin Infect Dis 2007;44(Suppl 2):S27–72.
5. Woodhead MA. Community-acquired pneumonia guidelines an international comparison: a view from Europe. Chest 1998;113:183s–7s.
6. Carratala J, Fernandez-Sabe N, Ortega L, et al. Outpatient care compared with hospitalization for community-acquired pneumonia: a randomized trial in low-risk patients. Ann Intern Med 2005;142:165–72.
7. Fine MJ, Auble TE, Yealy DM, et al. A prediction rule to identify low-risk patients with community-acquired pneumonia. N Engl J Med 1997;336:243–50.
8. Roson B, Carratala J, Dorca J, et al. Etiology, reasons for hospitalization, risk classes, and outcomes of community-acquired pneumonia in patients hospitalized on the basis of conventional admission criteria. Clin Infect Dis 2001;33:158–65.
9. Dambrava PG, Torres A, Valles X, et al. Adherence to guidelines' empirical antibiotic recommendations and community-acquired pneumonia outcome. Eur Respir J 2008;32:892–901.
10. Niederman MS, Mandell LA, Anzueto A, et al. Guidelines for the management of adults with community-acquired pneumonia. Diagnosis, assessment of severity, antimicrobial therapy, and prevention. Am J Respir Crit Care Med 2001;163:1730–54.
11. Cilloniz C, Ewig S, Polverino E, et al. Microbial aetiology of community-acquired pneumonia and its relation to severity. Thorax 2011;66(4):340–6.
12. Valencia M, Badia JR, Cavalcanti M, et al. Pneumonia Severity Index class V patients with community-acquired pneumonia: characteristics, outcomes, and value of severity scores. Chest 2007;132:515–22.
13. von Baum H, Welte T, Marre R, et al. Community-acquired pneumonia through Enterobacteriaceae and *Pseudomonas aeruginosa*: diagnosis, incidence and predictors. Eur Respir J 2010;35:598–605.
14. Stralin K, Goscinski G, Hedlund J, et al. Management of adult patients with community-acquired pneumonia. Evidence-based guidelines from the Swedish Infectious Diseases Association. Lakartidningen 2008;105:2582–7 [in Swedish].
15. Davey PG, Marwick C. Appropriate vs. inappropriate antimicrobial therapy. Clin Microbiol Infect 2008;14(Suppl 3):15–21.
16. Falguera M, Ruiz-Gonzalez A, Schoenenberger JA, et al. Prospective, randomised study to compare empirical treatment versus targeted treatment on the basis of the urine antigen results in hospitalised patients with community-acquired pneumonia. Thorax 2010;65:101–6.
17. van der Eerden MM, Vlaspolder F, de Graaff CS, et al. Comparison between pathogen directed antibiotic treatment and empirical broad spectrum antibiotic treatment in patients with community acquired pneumonia: a prospective randomised study. Thorax 2005;60:672–8.
18. Bjerre LM, Verheij TJ, Kochen MM. Antibiotics for community acquired pneumonia in adult outpatients. Cochrane Database Syst Rev 2009;4:CD002109.
19. Gleason PP, Kapoor WN, Stone RA, et al. Medical outcomes and antimicrobial costs with the use of the American Thoracic Society guidelines for outpatients with community-acquired pneumonia. JAMA 1997;278:32–9.

20. Niederman MS, Bass JB, Campbell GD, et al. Guidelines for the initial management of adults with community-acquired pneumonia: diagnosis, assessment of severity, and initial antimicrobial therapy. American Thoracic Society. Medical Section of the American Lung Association. Am Rev Respir Dis 1993;148:1418–26.

21. Suchyta MR, Dean NC, Narus S, et al. Effects of a practice guideline for community-acquired pneumonia in an outpatient setting. Am J Med 2001; 110:306–9.

22. Menendez R, Ferrando D, Valles JM, et al. Influence of deviation from guidelines on the outcome of community-acquired pneumonia. Chest 2002;122: 612–7.

23. Menendez R, Torres A, Zalacain R, et al. Guidelines for the treatment of community-acquired pneumonia: predictors of adherence and outcome. Am J Respir Crit Care Med 2005;172:757–62.

24. Dean NC, Bateman KA, Donnelly SM, et al. Improved clinical outcomes with utilization of a community-acquired pneumonia guideline. Chest 2006;130:794–9.

25. Mortensen EM, Restrepo MI, Anzueto A, et al. Antibiotic therapy and 48-hour mortality for patients with pneumonia. Am J Med 2006;119:859–64.

26. Arnold FW, Summersgill JT, Lajoie AS, et al. A worldwide perspective of atypical pathogens in community-acquired pneumonia. Am J Respir Crit Care Med 2007;175:1086–93.

27. Menendez R, Torres A, Rodriguez de CF, et al. Reaching stability in community-acquired pneumonia: the effects of the severity of disease, treatment, and the characteristics of patients. Clin Infect Dis 2004;39:1783–90.

28. Arnold FW, Lajoie AS, Brock GN, et al. Improving outcomes in elderly patients with community-acquired pneumonia by adhering to national guidelines: community-acquired pneumonia organization international cohort study results. Arch Intern Med 2009;169:1515–24.

29. Orrick JJ, Segal R, Johns TE, et al. Resource use and cost of care for patients hospitalised with community acquired pneumonia: impact of adherence to Infectious Diseases Society of America guidelines. Pharmacoeconomics 2004;22:751–7.

30. Menendez R, Reyes S, Martinez R, et al. Economic evaluation of adherence to treatment guidelines in nonintensive care pneumonia. Eur Respir J 2007; 29:751–6.

31. Gora-Harper ML, Rapp RP, Finney JP. Development of a best-practice model at a university hospital to increase efficiency in the management of patients with community-acquired pneumonia. Am J Health Syst Pharm 2000;57(Suppl 3):S6–9.

32. Stahl JE, Barza M, DesJardin J, et al. Effect of macrolides as part of initial empiric therapy on length of stay in patients hospitalized with community-acquired pneumonia. Arch Intern Med 1999;159: 2576–80.

33. Dudas V, Hopefl A, Jacobs R, et al. Antimicrobial selection for hospitalized patients with presumed community-acquired pneumonia: a survey of nonteaching US community hospitals. Ann Pharmacother 2000;34:446–52.

34. Bodi M, Rodriguez A, Sole-Violan J, et al. Antibiotic prescription for community-acquired pneumonia in the intensive care unit: impact of adherence to Infectious Diseases Society of America guidelines on survival. Clin Infect Dis 2005;41:1709–16.

35. Martin-Loeches I, Lisboa T, Rodriguez A, et al. Combination antibiotic therapy with macrolides improves survival in intubated patients with community-acquired pneumonia. Intensive Care Med 2010;36:612–20.

36. Frei CR, Attridge RT, Mortensen EM, et al. Guideline-concordant antibiotic use and survival among patients with community-acquired pneumonia admitted to the intensive care unit. Clin Ther 2010; 32:293–9.

37. Shorr AF, Bodi M, Rodriguez A, et al. Impact of antibiotic guideline compliance on duration of mechanical ventilation in critically ill patients with community-acquired pneumonia. Chest 2006;130: 93–100.

38. Waterer GW, Kessler LA, Wunderink RG. Delayed administration of antibiotics and atypical presentation in community-acquired pneumonia. Chest 2006;130:11–5.

39. Yu KT, Wyer PC. Evidence-based emergency medicine/critically appraised topic. Evidence behind the 4-hour rule for initiation of antibiotic therapy in community-acquired pneumonia. Ann Emerg Med 2008;51:651–62, 662.

40. Cheng AC, Buising KL. Delayed administration of antibiotics and mortality in patients with community-acquired pneumonia. Ann Emerg Med 2009;53:618–24.

41. Barlow G, Nathwani D, Williams F, et al. Reducing door-to-antibiotic time in community-acquired pneumonia: controlled before-and-after evaluation and cost-effectiveness analysis. Thorax 2007;62:67–74.

42. Kumar A, Roberts D, Wood KE, et al. Duration of hypotension before initiation of effective antimicrobial therapy is the critical determinant of survival in human septic shock. Crit Care Med 2006;34: 1589–96.

43. Ferrer R, Artigas A, Suarez D, et al. Effectiveness of treatments for severe sepsis: a prospective, multicenter, observational study. Am J Respir Crit Care Med 2009;180:861–6.

44. Battleman DS, Callahan M, Thaler HT. Rapid antibiotic delivery and appropriate antibiotic selection reduce length of hospital stay of patients with

community-acquired pneumonia: link between quality of care and resource utilization. Arch Intern Med 2002;162:682–8.

45. Barlow G, Nathwani D, Myers E, et al. Identifying barriers to the rapid administration of appropriate antibiotics in community-acquired pneumonia. J Antimicrob Chemother 2008;61:442–51.

46. Cabana MD, Rand CS, Powe NR, et al. Why don't physicians follow clinical practice guidelines? A framework for improvement. JAMA 1999;282:1458–65.

47. Halm EA, Atlas SJ, Borowsky LH, et al. Understanding physician adherence with a pneumonia practice guideline: effects of patient, system, and physician factors. Arch Intern Med 2000;160: 98–104.

48. Schouten JA, Hulscher ME, Kullberg BJ, et al. Understanding variation in quality of antibiotic use for community-acquired pneumonia: effect of patient, professional and hospital factors. J Antimicrob Chemother 2005;56:575–82.

49. Rello J, Lorente C, Bodi M, et al. Why do physicians not follow evidence-based guidelines for preventing ventilator-associated pneumonia?: a survey based on the opinions of an international panel of intensivists. Chest 2002;122:656–61.

50. Dean NC, Silver MP, Bateman KA, et al. Decreased mortality after implementation of a treatment guideline for community-acquired pneumonia. Am J Med 2001;110:451–7.

51. Capelastegui A, Espana PP, Quintana JM, et al. Improvement of process-of-care and outcomes after implementing a guideline for the management of community-acquired pneumonia: a controlled before-and-after design study. Clin Infect Dis 2004; 39:955–63.

52. Blasi F, Iori I, Bulfoni A, et al. Can CAP guideline adherence improve patient outcome in internal medicine departments? Eur Respir J 2008;32: 902–10.

53. Marrie TJ, Lau CY, Wheeler SL, et al. A controlled trial of a critical pathway for treatment of community-acquired pneumonia. CAPITAL Study Investigators. Community-Acquired Pneumonia Intervention Trial Assessing Levofloxacin. JAMA 2000;283:749–55.

54. Meehan TP, Weingarten SR, Holmboe ES, et al. A statewide initiative to improve the care of hospitalized pneumonia patients: the Connecticut Pneumonia Pathway Project. Am J Med 2001;111: 203–10.

55. Frei CR, Restrepo MI, Mortensen EM, et al. Impact of guideline-concordant empiric antibiotic therapy in community-acquired pneumonia. Am J Med 2006; 119:865–71.

56. Torres A, Ewig S, Lode H, et al. Defining, treating and preventing hospital acquired pneumonia: European perspective. Intensive Care Med 2009;35:9–29.

57. Chastre J, Fagon JY. Ventilator-associated pneumonia. Am J Respir Crit Care Med 2002;165: 867–903.

58. Alvarez-Lerma F. Modification of empiric antibiotic treatment in patients with pneumonia acquired in the intensive care unit. ICU-acquired Pneumonia Study Group. Intensive Care Med 1996;22: 387–94.

59. American Thoracic Society. Hospital-acquired pneumonia in adults: diagnosis, assessment of severity, initial antimicrobial therapy, and preventative strategies. A consensus statement. Am J Respir Crit Care Med 1996;153:1711–25.

60. American Thoracic Society, Infectious Diseases Society of America. Guidelines for the management of adults with hospital-acquired, ventilator-associated, and healthcare-associated pneumonia. Am J Respir Crit Care Med 2005;171:388–416.

61. Trouillet JL, Chastre J, Vuagnat A, et al. Ventilator-associated pneumonia caused by potentially drug-resistant bacteria. Am J Respir Crit Care Med 1998;157:531–9.

62. Leroy O, Giradie P, Yazdanpanah Y, et al. Hospital-acquired pneumonia: microbiological data and potential adequacy of antimicrobial regimens. Eur Respir J 2002;20:432–9.

63. Ioanas M, Cavalcanti M, Ferrer M, et al. Hospital-acquired pneumonia: coverage and treatment adequacy of current guidelines. Eur Respir J 2003; 22:876–82.

64. Ferrer M, Liapikou A, Valencia M, et al. Validation of the American Thoracic Society–Infectious Diseases Society of America guidelines for hospital-acquired pneumonia in the intensive care unit. Clin Infect Dis 2010;50:945–52.

65. Ibrahim EH, Ward S, Sherman G, et al. Experience with a clinical guideline for the treatment of ventilator-associated pneumonia. Crit Care Med 2001;29:1109–15.

66. Soo Hoo GW, Wen YE, Nguyen TV, et al. Impact of clinical guidelines in the management of severe hospital-acquired pneumonia. Chest 2005;128:2778–87.

67. Kett DH, Cano E, Quartin AA, et al. Implementation of guidelines for management of possible multidrug-resistant pneumonia in intensive care: an observational, multicentre cohort study. Lancet Infect Dis 2011;11:181–9.

68. Ewig S. Nosocomial pneumonia: de-escalation is what matters. Lancet Infect Dis 2011;11(3):155–7.

69. Yu VL. Guidelines for hospital-acquired pneumonia and health-care-associated pneumonia: a vulnerability, a pitfall, and a fatal flaw. Lancet Infect Dis 2011;11:248–52.

70. Iregui M, Ward S, Sherman G, et al. Clinical importance of delays in the initiation of appropriate antibiotic treatment for ventilator-associated pneumonia. Chest 2002;122:262–8.

71. Paladino JA, Sunderlin JL, Forrest A, et al. Characterization of the onset and consequences of pneumonia due to fluoroquinolone-susceptible or -resistant Pseudomonas aeruginosa. J Antimicrob Chemother 2003;52:457–63.

72. Rello J, Sa-Borges M, Correa H, et al. Variations in etiology of ventilator-associated pneumonia across four treatment sites: implications for antimicrobial prescribing practices. Am J Respir Crit Care Med 1999;160:608–13.

73. Beardsley JR, Williamson JC, Johnson JW, et al. Using local microbiologic data to develop institution-specific guidelines for the treatment of hospital-acquired pneumonia. Chest 2006;130: 787–93.

74. Sopena N, Sabria M. Multicenter study of hospital-acquired pneumonia in non-ICU patients. Chest 2005;127:213–9.

75. Esperatti M, Ferrer M, Theessen A, et al. Nosocomial pneumonia in the intensive care unit acquired during mechanical ventilation or not. Am J Respir Crit Care Med 2010;182:1533–9.

76. Bouza E, Torres MV, Radice C, et al. Direct E-test (AB Biodisk) of respiratory samples improves antimicrobial use in ventilator-associated pneumonia. Clin Infect Dis 2007;44:382–7.

Healthcare-Associated Pneumonia: Approach to Management

Andrew Labelle, MD, Marin H. Kollef, MD*

KEYWORDS

- Pneumonia • Healthcare-associated • Community-acquired
- Risk factors • Antibiotic therapy

Recently, a new classification of pneumonia, healthcare-associated pneumonia (HCAP), was introduced.[1] HCAP was created to identify patients with community-acquired pneumonia (CAP) at risk for developing infections from multidrug-resistant (MDR) pathogens, such as methicillin-resistant *Staphylococcus aureus* (MRSA) and *Pseudomonas aeruginosa* who need empiric treatment modification based on specific risk factors.[2–5] The 2005 American Thoracic Society (ATS) and the Infectious Disease Society of America (IDSA) nosocomial pneumonia guidelines[1] recognized HCAP as a distinct clinical entity and defined HCAP risk factors as: (1) hospitalization for 2 or more days in an acute care facility within 90 days of infection, (2) presentation from a nursing home or long-term care facility (LTCF), (3) attending a hospital or hemodialysis clinic, and (4) receiving intravenous antibiotic therapy, chemotherapy, or wound care within 30 days of infection.[1] The 2007 ATS-IDSA CAP guidelines[6] also recognized HCAP as a clinical entity but cautioned that some overlap still occurs between CAP and HCAP.

Healthcare-associated bloodstream infections were first described in a 2002 study by Friedman and colleagues.[7] The microbiology differed between patients with healthcare-associated infections and those with community-acquired infections. The predominant organism isolated from patients with a HCAI was MRSA, and *Escherichia coli* and *Streptococcus pneumoniae* were the predominant organisms isolated in community-acquired infections. In 2005, Kollef and colleagues[3] first described HCAP using a large, retrospectively collected administrative database of 4,543 patients in 59 hospitals in the United States. All of the patients identified had positive cultures, and the infections were classified as CAP, HCAP, hospital-acquired pneumonia (HAP), or ventilator-associated pneumonia (VAP). Patients with HCAP had a mortality (19.8%) similar to patients with HAP (18.8%) but higher than those with CAP (10.0%, *P*<0.0001). Subsequent cohort studies of culture-positive HCAP and CAP patients from St Louis, MO, USA[4] Spain,[8] Italy,[9] and Japan[10] have confirmed the higher mortality associated with HCAP. In an analysis of long-term outcomes of patients with HCAP and CAP in Seattle, WA, USA, those with CAP had a better survival 8 years after their pneumonia (78.8% CAP vs 44.5% HCAP, *P*<0.001).[11] Finally, patients without a positive respiratory culture have a lower severity of illness and better survival than those with a positive culture (7.4% mortality culture negative vs 24.6% culture positive, *P*<0.001).[12]

MICROBIOLOGY

The 2005 analysis by Kollef and colleagues[3] showed that the microbiology of HCAP was similar to HAP and VAP but distinct from CAP. The most common organism isolated in all pneumonia subtypes was *S aureus*, found in 25.5% of those with CAP and 46.7% of those with HCAP (*P*<0.001) (**Table 1**). MRSA and *P aeruginosa* were more common in patients with HCAP while

The authors have nothing to disclose.

Division of Pulmonary and Critical Care, Washington University School of Medicine, 660 South Euclid Avenue, Campus Box 8052, St Louis, MO 63110, USA

* Corresponding author.

E-mail address: mkollef@dom.wustl.edu

Clin Chest Med 32 (2011) 507–515

doi:10.1016/j.ccm.2011.05.003

Table 1
Pathogen distribution according to geographic region

| Study | United States | | | | | | Europe | | | | Japan | |
| | Kollef et al,[3] 2005 | | Micek et al,[4] 2007 | | Schreiber et al,[13] 2010 | | Carratala et al,[8] 2007 | | Venditti et al,[14] 2009 | | Shindo et al,[10] 2009 | |
	CAP	HCAP	CAP	HCAP	CAP	HCAP	CAP	HCAP	CAP	HCAP	CAP	HCAP
Gram-positive Pathogens (%)												
Streptococcus pneumoniae	16.6	5.5	40.9	10.4	21.9	6.4	33.9	27.8	43.9	7.1	19.1	13.5
Staphylococcus aureus	25.5	46.7	25.5	49.9	29.2	32.9	2.4	0	17.1	39.3	6.1	9.9
MRSA	8.9	26.5	12.0	36.0	14.6	22.3	—	—	6.4	25.0	0.9	3.5
MSSA	17.2	21.1	13.5	13.9	14.6	10.6	—	—	10.7	14.3	5.2	6.4
Gram-negative Pathogens (%)												
Pseudomonas aeruginosa	17.1	25.3	4.8	25.5	3.1	23.4	0.5	1.6	9.7	7.1	1.7	5.7
Haemophilus spp	16.6	5.8	17.3	4.2	—	—	6.0	11.9	—	—	7.4	2.8
Klebsiella spp	9.5	7.6	3.4	6.5	4.2	10.6	0.2	0	—	—	1.7	7.1
Escherichia coli	4.8	5.2	5.8	4.2	4.2	12.8	0.3	2.4	—	—	0.4	3.5
Other Nonfermenting GNB[a]	1.6	2.6	1.9	10	—	—	—	—	—	—	0	2.1
Other Enterobacteriaceae[b]	7.0	13.0	2.4	9.0	—	—	—	—	—	—	1.3	2.8

Abbreviations: GNB, gram-negative bacteria; MSSA, methicillin-susceptible *Staphylococcus aureus*.
[a] *Acinetobacter* species, *Stenotrophomonas maltophilia*, *Alcaligenes xylosoxidans*, *Burkholderia* species.
[b] *Enterobacter* species, *Citrobacter* species, *Serratia marcescens*, *Proteus* species, *Morganella* species.

S pneumoniae and *Hemophilus* species were more common in patients with CAP. In 2007, Micek and colleagues[4] confirmed these findings in a cohort of 639 patients from a single United States institution. The most common organisms were MRSA (30.6%) and *P aeruginosa* (25.5%), and the most common CAP organisms were *S pneumoniae* (40.9%) and *Hemophilus* species (17.3%). Finally, in a separate United States cohort, Schreiber and colleagues[13] confirmed the finding that MRSA and *P aeruginosa* were the most common organisms isolated from HCAP patients.

P aeruginosa and MRSA are the most common organisms causing HCAP in the United States, but cohorts from Europe and Japan have found differing results. In a prospective analysis of 727 patients presenting with pneumonia in Spain,[8] CAP was more common than HCAP (82.7% CAP vs 17.3% HCAP). In patients with HCAP, the most prevalent organism was *S pneumoniae* (27.8%) followed by *H influenzae* (11.9%). *P aeruginosa* (1.6%) and *S aureus* (2.4%) were more common in those with HCAP but were not frequently isolated. In a multicenter cohort study from Italy, *S aureus* was the most common HCAP organism (39.3%), but *P aeruginosa* was not frequently isolated (5.7%).[14] In a cohort of patients from Japan,[10] *S pneumoniae* was the most common organism in HCAP patients (13.5%), but gram-negative bacteria (24.1%), *P aeruginosa* (5.7%), and MRSA (3.5%) were more common in HCAP than CAP.

HCAP RISK FACTORS

The HCAP definition varies between the published clinical studies and the ATS-IDSA guidelines. All of the published studies include hemodialysis and residence in a LTCF as HCAP risk factors. Hospitalization for 2 or more days in the prior 90 days is used in the ATS-IDSA guidelines[1] and is the most commonly used definition[8,10,11,13,15,16] for prior hospitalization. However, time intervals as short as 30 days[3,17] and as long as 180 to 360[4,9] days have been used. Although not included in the ATS-IDSA guidelines, immunosuppression is frequently listed as an additional HCAP risk factor.[4,8,9,11,13,15–17] In addition, the individual risk factors do not carry an equivalent risk of infection with MDR pathogens. The lack of a consistent definition and the different weight each risk factor carries for infection with resistant organisms have lead some to question whether the HCAP definition is too broad and results in over-treatment.[18]

Hospitalization places patients at risk for colonization of the upper respiratory and gastrointestinal tract with pathogens that are not commonly found in the community. Microaspiration of these organisms has been proposed as a mechanism for development of HCAP. Admission to an ICU room where the previous patient was colonized with MRSA or vancomycin-resistant *Enterococcus* (VRE) increases one's odds (odds ratio [OR] 1.4, $P = 0.04$) of becoming colonized with MRSA or VRE.[19] Hospitalization also increases the risk of colonization by resistant gram-negative organisms. In a cohort of 167 patients in at single institution, 21% of the patients became new rectal carriers of extended spectrum β-lactamase (ESBL)-producing Enterobacteriaceae and 7% became nasal carriers of MRSA.[20] In a multivariate analysis of this cohort, age older than 65 and treatment with broad spectrum antibiotic therapy were risk factors for acquisition of ESBL-producing Enterobacteriaceae. Patients colonized with MDR pathogens are at risk for prolonged carriage. Of those who acquire MRSA during a hospitalization, 40% develop prolonged colonization for an average duration of 8.5 months.[21] Prolonged colonization was confirmed in subsequent studies showing an average MRSA colonization time of 7.4 months[22] and median colonization time of 132 days for ESBL-producing Enterobacteriaceae.[23]

Nursing-home–associated pneumonia (NHAP) is a clinical entity that was described prior to HCAP and was reported in the 2001 ATS-CAP guidelines as a risk factor for infection with MDR pathogens.[24] Originally published 20 years ago, MRSA colonization rates ranged from 13% to 35% among nursing home residents in the Veterans Administration medical system.[25,26] MDR gram-negative bacteria are also prevalent in nursing home residents. In a 648 bed facility, 51% of the residents were colonized with MDR gram-negative bacteria and 28% were colonized with MRSA.[27] In 2001, El-Solh and colleagues[28] examined a cohort of 104 elderly patients ($\geq$75 years old) requiring mechanical ventilation for pneumonia admitted from both the community and nursing homes. The most prevalent organisms in those admitted from the community were *S pneumoniae* (14%), *Legionella* sp (9%), *H influenza* (7%), and *S aureus* (7%). *S aureus* (29%), enteric gram-negative bacilli (15%), *S pneumoniae* (9%), and *P aeruginosa* (4%) were the predominant organisms in those admitted from a LTCF. In a multicenter prospective study from Germany of patients admitted to the hospital with pneumonia, those from a nursing home had an increased risk of infection with gram-negative bacilli (18.8% from nursing home vs 5.5% from community, $P = 0.02$) and worse mortality (OR 2.38, 95%, CI 1.36–4.15).[29] Among nursing home patients, the presence of foreign bodies, chronic wounds, and recent hospitalization are risk factors for colonization with MDR bacteria.[30] In a further analysis of NHAP, El-Solh and colleagues[31] found functional dependence and receipt of antibiotics in the past 6 months to be predictors of infection with MDR bacteria.

Nursing home residents are at risk for colonization and infection with multidrug-resistant organism, but not all patients carry the same risk. El-Solh and colleagues[32] studied a cohort of 334 patients admitted to a general medical ward in a single institution from a nursing home. Patients who had been hospitalized within the previous 30 days, admitted to the ICU, or immunosuppressed were excluded from the analysis, and most of the patients were culture negative. The investigators found no difference in outcomes between those treated with an HCAP regimen targeting MDR organisms and those that received a treatment regimen targeting typical CAP organisms (77% of total patients).

Colonization and infection with MDR bacteria is frequent in hemodialysis (HD) and immunosuppressed patients. In a multicenter prospective study, patient receiving inpatient HD had a MRSA colonization rate of 15%, and those receiving HD as an outpatient had a colonization rate of 14%.[33] Despite the high incidence of colonization with MDR bacteria, limited evidence is available regarding pneumonia in HD patients. In a cohort of all HD patients who developed a microbiologically confirmed infection at a single institution, 13% of the infections were pneumonia. Gram-negative bacilli were isolated in 55% of the cases of CAP, *Pseudomonas* in 21%, MRSA in 12%, and *S pneumoniae* in 6%.[34] In immunosuppressed patients, especially those with a hematologic malignancy, atypical organisms such as fungi or viruses are frequent causes of pneumonia. In a study of immunosuppressed patients with clinical pneumonia, defined as hematologic malignancy, receipt of solid organ or bone marrow transplant, and chronic prednisone use, bacterial pneumonia accounted for 24% of the cases. The most commonly isolated organisms were *S aureus*, *P aeruginosa*, and *E coli*.[35]

The individual HCAP risk factors do not carry an equivalent risk for infection with an MDR organism. Shorr and colleagues[15] analyzed a cohort of 289 HCAP patients, and MDR pathogens were identified in 45.2%. The HCAP definition was not specific in identifying an infection with a resistant organism (48.9% specificity). In a multivariate analysis, long-term HD (OR 2.11), nursing home residence (OR 2.75), admission to an ICU (OR 1.62), and hospitalization in the previous 90 days (OR 4.21) were significantly associated with infection by an MDR pathogen. A separate cohort of 190 HCAP patients with 32.6% MDR pathogens was analyzed. The HCAP criteria had a negative predictive value of 84.9% and a positive predictive value of 45.2%. A multivariate model identified immunosuppression (OR 4.85), nursing home residence (OR 2.36), and prior antibiotic use (OR 2.12) as independent predictors of infection with a resistant organism. The investigators created a scoring system to predict MDR bacteria based on this analysis, but 17% of the patients with a score of zero were infected with resistant bacteria.[13]

TREATMENT
Appropriate Therapy

Therapy for any serious infection requires early, effective treatment. Inappropriate initial antimicrobial therapy, defined as in vitro resistance to an antimicrobial agent used to treat the infection, has been implicated as an independent predictor of poor outcomes in serious hospital infections and bloodstream infections.[36–41] In an international cohort of 5,715 patients with septic shock, inappropriate therapy was associated with an increased mortality in the entire cohort and within all subgroups studied, including all major infection sites and organisms.[42] In a multivariate analysis, inappropriate therapy was strongly associated with mortality (OR 8.99). Appropriate therapy is also a cornerstone of effective therapy in VAP.[43–46] The bacteria most commonly associated with inappropriate treatment in VAP are frequently MDR and include P aeruginosa, Acinetobacter species, Klebsiella pneumoniae, Enterobacter species, and MRSA.[5]

Initial inappropriate therapy is frequent in healthcare-associated infections. In 2005, McDonald and colleagues[2] analyzed a cohort of patients with bloodstream infections and found that, compared to community-acquired infections, healthcare-associated infections were associated with an increased risk of inappropriate therapy (adjusted odds ratio [AOR] 3.1, 95% CI 1.6–6.1). Until recently, HCAP was classified and treated as CAP,[47] but it has distinct microbiologic characteristics and requires different therapy. Patients with HCAP have been shown to receive inappropriate antibiotic therapy in multiple studies,[4,9,10,48] and some have postulated that the increased mortality associated with HCAP is secondary to inappropriate initial therapy. Micek and colleagues[4] found that 28.3% of HCAP patients received inappropriate initial antibiotic therapy compared to 13.0% of CAP patients (P<0.001). In a multivariate analysis, inappropriate initial antibiotic therapy was an independent risk factor for hospital mortality (AOR 2.19, 95%, CI 1.27–3.78). The pathogens most associated with inappropriate therapy were S aureus, P aeruginosa, other nonfermenting gram-negative bacilli, and other Enterobacteriaceae.[4]

Early Therapy

Early antimicrobial therapy in serious infections, including CAP,[49] VAP,[50] and bacteremia,[51,52] is associated with improved mortality. Kumar and colleagues[53] analyzed a cohort of 2,731 critically ill patients with septic shock from multiple causes. The survival for patients who received appropriate therapy in the first hour of hypotension was 79.9%. In the first 6 hours of shock, each hour delay in therapy was associated with a decrease in survival of 7.6%, and in a multivariate analysis early therapy was the strongest predictor of survival. Early therapy is also important in HCAP. A retrospective analysis was performed in patients with HCAP to determine if escalation of therapy in those who received initial inappropriate therapy would improve patient outcomes.[48] Of the patients who received initial inappropriate therapy, 40.2% had therapy escalated based on in vitro culture data. The in-hospital mortality was the same for those who received therapy escalation compared to those who continued to receive inappropriate therapy (27.9% escalation and 30.2% no change, P = 0.802).

De-Escalation of Therapy

After a patient has received appropriate initial antibiotics, the next step in HCAP treatment is tailoring antibiotic therapy to the specific isolated organism.[54] This involves switching therapy to an antibiotic that is active against the isolated organism in vitro and frequently involves changing to monotherapy. The elimination of redundant therapy enables more effective targeting of the causative organism while avoiding increased antibiotic exposure and subsequent selection pressure for the development of antibiotic resistance. An important aspect of de-escalation is obtaining adequate respiratory cultures. Cultures can be obtained from a bronchoalveolar lavage, protected specimen brushes, tracheal aspirate, or adequate sputum cultures.[55] In intubated patients, one should consider performing a bronchoalveolar lavage or protected specimen brushing if there is a strong clinical concern for MRSA or *P aeruginosa*.[56]

In a clinically stable patient, the decision to de-escalate therapy should be made on day 2 to 3 as this is when culture data usually returns.[1] In a prospective study of patients with severe CAP, 31% of the patients did not initially respond to therapy. Variables associated with a poor response included respiratory rate less than 25, oxygen saturation less than 90%, and confusion.[57] Patients who are not responding should be evaluated for unsuspected or resistant organisms, noninfectious mimics of pneumonia, or extrapulmonary manifestations of pneumonia.[5] In a retrospective study by Schlueter and colleagues,[58] HCAP patients whose therapy was de-escalated had a shorter length of stay in the hospital and lower mortality. Approximately half of the patients admitted with HCAP have negative respiratory cultures.[12] Culture-negative patients have a lower severity of illness and mortality than culture-positive patients, and because of this, one can consider limiting the course of antibiotics. Schlueter and colleagues[58] also found that 70% of the culture-negative patients were successfully de-escalated to a fluoroquinolone, implying that culture-negative HCAP patients may have a different microbiology than culture-positive patients.

Duration of Therapy

Limiting antibiotic exposure in patients who are improving clinically is one strategy to reduce the incidence of antibiotic resistance. There are no current studies examining antibiotic treatment duration for HCAP, and recommendations are taken from studies of VAP and CAP. In a 2003 randomized, controlled trial comparing 8 versus 15 days of antibiotics for microbiologically confirmed VAP, there was no difference in recurrent pneumonia, time on the ventilator, ICU length of stay, or mortality between the groups, and patients in the 8-day group had a lower incidence of subsequent development of resistant organisms. Patients infected with *P aeruginosa* had a higher infection-recurrence rate when treated for 8 days but did not have a difference in length of mechanical ventilation, ICU length of stay, or mortality.[59] Based on the results of the above study, the latest ATS-IDSA guidelines recommend a 7 to 8 day course of antibiotics for VAP, HAP, and HCAP with consideration of a longer course for patients

infected with *P aeruginosa*.[1] In several studies investigating a procalcitonin based antibiotic discontinuation protocol, antibiotic courses have been successfully shortened to 7.2 days for VAP and 5.5 to 7.2 days for CAP.[60,61]

Treatment Recommendations

The initial goal of HCAP treatment is to provide an early, appropriate empiric treatment regimen that targets the most commonly isolated organisms. As shown above, the organisms isolated from HCAP patients vary by region and hospital.[4,8,10] Not all HCAP patients carry the same risk for infection with MDR organisms. Nursing home patients without other HCAP risk factors and not admitted to the ICU have been successfully treated with a CAP regimen. In addition, culture negative patients appear to have a lower risk of infection with MDR organisms,[12,32,58] have better outcomes, and can be de-escalated to a CAP treatment regimen. Treatment should be tailored to a specific patient, and hospitals should keep updated antibiograms to assist clinicians in treating infections. However, MDR organisms, including MRSA and *P aeruginosa* are more prevalent in HCAP than CAP in all regions. Unlike CAP, the organisms isolated in those with HCAP do not appear to depend on severity of illness.[10] In the absence of initial culture data, an empiric regimen should be selected that is active against MRSA and *P aeruginosa*. One should also consider a regimen that covers *Acinetobacter* species and ESBL-positive strains of Enterobacteriaceae if these organisms are prevalent in a specific region or hospital **Fig. 1** describes a management strategy for HCAP.

The 2005 IDSA-ATS guidelines for VAP, HAP, and HCAP provided recommendations for treatment of HCAP,[1] which include empiric broad spectrum antibiotics and tailoring of therapy once a specific organism is isolated. All patients should be treated with a β-lactam that is active against *Pseudomonas*. The initial choices are an antipseudomonal cephalosporin (cefepime), carbapenem (imipenem or meropenem), or penicillin–β-lactamase inhibitor (pipercillin-tazobactam). In addition, one can consider including in the treatment regimen a second agent active against *Pseudomonas*, such as an antipseudomonal fluoroquinolone or an aminoglycoside, especially in hemodynamically unstable patients. The rational for double coverage of *Pseudomonas* is to improve the odds that the initial empiric regimen will be appropriate.[41] Thus, the second agent can be discontinued if the chosen β-lactam is active against the isolated organism. Finally, either vancomycin or linezolid should be added for coverage against

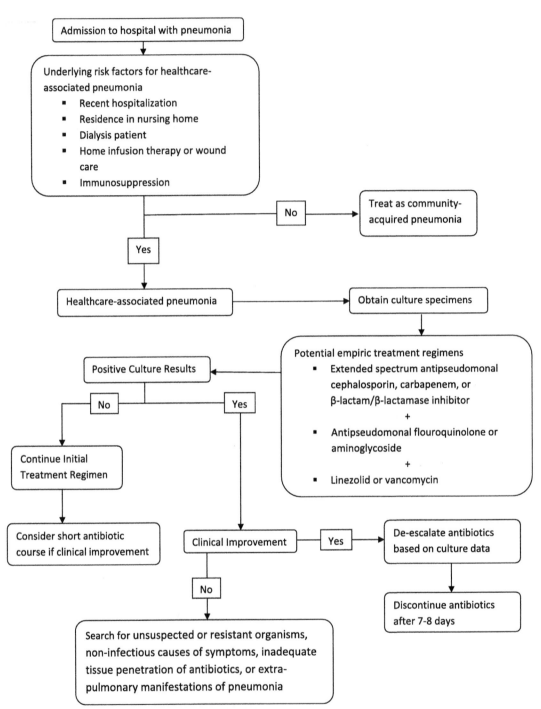

Fig. 1. Treatment strategy for patients with HCAP presenting from the Emergency Department

MRSA. For patients with MRSA pneumonia not re-sponding to vancomycin, one should consider switching to linezolid because increasing minimal inhibitory concentrations for vancomycin still within the susceptible range has been associated with worse outcomes[62,63] and linezolid achieves better lung penetration than vancomycin.[64–66] For patients with Panton Valentine leukocidin producing strains of community-acquired MRSA, one should also consider treatment with linezolid as it has been shown to decrease toxin production in an in vitro model.[67]

SUMMARY

This article provides evidence that HCAP is a distinct clinical entity from CAP. HCAP is associated with worse outcomes and a different microbiologic cause than CAP and more closely resembles HAP. However, the incidence and microbiology of HCAP vary by region, and physicians should ensure that their local practice is similar to published studies. Although patients with HCAP risk factors are at a greater risk for infection with MDR organisms, the HCAP definition itself is not a specific marker for infection with drug-resistant bacteria. In addition, the individual risk factors themselves do not carry equal weight in predicting MDR bacteria and vary in different study populations. Further study is needed to better define which patients are at risk for MDR bacteria and which patients do not need broad-spectrum antibiotic therapy tailored for resistant infections. The goals of therapy should be to provide an early, appropriate initial antibiotic regimen based on local microbiologic data and patient risk factors. Cultures should be obtained, and in responders, antibiotic therapy should be de-escalated and antibiotic course limited. Further awareness of HCAP as a distinct clinical entity and further study of the pathogens associated with and risk factors for HCAP may help to advance and tailor therapy.

REFERENCES

1. American Thoracic Society. Infectious Diseases Society of America. Guidelines for the management of adults with hospital-acquired, ventilator-associated, and healthcare-associated pneumonia. Am J Respir Crit Care Med 2005;171:388–416.

2. McDonald JR, Friedman ND, Stout JE, et al. Risk factors for ineffective therapy in patients with bloodstream infections. Arch Intern Med 2005;165:308–13.

3. Kollef MH, Shorr A, Tabak YP, et al. Epidemiology and outcomes of health care-associated pneumonia: results from a large US database of culture-positive pneumonia. Chest 2005;128:3854–62.

4. Micek ST, Kollef KE, Reichley RM, et al. Health care-associated pneumonia and community-acquired pneumonia: a single center experience. Antimicrob Agents Chemother 2007;51:3568–73.

5. Amin A, Kollef MH. Health care-associated pneumonia. Hosp Pract 2010;38:1–12.

6. Mandell LA, Wunderink RG, Anzueto A, et al. Infectious Diseases Society of America/American Thoracic Society consensus guidelines on the management of community-acquired pneumonia in adults. Clin Infect Dis 2007;44:S27–72.

7. Friedman NB, Kaye KS, Stout JE, et al. Health care-associated bloodstream infections in adults: a reason to change the accepted definition of community-acquired infections. Ann Intern Med 2002;137:791–7.

8. Carratalà J, Mykietiuk A, Fernández-Sabé N, et al. Healthcare-associated pneumonia requiring hospital admission: epidemiology, antibiotic therapy, and clinical outcomes. Arch Intern Med 2007;167: 1393–9.

9. Venditti M, Falcone M, Corrao S, et al. Study Group of the Italian Society of Internal Medicine. Outcomes of patients hospitalized with community-acquired, health care-associated, and hospital-acquired pneumonia. Ann Intern Med 2009;150:19–26.

10. Shindo Y, Sato S, Maruyama E, et al. Healthcare-associated pneumonia among hospitalized patients in a Japanese community hospital. Chest 2009;135: 633–40.

11. Cecere LM, Rubenfeld GD, Park DR, et al. Long-term survival after hospitalization for community-acquired and healthcare-associated pneumonia. Respiration 2010;79:128–36.

12. Labelle AJ, Arnold H, Reichley RM, et al. A comparison of culture-positive and culture-negative healthcare-associated pneumonia. Chest 2010;137:1130–7.

13. Schreiber MP, Chan CM, Shorr AF. Resistant pathogens in non-nosocomial pneumonia and respiratory failure: is it time to refine the definition of healthcare-associated pneumonia? Chest 2010;137:1283–8.

14. Falcone M, Venditti M, Corrao, et al. Role of multidrug-resistant pathogens in health care-associated pneumonia. Lancet Infect Dis 2001;11:11–2.

15. Shorr AF, Zilberberg MD, Micek ST, et al. Prediction of infection due to antibiotic-resistant bacteria by select risk factors for healthcare-associated pneumonia. Arch Intern Med 2008;168:2205–10.

16. Rello J, Luján M, Gallego M, et al. Why mortality is increased in Healthcare-associated Pneumonia: lessons from pneumococcal bacteremic pneumonia. Chest 2010;137:1138–44.

17. Webster D, Chui L, Tyrrell GJ, et al. Healthcare-associated *Staphylococcus aureus* pneumonia. Can J Infect Dis Med Microbiol 2007;18:181–8.

18. Ewig S, Welte T, Chastre J, et al. Rethinking the concepts of community-acquired and health-care-associated pneumonia. Lancet Infect Dis 2010;10: 279–87.

19. Huang SS, Datta R, Platt R. Risk of acquiring antibiotic-resistant bacteria from prior room occupants. Arch Intern Med 2006;166:1945–51.

20. Friedmann R, Raveh D, Zartzer E, et al. Prospective evaluation of colonization with extended-spectrum beta-lactamase (ESBL)-producing enterobacteriaceae among patients at hospital admission and of subsequent colonization with ESBL-producing enterobacteriaceae among patients during hospitalization. Infect Control Hosp Epidemiol 2009;30: 534–42.

21. Scanvic A, Denic L, Gaillon S, et al. Duration of colonization by methicillin-resistant *Staphylococcus aureus* after hospital discharge and risk factors for prolonged carriage. Clin Infect Dis 2001;32:1393–8.

22. Marschall J, Mühlemann K. Duration of methicillin-resistant *Staphylococcus aureus* carriage, according to risk factors for acquisition. Infect Control Hosp Epidemiol 2006;27:1206–12.

23. Zahar JR, Lanternier F, Mechai F, et al. Duration of colonisation by Enterobacteriaceae producing extended-spectrum beta-lactamase and risk factors for persistent faecal carriage. J Hosp Infect 2010; 75:76–8.

24. Niederman MS, Mandell La, Anzueto A, et al, American Thoracic Society. Guidelines for the management of adults with community-acquired pneumonia. Diagnosis, assessment of severity, antimicrobial therapy, and prevention. Am J Respir Crit Care Med 2001;163:1730–54.

25. Bradley SF, Terpenning MS, Ramsey MA, et al. Methicillin-resistant *Staphylococcus aureus*: colonization and infection in a long-term-care facility. Ann Intern Med 1991;115:417–22.

26. Muder RR, Brennen C, Wagener MM, et al. Methicillin-resistant staphylococcal colonization and infection in a long-term care facility. Ann Intern Med 1991;114:107–12.

27. Pop-Vicas A, Mitchell SL, Kandel R, et al. Multidrug-resistant gram-negative bacteria in a long-term care facility: prevalence and risk factors. J Am Geriatr Soc 2008;56:1276–80.

28. El-Solh AA, Sikka P, Ramadan F, et al. Etiology of severe pneumonia in the very elderly. Am J Respir Crit Care Med 2001;163:645–51.

29. Kothe H, Bauer T, Marre R, et al. Outcome of community-acquired pneumonia: influence of age, residence status and antimicrobial treatment. Eur Respir J 2008;32:139–46.

30. El Solh AA, Niederman NS, Drinka P. Management of pneumonia in the nursing home. Chest 2010;138: 1480–5.

31. El Solh AA, Pietrantoni C, Bhat A, et al. Indicators of potentially drug-resistant bacteria in severe nursing home-acquired pneumonia. Clin Infect Dis 2004; 39:474–80.

32. El Solh AA, Akinnusi ME, Alfarah Z, et al. Effect of antibiotic guidelines of hospitalized patients with nursing home-acquired pneumonia. J Am Geriatr Soc 2009;57:1030–5.

33. Mermel LA, Eells SJ, Acharya MK, et al. Quantitative analysis and molecular fingerprinting of methicillin-resistant *Staphylococcus aureus* nasal colonization in different patient populations: a prospective, multicenter study. Infect Control Hosp Epidemiol 2010; 31:592–7.

34. Berman SJ, Johnson EW, Nakatsu C, et al. Burden of infection in patients with end-stage renal disease requiring long-term dialysis. Clin Infect Dis 2004;39: 1747–53.

35. Rañó A, Agustí C, Jimenez P, et al. Pulmonary infiltrates in non-HIV immunocompromised patients: a diagnostic approach using noninvasive and bronchoscopic procedures. Thorax 2001;56:379–87.

36. Ibrahim EH, Sherman G, Ward S, et al. The influence of inadequate antimicrobial treatment of bloodstream infections on patient outcomes in the ICU setting. Chest 2000;118:146–55.

37. Kollef MH. Inadequate antimicrobial treatment: an important determinant of outcome for hospitalized patients. Clin Infect Dis 2000;31:S131–8.

38. Kollef MH, Sherman G, Ward S, et al. Inadequate antimicrobial treatment of infections: a risk factor for hospital mortality among critically ill patients. Chest 2000;115:462–74.

39. Micek ST, Loyd AE, Ritchie DJ, et al. *Pseudomonas aeruginosa* bloodstream infection: importance of appropriate initial antimicrobial treatment. Antimocrob Agents Chemother 2005;49:1306–11.

40. Schramm GE, Johnson JA, Doherty JA, et al. Methicillin-resistant *Staphylococcus aureus* sterile-site infection: the importance of appropriate initial antimicrobial treatment. Crit Care Med 2006;34: 2069–74.

41. Micek ST, Welch EC, Khan J, et al. Empiric combination antibiotic therapy is associated with improved outcome against sepsis due to Gram-negative bacteria: retrospective analysis. Antimicrob Agents Chemother 2010;54:1742–8.

42. Kumar A, Ellis P, Arabi Y, et al. Initiation of inappropriate antimicrobial therapy results in a five-fold reduction of survival in human septic shock. Chest 2009;135:1237–48.

43. Ibrahim EH, Ward S, Sherman G, et al. Experience with a clinical guideline for the treatment of ventilator-associated pneumonia. Crit Care Med 2001;29: 1109–15.

44. Kollef MH, Ward S. The influence of mini-BAL cultures on patient outcomes: implications for the antibiotic management of ventilator-associated pneumonia. Chest 1998;113:412–20.

45. Luna CM, Vujacich P, Niederman MS, et al. Impact of BAL data on the therapy and outcome of ventilator-associated pneumonia. Chest 1997;111:676–85.

46. Rello J, Gallego M, Mariscal D, et al. The value of routine microbial investigation in ventilator-associated pneumonia. Am J Respir Crit Care Med 1997;156: 196–200.

47. Niederman MS, Mandell LA, Anzueto A, et al. Guidelines for the management of adults with community-acquired pneumonia: diagnosis, assessment of severity, antimicrobial therapy, and prevention. Am J Respir Crit Care Med 2001;163:1730–54.

48. Zilberberg MD, Shorr AF, Micek ST, et al. Antimicrobial therapy escalation and hospital mortality among

patients with healthcare-associated pneumonia: a single-center experience. Chest 2008;134:963–8.

49. Houck PM, Bratzler DW, Nsa W, et al. Timing of antibiotic administration and outcomes for Medicare patients hospitalized with community-acquired pneumonia. Arch Intern Med 2004;164:637–44.

50. Iregui M, Ward S, Sherman G, et al. Clinical importance of delays in the initiation of appropriate antibiotic treatment for ventilator-associate pneumonia. Chest 2002;122:262–8.

51. Kang CI, Kim SH, Kim HB, et al. *Pseudomonas aeruginosa* bacteremia: risk factors for mortality and influence of delayed receipt of effective antimicrobial therapy on clinical outcome. Clin Infect Dis 2003;37:745–51.

52. Lodies TP, McKinnon PS, Swiderski L, et al. Outcomes analysis of delayed antibiotic treatment for hospital-acquired *Staphylococcus aureus* bacteremia. Clin Infect Dis 2003;36:1418–23.

53. Kumar A, Roberts D, Wood KE, et al. Duration of hypotension before initiation of effective antimicrobial therapy is the critical determinant of survival in human septic shock. Crit Care Med 2006;34:1589–96.

54. Niederman MS. The importance of de-escalating antimicrobial therapy in patients with ventilator-associated pneumonia. Semin Respir Crit Care Med 2006;27:45–50.

55. Canadian Critical Care Trials Group. A randominzed trial of diagnostic techniques for ventilator-associated pneumonia. N Engl J Med 2006;355: 2619–30.

56. Kollef MH. Diagnosis of ventilator-associated pneumonia. N Engl J Med 2006;355:2691–3.

57. Hoogewerf M, Oosterheert JJ, Hak E, et al. Prognostic factors for early clinical failure in patients with severe community-acquired pneumonia. Clin Microbiol Infect 2006;12:1097–104.

58. Schlueter M, James C, Dominguez A, et al. Practice patterns for antibiotic de-escalation in culture-negative healthcare-associated pneumonia. Infection 2010;38:357–62.

59. Chastre J, Wolff M, Fagon JY, et al. Comparison of 8 vs 15 days of antibiotic therapy for ventilator-associated pneumonia in adults: a randomized controlled trial. JAMA 2003;290:2588–98.

60. Schuetz P, Christ-Crain M, Thomann R, et al. Effect of procalcitonin-based guidelines vs standard guidelines on antibiotic use in lower respiratory tract infections: the ProHOSP randomized controlled trial. JAMA 2009;302:1059–66.

61. Bouadma L, Luyt CE, Tubach F, et al. Use of procalcitonin to reduce patient's exposure to antibiotics in intensive care units (PRORATA trial): a multicenter randomized controlled trial. Lancet 2010;375: 463–74.

62. Soriano A, Marco F, Martinez JA, et al. Influence of vancomycin minimum inhibitory concentration on the treatment of methicillin-resistant *Staphylococcus aureus* bacteremia. Clin Infect Dis 2008;46:193–200.

63. Haque NZ, Cahuayme Zaniga L, Peyrani P, et al. Relationship of vancomycin minimum inhibitory concentration to mortality in patients with methicillin-resistant Staphylococcus aureus hospital-acquired, ventilator-associated, or health-care- associated pneumonia. Chest 2010;138:1356–62.

64. Lamer C, de beco V, Soler P, et al. Analysis of vancomycin entry into pulmonary lining fluid by bronchoalveolar lavage in critically ill patients. Antimicrob Agents Chemother 1993;37:281–6.

65. Cruciani M, Gattr G, Lazzarini L, et al. Penetration of vancomycin into human lung tissue. J Antimicrob Chemother 1996;38:865–9.

66. Boselli E, Breilh D, Rimmelé T, et al. Pharmacokinetics and intrapulmonary concentrations of linezolid administered to critically ill patients with ventilator-associated pneumonia. Crit Care Med 2005;33: 1529–33.

67. Stevens DL, Ma Y, Salmi DB, et al. Impact of antibiotics on expression of virulence-associated exotoxin genes in methicillin-sensitive and methicillin-resistant *Staphylococcus aureus*. J Infect Dis 2007; 195:202–11.

De-Escalation Therapy: Is It Valuable for the Management of Ventilator-Associated Pneumonia?

Michael S. Niederman, MD[a,b,c,]*, Vasiliki Soulountsi, MD[c,d]

KEYWORDS

- De-Escalation • Antimicrobial resistance
- Ventilator-associated pneumonia (VAP) therapy
- Therapeutic protocols

Ventilator-associated pneumonia (VAP) is a common ICU infection and, in one large epidemiologic study, a frequent reason for empiric antibiotic use among critically ill patients.[1] As is the case with bacteremia, the use of inappropriate initial antibiotic therapy is a risk factor for mortality in patients with VAP, emphasizing the importance of timely and accurate therapy for this infection.[2,3] To achieve appropriate therapy, it is often necessary to use multiple broad-spectrum antibiotics, directed against both gram-positive and gram-negative pathogens, because VAP can be a polymicrobial infection and up to half of all ICU infections can be caused by antibiotic-resistant varieties of these pathogens.[4] The use of aggressive, broad-spectrum empiric therapy, however, although increasing the likelihood of initial appropriate therapy, could also lead to the indiscriminate use of the most effective antibiotics, and it is well-known that the excessive use of antibiotics can further increase the prevalence of infection with multidrug-resistant (MDR) bacteria,[5] possibly leading to a vicious cycle of antibiotic resistance, driving the aggressive use of antibiotics and the excessive use of antibiotics, creating even more resistance.

Several approaches have been proposed to promote the appropriate use of antibiotics, including improved diagnosis, antibiotic restriction, and de-escalation. De-escalation involves the practice of starting with a broad-spectrum empiric therapy regimen designed to avoid inappropriate therapy combined with a commitment to change from broad-spectrum to narrow-spectrum therapy, reduce the number of drugs and the duration of therapy, and even stop therapy in selected patients.[6] These changes are usually made on day 2 or 3 of therapy, as dictated by a patient's clinical response and the data collected from lower respiratory tract cultures obtained at the time of pneumonia diagnosis. The Infectious Diseases Society of America published antimicrobial stewardship guidelines in 2007 and emphasized the importance of de-escalation along with the use of prospective audit and physician feedback on antibiotic usage patterns, dose optimization, and the use of antibiotic treatment guidelines that have been modified with knowledge of local microbiologic patterns. Formulary restriction and preauthorization were not regarded as highly effective strategies to control antibiotic resistance.[7]

In this review, the focus is on de-escalation, a strategy recommended in the 2005 guidelines for the management of nosocomial pneumonia published by the American Thoracic Society (ATS)

[a] Department of Medicine, Winthrop-University Hospital, 222 Station Plaza North, Suite 509, Mineola, NY 11501, USA
[b] Department of Medicine, SUNY at Stony Brook, Stony Brook, NY, USA
[c] Department of Pulmonary and Critical Care Medicine, Winthrop-University Hospital, Mineola, NY, USA
[d] Department of A'ICU, General Hospital G.Papanikolaou, Eliti 2, 54248 Kifisia Thessaloniki, Greece
* Corresponding author. 222 Station Plaza North, Suite 509, Mineola, NY 11501.
E-mail address: mniederman@winthrop.org

Clin Chest Med 32 (2011) 517–534
doi:10.1016/j.ccm.2011.05.009
0272-5231/11/$ – see front matter © 2011 Elsevier Inc. All rights reserved.

and the Infectious Diseases Society of America.[5] Since that publication, there have been several reviews and studies that have examined the utility of de-escalation and the clinical factors that promote the effective use of this strategy as well as the potential benefits and harm of using this approach.[8–22] The data show that de-escalation is a safe strategy that can effectively reduce the use of prolonged broad-spectrum, multidrug therapy, without harm to patients and potentially with clinical benefit. The approach is not used as much as it could be, however, and the rate of de-escalation has varied from 22% to 74%, depending on a variety of clinical factors. Based on findings from these studies, the authors believe that there are opportunities for more widespread use of de-escalation and that there is a better understanding of how to optimize this practice.

HOW TO ACCOMPLISH DE-ESCALATION

To effectively practice a de-escalation strategy, it is necessary to meet several requirements. Ideally, each ICU should have a protocol for initial empiric therapy that is based on established and accepted guidelines but modified by knowledge of the local prevalence of common MDR pathogens and an awareness of their antimicrobial susceptibility patterns. It is also important to make sure that all patients have a deep lower respiratory tract sample (endotracheal aspirate, bronchoscopic or non-bronchsocopic bronchoalveolar lavage, or protected brush) collected for culture before starting empiric therapy. This information needs to be supplemented by daily patient assessment of clinical response; thus, it is important to be able to define a favorable or unfavorable response to therapy. In some studies, this has been facilitated by the serial measurement of inflammatory biomarkers, such as procalcitonin (PCT), and clinical infection scores, such as the Clinical Pulmonary Infection Score (CPIS).[20–24] Ultimately, even with this information, it is only possible to de-escalate if clinicians have confidence that it is a safe and effective practice and if they have a protocolized approach for how to do de-escalation.

The Need for a Protocol for Initial Therapy

The best way to achieve effective empiric therapy for patients with VAP is to have a protocol for which drugs to start and have the choice dictated by awareness of individual risk factors for infection with specific pathogens combined with a knowledge of local microbiologic patterns, including the prevalence of specific organisms and their susceptibility to antibiotics. In defining which patients are at risk for infection with MDR pathogens, it is important

to assess time of pneumonia onset (before day 5 of hospital stay or later) and the prior use of antibiotics. Patients with both risk factors may have a frequency of infection by MDR pathogens of at least 60%, but when choosing therapy for these patients, some studies have shown that it is possible to devise an empiric therapy regimen that was 80% to 95% effective, depending on if multiple agents were used and if the choices were modified with a knowledge of local microbiology patterns.[25,26]

For example, Trouillet and colleagues[25] could achieve a high degree of appropriate therapy if they used 3 different broad-spectrum agents, specifically, imipenem or piperacillin/tazobactam, combined with amikacin and vancomycin. Alternatively, Beardsley and colleagues[26] found that the most active β-lactam agents were only approximately 80% active against the gram-negative pathogens in their ICU when used as monotherapy. To achieve coverage above 95%, it was necessary to combine one of these agents with amikacin, but similar efficacy was not achieved if these agents were combined with other aminoglycosides or with ciprofloxacin.

Each ICU has its own unique microbiologic patterns, and it is necessary to know this information in order to design a protocol for effective empiric therapy. Studies have demonstrated the predominant resistant organisms can vary from hospital to hospital, even if patients with the same risk factors are evaluated, and the predominant pathogen can change over time.[27] In addition, within a given hospital, the patterns of antimicrobial resistance are often unique to a specific ICU, with medical and surgical units often having different flora and antimicrobial susceptibility patterns.[28] One way to update and enhance the knowledge of local microbiology is to collect surveillance cultures on a regular basis and to base initial empiric therapy decisions on this information. The value of surveillance cultures is enhanced if they are collected often, generally at least 2 to 3 times per week. In one study of intubated patients, samples of endotracheal aspirates were cultured twice weekly in a group of 299 mechanically ventilated patients.[29] When empiric therapy was chosen based on these data in the 41 patients with VAP, it was accurate 95% of the time; yet, the therapy itself involved broad-spectrum antibiotics only 45% of the time.

When empiric therapy is given, it must be both appropriate and adequate. Although most studies of de-escalation have only focused on achieving appropriate therapy, it is also important to use adequate therapy, which requires not only using the right antibiotic but also using it at the correct dose, with good penetration to the site of infection and in combination (if necessary).[5] Recently, investigators have examined the use of a protocol for VAP therapy that focused on maximizing antibiotic dosing, and using prolonged infusion of certain β-lactam antibiotics. With this approach to dose optimization, infection-related mortality and length of stay were reduced, and nonsusceptible organisms that were not ordinarily able to be treated were managed effectively by using higher doses of effective antibiotics.[30] In studies of de-escalation, the best opportunities for narrowing and focusing empiric therapy come when there is a high rate of appropriate empiric therapy, usually by employing a protocol that recommends specific antimicrobial agents.

The Need for Culture Data

To effectively modify antibiotic therapy, it is necessary to have bacteriologic data collected at the time of initial empiric therapy. It may not matter, however, which diagnostic method is used. In the Canadian Clinical Trials study of VAP, "targeted therapy" was defined as stopping antibiotics if cultures were negative or narrowing the spectrum and number of drugs if the cultures indicated this was possible.[15,16] In the study, 2 diagnostic methods were compared in a randomized fashion, bronchoalveolar lavage (BAL) and endotracheal aspirate, and the investigators found that targeted therapy was used more than 70% of the time, regardless of which diagnostic method was used. Thus, the collection of a culture, of any type, can facilitate de-escalation, but it is much harder if no cultures are collected. One study from Greece suggested a higher rate of de-escalation with the use of BAL than endotracheal aspirate (66% vs 21%), but there was no systematic randomization to which diagnostic method was used.[17]

Although a culture is necessary before therapy in order to modify antibiotic management, in some patients, diagnostic cultures are negative, and this is often used as a reason not to de-escalate. Patients with negative cultures, however, may still be good candidates for antibiotic modification, because in retrospect, some of these patients will be deemed to have had congestive heart failure, atelectasis, or nonrespiratory sources of fever, and a negative culture may give impetus to stop therapy completely in such patients. The finding of a negative culture could have limited value if a patient were on antimicrobial therapy when collected, unless the therapy had been continued unchanged for at least 72 hours. Even in the setting of negative cultures, antibiotic modification may be possible.[31] In one study, 101 episodes of clinically suspected VAP with culture-negative BAL were

evaluated to determine the safety of stopping antibiotics.[14] In the study, only 19 patients were on antibiotics at the time of BAL, but after the sampling, antibiotics were started in 65 episodes. Based on clinical observations, in conjunction with the BAL data, all patients had antibiotics stopped within 3 days, and outcomes were excellent, with only 6 patients having a second episode of suspected pneumonia. Thus, it does seem safe to stop antibiotics in patients with negative cultures, if the clinical course supports the microbiologic data, even if the patient were on antibiotic therapy at the time of culture collection. Overall, of the culture negative patients, 66% who had been treated with antibiotics and 69% of those who who were not treated with antibiotics had a specific noninfectious diagnosis, including processes, such as atelectasis, pulmonary embolus, pulmonary hemorrhage, or congestive heart failure.

Using Clinical Assessment to Evaluate Response to Therapy

In making the decision to narrow and/or focus antibiotic therapy, it is necessary to determine if a patient has responded to initial therapy. If so, then it may be possible to de-escalate antibiotic therapy. One study of 63 mechanically ventilated patients examined the time course of VAP resolution and the clinical parameters that reflected a favorable response to therapy.[24] In that study, investigators examined serial measurements of a modified CPIS, including fever, white blood cell count, leukocytosis, radiographic patterns, and oxygenation. Patients who survived had a rapid drop in CPIS, which occurred by day 3, in contrast to no significant change in patients who did not survive. In addition, of all the CPIS components, the one to change most rapidly in those receiving appropriate therapy was oxygenation. Thus, day 3 seems a good time point to recognize patients who are responding to therapy and in whom de-escalation could be considered.

In another study, Micek and colleagues[32] were able to significantly reduce the duration of antibiotic therapy in VAP patients by combining a protocol for initial therapy, based on local microbiologic data that led to 93.5% of patients receiving effective empiric therapy, with a clinical algorithm for early cessation of therapy. Therapy was stopped as soon as patients were found to have a noninfectious cause of lung infiltrate or had resolution of clinical signs of pneumonia. In this study, resolution was defined as normalization of fever, white blood cell count, oxygenation, purulence of sputum, and a lack of radiographic progression. They also found that the overall duration of therapy was related to the magnitude of clinical findings initially present, as reflected by the CPIS. When the initial CPIS was 6 or lower, the duration of therapy was less than if the score were above 6. Older studies, including the randomized trial by Singh and colleagues,[33] have also shown that if the clinical suspicion of VAP is low (as reflected by a modified CPIS $\leq$6), it is safe to stop therapy after only 3 days, unless the clinical findings worsen, as reflected by a rising CPIS score. Thus, the CPIS, or its components, in particular, serial measurements of oxygenation, can be used to define whether or not a patient is responding to empiric therapy and if the patient is a good candidate for focused therapy or for a reduced duration of therapy.

Using Biomarkers to Evaluate Response to Therapy

A variety of biomarkers, notably procalcitonin, have been used in studies of infection to define when to start therapy, when bacterial infection (vs viral infection) is present, and when to stop antibiotic therapy.[20,21,23,34,35] In the management of VAP, Luyt and colleagues[34] demonstrated that measurement of serum PCT at days 1, 3, and 7 could distinguish patients with favorable outcomes from those with unfavorable outcomes, with the levels lower in those with favorable outcomes. At day 3, the chance for an unfavorable outcome was nearly 25 times higher when PCT values were elevated. Serial measurements of serum biomarkers may also help define prognosis and identify patients who are receiving appropriate antibiotic therapy. Povoa and colleagues[35] measured C-reactive protein (CRP) daily during the therapy for VAP. They observed that if the CRP value exceeded 60% of its initial value at day 4, then the prognosis was poor, and patients who received appropriate therapy had a drop in CRP, whereas those receiving inappropriate therapy did not. Thus, the concept was established that biomarkers could potentially guide the duration of VAP therapy and that those with declining levels, as a consequence of appropriate therapy, could potentially have antibiotic therapy stopped at an early time point.

Three intervention trials have used PCT levels to guide the duration of therapy in critically ill patients with ICU infections, including VAP.[20,21,23] In one study, Nobre and colleagues[20] evaluated the impact of a PCT-guided antibiotic discontinuation policy in 39 patients, comparing them with 40 patients treated with standard care. Patients in the PCT group were re-evaluated on days 3 and 5 with the use of a specific protocol. In that study, 81% of the patients in the PCT-guided group had antibiotics stopped (de-escalated) as suggested by the protocol, whereas in the remaining patients, the physician did not de-escalate in spite of the PCT findings. With the implementation of this protocol, there was a statistically significant decrease in the duration of the therapy for the first episode of sepsis (P = .003) and for the total antibiotic exposure days per 1000 inpatient days (P = .0002) and an increase in the days alive and without antibiotics (P = .04) in favor of the PCT per protocol group. In the intention-to-treat analysis, however, although the duration of antibiotic therapy (6 days vs 9.5 days) and the total exposure days to antibiotics (541/1000 days vs 644 days/1000 days) were lower in the PCT group, the differences were not statistically significant. Mortality at 28 days and in-hospital mortality were similar in both groups (P = .74 and P = .79, respectively) in the per protocol group. Similarly, Stolz and colleagues[21] randomized 101 patients to antibiotic discontinuation for VAP to be determined by serial measurements of PCT or by clinical evaluation. PCT guidance led to a 27% reduction in duration of antibiotic therapy, with no adverse effect on mortality or length of stay.

In another study, 307 patients were managed by a PCT protocol for a mixture of infections in the ICU, whereas 314 patients were managed by clinical data and protocols for antibiotic duration. More than 90% of patients in both groups received appropriate empiric therapy, and in general almost all patients in both groups received empiric therapy for suspected infection, with antibiotics withheld in only 28 patients in the PCT group and in 15 patients in the control group. Although the PCT guidance was not always followed and was often overruled by clinical evaluation, the use of PCT guidance led to an absolute reduction in duration of therapy by a mean of 2.7 days, with no adverse effect on mortality.[23] In that study, there were 141 patients with VAP, and the 75 with PCT guidance had an absolute reduction in duration of therapy of 3.1 days. In spite of using less antibiotic therapy with PCT guidance, this group did not have a lower frequency of the emergence of resistance than patients who did not have this guided approach. The sum of all these studies does suggest that in critically ill patients, the decision to start antibiotic therapy should be a clinical one, made by an ICU physician. Biomarkers can be used, however, with clinical assessment to guide duration of therapy and help define a safe and early time point for discontinuation of antibiotic therapy, a key component of de-escalation.

Using a Protocol to De-Escalate

In most studies of de-escalation, the investigators have defined a protocol for when to de-escalate and which criteria should be used to permit narrowing and focusing of antibiotic therapy. When this has been done, the rates of de-escalation can be as high as 74%.[11,15] In one study that compared the frequency of de-escalation in 50 patients before and in 50 patients after a protocol that was implemented by clinical pharmacists, the use of a protocol increased the rate of appropriate de-escalation from 42% to 72% ($P = .002$), and use of a protocol was associated with a significant reduction in total duration of antibiotic therapy.[11] In another before and after study, the use of a protocol for de-escalation led to a significant reduction in the duration of antibiotic therapy and an increase in the use of therapy tailored to the results of respiratory tract cultures.[13] The protocol used recommended discontinuation of therapy at 8 days unless the patient had infection with a non-fermenting gram-negative organism or if the CPIS remained greater than 6 at day 8. In another study, when all patients were managed with a protocol for focused therapy that directed therapy to be focused or stopped on the basis of deep lower respiratory tract cultures, more than 70% had targeted therapy initiated.[15] In all of these studies, the use of a de-escalation regimen was generally early in the course of therapy as soon as culture and clinical data became available.

Going from Combination Therapy to Monotherapy

One form of de-escalation is to change from multiple agents to a single agent. This can generally be done when cultures show a single organism or organisms that are sensitive to a single antibiotic that ideally is not a broad-spectrum agent. The use of some of the protocols (discussed previously) has generally been helpful in promoting such a narrowing of therapy. For example, in the study of Stolz and colleagues,[21] the use of PCT guidance led to 54% of patients getting monotherapy at 72 hours compared with only 28% without PCT guidance. Alternatively, if initial empiric therapy involves a combination of agents, then the possibility of de-escalation is greater than if initial therapy is only with a single agent. Similarly, if initial therapy is for early-onset infection, in one study the frequency of de-escalation was lower than if initial therapy was for late-onset infection.[18] In that study, when initial therapy was narrow spectrum, de-escalation was done in 42 % of the time, whereas it was done 44% of the time if the initial therapy was broad spectrum. Escalation

was done, however, 26% of the time when initial therapy was narrow spectrum but only 11% of the time when it was broad-spectrum. When therapy was given for early-onset infection, de-escalation was done 26% of the time compared with 72% of the time during the therapy for late-onset infection. In general in this study, when de-escalation was done, it usually involved stopping a combination regimen and/or using a narrow-spectrum agent.

Initially, if a patient has risk factors for MDR pathogens, guidelines recommend using an initial empiric therapy with a combination regimen, not for the purpose of administering synergistic therapy (β-lactam with an aminoglycoside) or to prevent the emergence of resistance that is common with monotherapy, rather to simply provide therapy that is likely to cover the suspected MDR pathogens. In general, it is difficult to prove the value of combination therapy for VAP beyond its ability to increase the likelihood of initially appropriate antibiotic therapy.

In the setting of bacteremic pseudomonal pneumonia, however, combination therapy may reduce mortality compared with monotherapy.[36,37] In nonbacteremic VAP, combination therapy does increase the likelihood that initial therapy covers the etiologic organism, but it may also increase

---

Box 1
Possible reasons for not using de-escalation more often in patients with VAP

- Want to start with a narrow-spectrum regimen and then broaden therapy only if needed
  - An ecologic policy that puts patients at risk
- Lower respiratory tract cultures were negative
  - Still can de-escalate
- Afraid to change a winning hand
  - Not justified as a concern
- Unable to reduce number of drugs
  - May need continued combination therapy for pseudomonal bacteremia, not for nonbacteremic infection
- Unable to reduce spectrum of activity of drugs
  - Occasionally, when certain MDR pathogens are present (eg, Acinetobacter spp)
- Unable to reduce duration of therapy
  - Rarely (g, S aureus bacteremia and/or endocarditis)

Table 1
General characteristics of recent studies of de-escalation in VAP

Study (Reference Number)	Year of Publication	Design of Study/Origin Country/No. of Patients/ Specific Characteristics	Diagnosis of VAP in Addition to Clinical Criteria (Fever, New or Persistent Infiltrates, Leukocytosis/ Leukopenia, Purulent Sputum)	Criteria for Initial/Empiric Therapy	Day and Strategy of De-Escalation
1. Soo Hoo et al[10]	2005	• Before and after protocol development • Observational, cohort • United States • Total 106 patients • HAP (VAP) • Included second episodes of pneumonia	• BAL bronchoscopic or nonbronchoscopic (10^4 CFU/mL) OR • TA when intubation <24 h	• Usual care versus • Specific protocol with 2–3 drugs based on ATS guidelines, local microbiologic data, severity status	ON DAY 3 based on microbiologic data • Narrow OR • Discontinue specific agents
2. Lancaster et al[11]	2008	• Before and after protocol development • Observational • United States • 100 patients: 37 VAP patients and 63 HAP patients • Only first episode of VAP/HAP was considered • Excluded patients receiving immunosuppressants, corticosteroids, those with neutropenia, and HIV infection	• BAL (3.6% of the cultures) • Mini-BAL (18.11% of the cultures) • Sputum cultures (78.26% of the cultures) • No cultures (25% of the patients)	• Usual care versus • Specific protocol based on ATS guidelines, institutional antibiograms, time of onset of pneumonia, physician preference	Microbiologic data + clinical response • Continue if there was no alternative agent • Narrow • Discontinue specific agents
3. Dellit et al[13]	2008	• Before and after protocol development • Retrospective • United States • 819 VAP patients • Included second episodes of VAP • Excluded patients receiving therapy for infection other than VAP	Quantitative cultures of • BAL (10^4 CFU/mL) or mini-BAL OR • PSB (10^3 CFU/mL)	• Usual care versus • Specific protocol defined by time of onset of pneumonia (early vs late), including multidrug antibiotic choice + duration of therapy)	Microbiologic data + clinical response • Narrow • Discontinue specific agents • Duration of therapy

	Year				
4. Leone et al[18]	2007	• Protocol development without control group • Prospective, observational • European • 115 VAP patients • Excluded septic shock patients	• BAL ≥10^4 CFU/mL OR • TA ≥10^5 CFU/mL	Specific antibiotic protocol defined by time of onset of pneumonia + local microbiologic data + patient comorbidities + clinical status	*ON DAY 2–3 Microbiologic data + CPIS to* • Narrow +/or • Discontinue specific agents
5. Alvarez-Lerma et al[19]	2006	• Protocol development without control group • Prospective, observational • Multicenter (24 ICUS) • European • 258 VAP/HAP patients • Only first episode of VAP/HAP • Excluded patients with previous carbapenem administration, renal insufficiency (CLcr <20 mL/min), HIV patients, development of pneumonia on days 1–4 postadmission without concomitant risk factors	• Quantitative BAL ≥10^4 CFU/mL (4.1%) OR • Quantitative TA ≥10^5 CFU/mL (81.6%) OR • PSB ≥10^3 CFU/mL (32.8%) ± • Blood pleural cultures with the same pathogen as respiratory samples OR • Histopathologic evidence of pneumonia OR • Serology identification of Legionella	Specific protocol: carbapenem-based multidrug protocol	*On days 3–5 microbiologic data + clinical response to* • Narrow • Discontinue specific agents

6. Giantsou et al[17]	2007	• Compare diagnostic strategies for the purpose of de-escalation
		• Prospective, observational
		• European
		• 143VAP patients
		• Only first episode of VAP for each patient
		• Excluded HIV /transplant patients
			• Quantitative BAL and TA (IN ALL PATIENTS)
			Protocol assignment to de-escalation based on:
			  BAL: 62 patients
			  TA: 81 patients
				Antibiotic protocol based on local microbiologic data, risk factors, Gram stain, physician preference	*On day 3 microbiologic data + clinical response to*
					• Narrow
					+/or
					• Discontinue specific agents

(continued on next page)

Table 1
(continued)

Study (Reference Number)	Year of Publication	Design of Study/Origin Country/No. of Patients/ Specific Characteristics	Diagnosis of VAP in Addition to Clinical Criteria (Fever, New or Persistent Infiltrates, Leukocytosis/ Leukopenia, Purulent Sputum)	Criteria for Initial/Empiric Therapy	Day and Strategy of De-Escalation
7. Canadian Critical Trials Group[15] and 8. Joffe et al[16]	2006 and 2008	• Compare diagnostic strategies for the purpose of de-escalation • Prospective, randomized • Canada • Multicenter (28 ICUs) • 740 VAP patients • Excluded immunocompromised patients, patients infected or colonized with Pseudomonas species or MRSA, recent recipients of study drugs	• Quantitative BAL (n = 365) OR • Nonquantitative TA (n = 374)	*Standardized antibiotic administration randomly assigned* Monotherapy (meropenem) versus Combination (both meropenem based)	*WITHIN 5 DAYS of enrollment when microbiologic data available* • Narrow • Discontinue specific agents
9. Kollef and Kollef[14]	2005	• Prospective, observational • United States • 101 Patients with suspected VAP • ALL with (-) BAL • Only first episode of VAP • Included immunosuppressed patients	• Quantitative BAL ≥10^4 CFU/mL (all patients)	Specific multidrug therapy chosen based on local susceptibility data	*WITHIN 3 DAYS based on clinical criteria* • Discontinue specific agents • Shorten duration of therapy

	Year			
10. Kollef et al[12]	2006	• Prospective, observational • United States • Multicenter (20 ICUs) • 398VAP patients • Only first episode of VAP • Excluded lung transplant patients	• TA (58.3%) • BAL quantitative bronchoscopic or nonbronchoscopic (33.7%) • Both TA and BAL (1.8%) • No cultures (6.3%)	>100 Different prescriptions • One-drug regimen (27.9%) • Two-drug regimens (46.2%) • Three-drug regimens (22.6%)	• Narrow • Discontinue specific agents
11. Nobre et al[20]	2008	• Intervention based on PCT • Randomized, controlled • European • 79 Patients; 69% pulmonary sepsis (community and nosocomial) • Excluded immunocompromised patients • Excluded MDR pathogens (and P aeruginosa)	• BAL • Tracheal aspirates • Blood cultures	• Local guidelines and susceptibility patterns, physician discretion	• On day 5 or • On day 3 In intervention group PCT depending on PCT values and physician discretion • Discontinue antibiotics
12. Eachempati et al[22]	2009	• Retrospective, observational • Protocol for de-escalation • United States • 138 Surgical Patients with VAP	• Bronchoscopic BAL >10^4 CFU/mL	• Local protocol of at least 2 antibiotics, active against gram positives and gram negatives (rotate agents)	• 48–72 Hours, can narrow and/or discontinue agents based on cultures
13. Stolz et al[21]	2009	• Prospective, randomized intervention, contolled, based on serial PCT data • United States and Switzerland • 101 Patients with VAP • Excluded immune compromised	• Bronchoscopic or endotracheal aspirates in 96%, with 73% positive results • CPIS calculated	• All given initial empiric therapy, no protocol, with knowledge of local microbiology	• At 72 hours based on serial levels of PCT, with an algorithm guiding use of antibiotics • Protocol to impact duration of therapy, and to reduce the number of drugs

Abbreviations: CFU, colony-forming unit; CLcr, creatinine clearance; HAP, hospital-acquired pneumonia; PSB, protected specimen brush; TA, tracheal aspirates.

the rate of bacterial killing, which can translate into a reduced mortality.[38,39] In one large multicenter study, the use of combination therapy led to appropriate therapy for MDR gram-negative organisms 84% of the time compared with only 11% of the time when monotherapy was used for these organisms.[38] In another study of patients with septic shock, the use of combination therapy led to reduced mortality compared with monotherapy, even though both types of regimens in the study provided appropriate therapy. These findings suggest that the use of 2 agents has a benefit, beyond just providing appropriate therapy, possibly by increasing the rapidity of bacterial killing, and the benefit was particularly evident for patients with respiratory tract infection.[39]

If initial therapy is with a combination of agents, the regimen may not need to be continued for a prolonged period, and it may be possible to de-escalate to a single agent, once culture and clinical data become available. Meta-analyses have shown that the addition of an aminoglycoside to a β-lactam does not improve efficacy or prevent the emergence of resistance but may add to the risk of nephotoxicity.[40,41] Thus, even if a nonfermenting gram-negative organisms, like Pseudomonas aeruginosa is present, the maximal benefit of adding the aminoglycoside may have occurred during 5 days of combination therapy.[5,42] For these patients, de-escalation can be achieved by discontinuing the aminoglycoside part of the initial combination therapy after 5 days, especially if a patient is clinically improving.[5,42] If the cultures do not demonstrate a nonfermenting gram-negative organism, however, then the aminoglycoside can probably be stopped as soon as the sensitivity data become available (often by day 3), and therapy can be finished with a single agent that is active against the identified pathogen. When changing to a single agent, only 7 antimicrobials have been shown effective for critically ill mechanically ventilated patients with VAP: imipenem, meropenem, doripenem cefepime, piperacillin-tazobactam, ciprofloxacin, or high-dose levofloxacin (750 mg daily).[43–47]

WHY IS DE-ESCALATION NOT DONE MORE OFTEN?

As discussed previously, the frequency of de-escalation has varied in published studies from rates as low as 22 % to rates as high as 74% (**Box 1**).[10–22] There are several possible reasons for not doing de-escalation, some justifiable and others not. These include the following. (1) Using an initial empiric therapy regimen that is so narrow spectrum that initial therapy is not always accurate—thus, it is often necessary to add more agents (escalate) rather than to de-escalate when culture data become available. This situation arises when clinicians put an undue focus on using narrow-spectrum empiric therapy regimens and only use broad-spectrum agents when justified by culture data. This approach is an ecologic policy that has the putative benefit of preventing antibiotic overuse but can put specific patients at risk for a poor outcome. (2) If respiratory tract cultures are negative, some clinicians are reluctant to narrow and focus therapy, but as pointed out previously, de-escalation can be done safely in this setting and a negative culture is good evidence of the absence of a highly resistant pathogen (unless it was collected within 24–72 hours of starting appropriate therapy). (3) Sometimes, de-escalation is not done because there is fear of changing a "winning hand." This concern is not justified, however, and in one retrospective study, when de-escalation occurred (presumably because clinical and culture data justified this practice), mortality was lower than if no de-escalation had been done.[12] Although de-escalation may not have been the cause of a reduced mortality and may have been nothing more than a surrogate marker of a responding patient, the lower mortality in this group of patients suggests that the practice is a safe one, and one that does not harm patients. (4) In some settings, it may be justified not to de-escalate, but these situations are not present in the majority of patients. The inability to de-escalate could occur if Pseudomonas aeruginosa bacteremia is present, if infection is caused by such a highly resistant pathogen that only a combination of agents could be effective, if infection is polymicrobial with MDR gram-negatives and methicillin-resistant *Staphylococcus aureus* (MRSA), and if it is impossible to shorten the duration of therapy (as in MRSA pneumonia with bacteremia and endocarditis).

RECENT DATA ABOUT DE-ESCALATION
Factors Associated with De-Escalation

Since the guidelines for nosocomial pneumonia were published in 2005, several studies have examined the practice of de-escalation for patients with VAP and have demonstrated factors associated with successful implementation of this strategy. Between 2005 and 2009, there were 13 different publications that reported the use of de-escalation for patients with VAP (**Table 1**).[10–22] De-escalation was based in 7 studies on the application of a specific protocol; in 2 studies on the use of a specific diagnostic culture method (1 of which also used a protocol), in 2 studies on the positivity of initial respiratory cultures, and in 2 studies on the use of the biomarker PCT. The studies varied widely in their definition and methods of de-escalation, but when used, this practice led to the use of less broad-spectrum antibiotics, fewer antibiotics, and a shorter duration of antibiotic therapy. The rate of de-escalation varied between 22.3% and 74.42%, with higher rates reported when a protocol was followed (compared with usual care) and when initial therapy was appropriate. In general, the use of broad-spectrum, multidrug therapy for late-onset infection led to more de-escalation than the use of a narrow-spectrum monotherapy regimen for early-onset infection. In addition, de-escalation rates were lower in hospitals that had a high frequency of infection with MDR pathogens. De-escalation was applied as early as day 3[10,18–22] or up today 5,[15,19,20] considering clinical response,[14] or microbiologic data,[10,12,15,16,22] or both[11,13,17–19] or, in 2 studies, using PCT values (see **Table 1**).[20,21] In all studies, the de-escalation strategy included either change from broad-spectrum to narrow-spectrum antibiotics,[10–13,15,17–19] discontinuing antibiotics,[10–22] or both.[10–13,15,17–19,22] whereas shortening of duration of therapy was applied in 4 studies (see **Table 1**).[13,14,20,21]

In examining the available data it seems that de-escalation was done more often when patients received appropriate therapy and with positive culture data (**Table 2**). In general, however, in the studies that developed a protocol for initial empiric therapy that was based on guidelines and local microbiologic data, the use of a protocol led to more patients getting appropriate therapy, and this was associated with an increased rate of de-escalation when compared with the preprotocol period.[10,11] In one study, with the use of a protocol for initial therapy, the rate of de-escalation was 69% in patients with positive cultures compared with a 29% rate in those with negative cultures.[13] In that study, the use of a protocol for initial therapy led to a significant increase in the rate of de-escalation among those with positive cultures when compared with a period before a protocol was implemented. In other studies, the rate of de-escalation was higher in those with positive cultures than in those with negative cultures, demonstrating the reluctance to narrow and focus therapy in patients with no pathogen in the respiratory cultures.[12,15]

In 2 studies,[15,17] one of which also used a protocol, the impact of culture method (bronchoscopic vs tracheal aspirate) on the rate of de-escalation was evaluated. One study was a prospective, observational design whereas the other was a prospective randomized trial. In another study, the investigators used a subgroup analysis to compare de-escalation rates in relation to the diagnostic method used.[12] The findings were mixed with the largest study and the one that used a prospective, randomized design finding that the rates of de-escalation were high (>70%) and independent of the diagnostic method used.[15] In the other 2 studies, there was a higher rate of de-escalation for patients undergoing BAL than for those diagnosed with tracheal aspirate.[12,17] In both of the prospective trials,[15,17] almost all the patients received appropriate empiric therapy (89%–100%) but de-escalation rates differed significantly (40.5% vs 74.2%). In one of the prospective trials, the use of BAL was associated with a lower mortality at 15 and 28 days (11.29% and 20.96%, respectively, vs 28.39% and 38.27%, respectively, than in the tracheal aspirate group) ($P = .01$ and $P = .02$, respectively).[17] In the larger study, however, the investigators did not find any difference in mortality between the 2 diagnostic groups (18.9% vs 18.4%, $P = .94$).[15]

Impact of De-Escalation on Duration and Use of Antibiotic Therapy

In 3 studies[10,16,19] it was possible to compare the duration of therapy in patients with and without de-escalation. In all of them, the duration of therapy was shorter with de-escalation, being statistically significant in only 2 of them for certain patient subsets.[16,19] Alvarez-Lerma and colleagues[19] reported no change in the duration of therapy for patients who had de-escalation, compared with those who did not, but they did observe a significant reduction in the duration of imipenem use ($P<.001$) for those who had de-escalation. In the Canadian Critical Care group trial, de-escalation (vs no de-escalation) led to a significantly ($P<.001$) shorter duration of therapy with all antibiotics in patients with negative cultures but not in those with positive cultures.[16] There was also a significantly shorter duration of study antibiotics (meropenem and ciprofloxacin) when de-escalation was done, compared with when it was not, in those with negative cultures.

Many of the studies that used a protocol for initial empiric therapy reported a reduction in duration of therapy after initiating a protocol, but it was unclear if the benefit was the result of the initial therapy choices or the use of de-escalation. Soo Hoo and colleagues[10] demonstrated that after initiation of a protocol, appropriate use of imipenem occurred in 74% of patients, and with the incorporation of a de-escalation strategy there was a remarkable reduction in the duration of imipenem use compared with the preprotocol period.

Table 2
Rates of de-escalation and appropriate empiric therapy in relation to use of a protocol and to culture results

Study (Reference Number)	No Protocol	Protocol	P Value	Positive Cultures	Negative Cultures	MDR[a] or Major[b] Pathogens	No MDR[a] or Major[b] Pathogens
1. Soo Hoo et al,[10] 2005							
• Rate of de-escalation	NR	29.5%	—	—	—	—	—
• Use of culture-based therapy	NR	74%	—	—	—	—	—
• Appropriate initial empiric therapy	46%	81%	<0.01	—	—	—	—
2. Lancaster et al,[11] 2008							
• Rate of de-escalation	42%	72%	0.002	74%	30%	—	—
• Appropriate initial empiric therapy	34%	62%	0.005	—	—	—	—
• Appropriate definitive therapy	68%	82%	0.11	—	—	—	—
3. Dellit et al,[13] 2008							
• Rate of de-escalation in pts with positive cultures	61.3%	69.4%	0.034	Depends on protocol	Depends on Protocol	—	—
• Rate of de-escalation in pts with negative cultures	32.8%	29.2%	0.420	—	—	—	—
• Appropriate initial empiric therapy in pts with positive cultures	82.1%	75.5%	0.158	—	—	—	—
• Appropriate definitive therapy in pts with positive cultures	80.4%	89.4%	0.001	—	—	—	—
4. Leone et al,[18] 2007							
• Rate of de-escalation in all patients	No controls	42%	—	—	—	54%	39%
• Appropriate initial empiric therapy	No controls	87%	—	—	—	—	—

5. Alvarez-Lerma et al,[19] 2006							
• Rate of de-escalation in all patients	No controls	%	—	42.7%	0%	9/39[c] (23.1%)	47/69[d] (68.1%)[a]
• Exclusion of pts with inadequate therapy	No controls	25.3%	—	—	—	—	—
• Exclusion of pts with unknown etiology	No controls	42.7%	—	—	—	—	—
• Rate of de-escalation in pts with susceptible pathogen	No controls	51.9%	—	—	—	—	—
• Appropriate initial empiric therapy in pts with positive cultures	No controls	82.4%	—	—	—	—	—
6. Giantsou et al,[17] 2007							
• Rate of de-escalation, all patients had appropriate therapy to be included	—	40.5%	—	—	—	Not done if resistant to therapy	Done if sensitive to therapy, all pathogens
• Rate of de-escalation with BAL	—	66.1%	—	—	—	—	—
• Rate of de-escalation with tracheal aspirate	—	21%	—	—	—	—	—
7. Canadian Critical Trials Group,[15,16] 2006, 2008							
• Rate of appropriate therapy in patients with positive cultures (similar regardless of culture method)	No controls	89.5%	—	—	—	—	—
• Rate of de-escalation in all patients	All received protocol	74.4%	—	77.7%	70.3%	—	—
8. Kollef et al,[12] 2006							
• Rate of de-escalation, all patients	—	22.3%	—	—	—	26.8%[b]	6.5%[b]
• Rate appropriate therapy in patients with positive cultures	—	55%	—	—	—	—	—

(continued on next page)

Table 2
(continued)

Study (Reference Number)	No Protocol	Protocol	P Value	Positive Cultures	Negative Cultures	MDR[a] or Major[b] Pathogens	No MDR[a] or Major[b] Pathogens
9. Eachempati et al,[22] 2009							
• Rate of de-escalation in all patients	No controls	57%	—	—	—	—	—
• Rate of appropriate therapy in all patients	—	93%	—	—	—	—	—
10. Stolz et al,[21] 2009							
• Rate of de-escalation in all patients	28.6% Monotherapy after 72 h	54% Monotherapy after 72 h	0.008	Increased continued antibiotic use by odds ratio = 2.3	—	—	—
• Rate of appropriate therapy	86% for All patients	86% for All patients	—	—	—	Increased duration of antibiotics to 15 days	Duration of antibiotics of 7 days

Relevant data not available from studies in 21 and 27.

Abbreviations: NR, not reported; pts, patients.

[a] MDR pathogen isolated in cultures.
[b] MAJOR pathogen isolated in cultures.
[c] Patients with potentially multiresistant pathogens.
[d] Patients with remaining pathogens.

Lancaster and colleagues[11] and Dellit and colleagues[13] also demonstrated a statistically significant decrease in the duration of therapy in the postprotocol period compared with the baseline period ($P = .01$ and $P = .001$, respectively). In addition, Dellit and colleagues[13] described that with the use of a protocol, there was a reduction in the antibiotic days per patient (6.2 days vs 5.3 days, $P = .020$), in the duration of therapy for MRSA (10.7 days vs 12.4 days, $P = .042$) and in the total duration of use of broad-spectrum antibiotics. In the study by Leone and colleagues,[18] the use of a protocol resulted in a shorter duration of therapy (8 days vs 10 days, $P = .2$) for those who received appropriate therapy compared with those who did not. As discussed previously, the studies that used PCT guidance also had a reduction in the duration of therapy when this biomarker was measured.[20,21]

Impact of De-Escalation on Mortality

In most of the studies, mortality was reduced when appropriate therapy was used compared with inappropriate therapy, but (as discussed previously) there was also a relationship between the use of appropriate therapy and higher rates of de-escalation, so it is difficult to separate the impact on mortality of de-escalation and appropriate therapy. In one of the studies, however, Giantsou and colleagues[17] included only patients receiving appropriate therapy and observed a further significant reduction in mortality when de-escalation was done compared with when it was not (12% vs 43% at 28 days, $P<.05$).

In spite of this complex set of factors having an impact on mortality, in 8 studies, mortality data were reported in relation to whether de-escalation occurred (**Table 3**). In 2 of these studies, there was a significantly lower mortality in patients who had de-escalation than in those who did not.[12,17] In one of these studies, Kollef and colleagues[12] examined the practice of de-escalation in a multicenter study of patients who had de-escalation done on the basis of clinician preference and in the absence of a specific protocol. In that study, the mortality rate was significantly lower (17%) for those who received

Table 3
Mortality rates in relation to de-escalation status

Study (Reference Number)	De-Escalation	No De-Escalation	Escalation	P Value
1. SooHoo et al,[10] 2005				
• Mortality at 14 d, guided group	6.6%	13%	—	—
• Mortality at 30 d, guided group	20%	32%	—	—
2. Leone et al,[18] 2007				
• Mortality	18%	11%	—	0.15
3. Alvarez-Lerma et al,[19] 2006				
• Mortality	14.6%	20.4	33.3%	—
4. Giantsou et al,[17] 2007				
• Mortality at 15 d, all pts	5.1%	31.7%	—	<0.05
• Mortality at 28 d, all pts	12%	43.5%	—	<0.05
5. Joffe et al,[16] 2008				
• Mortality at 28 d in pts with				
Negative cultures	22.2%	19.6%	—	0.66
Positive cultures	17.2%	14.1%	—	0.53
• Hospital mortality in pts with				
Negative cultures	26.5%	33%	—	0.28
Positive cultures	22.8%	17.4%	—	0.32
6. Kollef et al,[12] 2006				
• Mortality at 30 d	17%	23.7%	42.6%	0.001
7. Eachempati et al,[22] 2009	33.8%	42.1%	—	0.324
8. Stolz et al,[21] 2009				
• Mortality at 28 d	16% with PCT protocol	24% without PCT protocol	—	0.327

Abbreviation: Pts, patients.

de-escalation than for those who did not (23.7%) and than for those who had escalation of therapy (42.6%). De-escalation, however, was probably only done in patients who were clinically responding to initial therapy; thus, it may have been only a surrogate marker of a good outcome and not the causal factor. In 4 additional studies, there was a trend to reduced mortality when de-escalation was used, compared with when it was not, but the differences were not significant.[10,19,21,22] In the other 2 studies, there was no reduction in mortality when de-escalation was used.[16,18]

SUMMARY

A de-escalation strategy aimed at controlling antibiotic prescription and subsequently minimizing the emergence of resistance should be part of antimicrobial stewardship in clinical practice.[7] The available data are limited and come from studies with heterogeneous design and patient characteristics, but they suggest that the rate of de-escalation can be increased and this could result in a potential benefit in antibiotic consumption. It is uncertain, however, if the improved mortality associated with de-escalation that has been reported in some studies is the direct result of this practice or whether it is simply the result of other associated processes, such as the more frequent use of initial appropriate therapy.

More information is needed to define the optimal duration of therapy for patients with VAP. Although 8 days of therapy has been shown effective for patients with nonresistant pathogens who are treated with initially appropriate therapy, the correct duration of therapy for MDR gram-negatives, such as P aeruginosa and Acinetobacter spp, is unknown.[48] The answer may not be prolonged duration, however, but rather the use of innovative adjunctive therapies, such as immune modulation or the addition of aerosolized antibiotics to initial therapy.[49] Another approach may even be to follow cultures serially as patients are managed, and at least one study has demonstrated that when a repeat lower respiratory tract culture, collected on days 2 through 5 of therapy, is sterile, the prognosis is better than if the culture is persistently positive.[50] This finding suggests that the safety of de-escalation needs to be studied in patients with persistently positive culture findings. Some investigators have been reluctant to de-escalate to fewer antibiotics when an organism like P aeruginosa is present. The need for prolonged combination therapy for these pathogens is not established, however, and the safety of de-escalation, even for this organism, has been shown in recent studies.[12]

To increase the use of de-escalation and to achieve good outcomes, a multifaceted approach is needed. The appropriateness of empiric therapy is fundamental, and protocols for initial therapy and for duration of therapy should be incorporated into practice and can have a significant benefit on rates of de-escalation rates, duration of antibiotics, and overall mortality.[10,11,13,15,18,19] The impact of protocols should be further investigated, however, in well-designed multicenter randomized studies with a standard protocol, a control group, and an evaluation of the adherence to recommended practices. The impact of invasive and noninvasive culture techniques on de-escalation should also be further studied because current findings are conflicting, but it is clear that de-escalation is most easily done if an effort is made to obtain cultures before starting antibiotic therapy. Although protocols provide guidance for duration of antibiotic treatment, this approach could be supplemented by biomarkers, which might help overcome the reluctance of clinicians to discontinue antibiotics in patients with negative cultures, a practice documented as safe in several studies.[14,16]

REFERENCES

1. Vincent JL, Rello J, Marshall J, et al. International study of the prevalence and outcomes of infection in intensive care units. JAMA 2009;302:2323–9.
2. Kollef MH, Sherman G, Ward S, et al. Inadequate antimicrobial treatment of infections: a risk factor for hospital mortality among critically ill patients. Chest 1999;115:462–74.
3. Luna CM, Vujacich P, Niederman MS, et al. Impact of BAL data on the therapy and outcome of ventilator-associated pneumonia. Chest 1997;111:676–85.
4. Gaynes R, Edwards JR, National Nosocomial Infections Surveillance System. Overview of infections caused by gram-negative bacilli. Clin Infect Dis 2005;41:848–54.
5. Niederman MS, Craven DE, Bonten MJ, et al. Guidelines for the management of adults with hospital-acquired, ventilator-associated, and healthcare-associated pneumonia. Am J Respir Crit Care Med 2005;171:388–416.
6. Hoffken G, Niederman MS. Nosocomial pneumonia: the importance of a de-escalating strategy for antibiotic treatment of pneumonia in the ICU. Chest 2002; 122:2183–96.
7. Dellit T, Owens R, McGowan J, et al. Infectious Diseases Society of America and the society for healthcare epidemiology of america guidelines for developing an institutional program to enhance antimicrobial stewardship. Clin Infect Dis 2007;44:159–77.
8. Niederman MS. The importance of de escalating antimicrobial therapy in patients with ventilator

associated pneumonia. Semin Respir Crit Care Med 2006;27:45–50.

9. Niederman MS. Use of broad spectrum antimicrobials for the treatment of pneumonia in seriously Ill patients: maximizing clinical outcomes and minimizing selection of resistant organisms. Clin Infect Dis 2006;42:S72–81.

10. Soo Hoo GW, Wen YE, Nguyen T, et al. Impact of clinical guideline in the management of severe hospital acquired pneumonia. Chest 2005;128:2778–87.

11. Lancaster JW, Lawrence KR, Fong JJ, et al. Impact of an institution-specific hospital-acquired pneumonia protocol on the appropriateness of antibiotic therapy and patient outcomes. Pharmacotherapy 2008;28(7):852–62.

12. Kollef MH, Morrow LE, Niederman MS, et al. Clinical characteristics and treatment patterns among patients with ventilator-associated pneumonia. Chest 2006;129:1210–8.

13. Dellit TH, Chan JD, Skerrett SJ, et al. Development of a guideline for the management of VAP based on local microbiological findings and impact of the guideline on antimicrobial use practices. Infect Control Hosp Epidemiol 2008;29(6):525–33.

14. Kollef MH, Kollef KE. Antibiotic utilization and outcomes for patients with clinically suspected ventilator-associated pneumonia and negative quantitative BAL culture results. Chest 2005;128: 2706–13.

15. The Canadian Critical Care Trials Group. A randomized trial of diagnostic techniques for ventilator-associated pneumonia. N Engl J Med 2006;355:2619–30.

16. Joffe AR, Muscedere J, Marshall JC, et al. The safety of targeted antibiotic therapy for ventilator-associated pneumonia: a multicenter observational study. J Crit Care 2008;23:82–90.

17. Giantsou E, Liratzopoulos N, Efraimidou E, et al. De-escalation therapy rates are significantly higher by bronchoalveolar lavage than by tracheal aspirate. Intensive Care Med 2007;33:1533–40.

18. Leone M, Garcin F, Bouvenot J, et al. Ventilator-associated pneumonia: breeaking the vicious circle of antibiotic overuse. Crit Care Med 2007;35:379–85.

19. Alvarez-Lerma F, Alvarez B, Luque P, et al. Empiric broad-spectrum antibiotic therapy of nosocomial pneumonia in the intensive care unit: a prospective observational study. Crit Care 2006;10:R78.

20. Nobre V, Harbarth S, Graf JD, et al. Use of procalcitonin to shorten antibiotic treatment duration in septic patients. Am J Respir Crit Care Med 2008; 177:498–505.

21. Stolz D, Smyrnios N, Eggimann P, et al. Procalcitonin for reduced antibiotic exposure in ventilator-associated pneumonia: a randomised study. Eur Respir J 2009;34:1364–75.

22. Eachempati SR, Hydo LJ, Shou J, et al. Does de-escalation of antibiotic therapy for ventilator-associated pneumonia affect the likelihood of recurrent pneumonia or mortality in critically ill surgical patients? J Trauma 2009;66:1343–8.

23. Bouadma L, Luyt CE, Tubach F, et al. Use of procalcitonin to reduce patients' exposure to antibiotics in intensive care units (PRORATA trial): a multicentre randomised controlled trial. Lancet 2010;375: 463–74.

24. Luna CM, Blanzaco D, Niederman MS, et al. Resolution of ventilator-associated pneumonia: prospective evaluation of the clinical pulmonary infection score as an early clinical predictor of outcome. Crit Care Med 2003;31:676–82.

25. Trouillet JL, Chastre J, Vuagnat A, et al. Ventilator-associated pneumonia caused by potentially drug-resistant bacteria. Am J Respir Crit Care Med 1998;157:531–9.

26. Beardsley JR, Willamson JC, Johnson JW, et al. Using local microbiologic data to develop institution-specific guidelines for the treatment of hospital-acquired pneumonia. Chest 2006;130:787–93.

27. Rello J, Sa-Borges M, Correa H, et al. Variations in etiology of ventilator-associated pneumonia across four treatment sites: implications for antimicrobial prescribing practices. Am J Respir Crit Care Med 1999;60:608–13.

28. Namias N, Samiian L, Nino D, et al. Incidence and susceptibility of pathogenic bacteria vary between intensive care units within a single hospital: implications for empiric antibiotic strategies. J Trauma 2000;49:638–45.

29. Michel F, Franceschini B, Berger P, et al. Early antibiotic treatment for BAL-confirmed ventilator-associated pneumonia: a role for routine endotracheal aspirate cultures. Chest 2005;127:589–97.

30. Nicasio AM, Eagye KJ, Nicolau DP, et al. Pharmaco-dynamic-based clinical pathway for empiric antibiotic choice in patients with ventilator-associated pneumonia. J Crit Care 2010;25:69–77.

31. Souweine B, Veber B, Bedos JP, et al. Diagnostic accuracy of protected specimen brush and bronchoalveolar lavage in nosocomial pneumonia: impact of previous antimicrobial treatments. Crit Care Med 1998;26:236–44.

32. Micek ST, Ward S, Fraser VJ, et al. A randomized controlled trial of an antibiotic discontinuation policy for clinically suspected ventilator-associated pneumonia. Chest 2004;125:1791–9.

33. Singh N, Rogers P, Atwood CW, et al. Short–course empiric antibiotic therapy for patients with pulmonary infiltrates in the intensive care unit: a proposed solution for indiscriminate antibiotic prescription. Am J Respir Crit Care Med 2000;162:505–11.

34. Luyt CE, Guerin V, Combes A, et al. Procalcitonin kinetics as a prognostic marker of ventilator-associated pneumonia. Am J Respir Crit Care Med 2005;171:48–53.

35. Povoa P, Coelho L, Almeida E, et al. C-reactive protein as a marker of ventilator-associated pneumonia resolution: a pilot study. Eur Respir J 2005; 25:804–12.

36. Hilf M, Yu VL, Sharp J, et al. Antibiotic therapy for Pseudomonas aeruginosa bacteremia: outcome correlations in a prospective study of 200 patients. Am J Med 1989;87:540–6.

37. Safdar N, Handelsman J, Maki DG. Does combination antimicrobial therapy reduce mortality in gram-negative bacteraemia? A meta-analysis. Lancet Infect Dis 2005;4:519–27.

38. Heyland DK, Dodek P, Muscedere J, et al. Randomized trial of combination versus monotherapy for the empiric treatment of suspected ventilator-associated pneumonia. Crit Care Med 2008;36:737–44.

39. Kumar A, Ellis P, Light BR, et al. Early combination antibiotic therapy yields improved survival compared with monotherapy in septic shock: a propensity-matched analysis. Crit Care Med 2010;38:1773–85.

40. Paul M, Benuri-Silbiger I, Soares-Weiser K, et al. Beta-lactam monotherapy versus beta-lactam-aminoglycoside combination therapy for sepsis in immunocompetent patients: systematic review and meta-analysis of randomizsed trials. BMJ 2004; 328:668.

41. Bliziotis IA, Samonis G, Vardakas KZ, et al. Effect of aminoglycoside and beta-lactam combination therapy versus beta-lactam monotherapy on the emergence of antimicrobial resistance: a meta-analysis of randomized, controlled trials. Clin Infect Dis 2005;15(41):149–58.

42. Gruson D, Hilbert G, Vargas F, et al. Strategy of antibiotic rotation: long-term effect on incidence and susceptibilities of Gram-negative bacilli responsible for ventilator-associated pneumonia. Crit Care Med 2003;31:1908–14.

43. Fink MP, Snydman DR, Niederman MS, et al. Treatment of severe pneumonia in hospitalized patients: results of a multicenter, randomized, double-blind trial comparing intravenous ciprofloxacin with imipenem-cilastatin. The Severe Pneumonia Study Group. Antimicrob Agents Chemother 1994;38: 547–57.

44. Sieger B, Berman SJ, Geckler RW, et al. Empiric treatment of hospital-acquired lower respiratory tract infections with meropenem or ceftazidime with tobramycin: a randomized study. Meropenem Lower Respiratory Infection Group. Crit Care Med 1997; 25:1663–70.

45. West M, Boulanger BR, Fogarty C, et al. Levofloxacin compared with imipenem/cilastatin followed by ciprofloxacin in adult patients with nosocomial pneumonia: a multicenter, prospective, randomized, open-label study. Clin Ther 2003;25:485–506.

46. Joshi M, Bernstein J, Solomkin J, et al. Piperacillin/tazobactam plus tobramycin versus ceftazidime plus tobramycin for the treatment of patients with nosocomial lower respiratory tract infection. Piperacillin/tazobactam Nosocomial Pneumonia Study Group. J Antimicrob Chemother 1999;43:389–97.

47. Chastre J, Wunderink R, Prokocimer P, et al. Efficacy and safety of intravenous infusion of doripenem versus imipenem in ventilator-associated pneumonia: a multicenter, randomized study. Crit Care Med 2008;36:1089–96.

48. ChastreJ WM, Wolff M, Fagon JY, et al. Comparison of 8 vs 15 days of antibiotic therapy for ventilator-associated pneumonia in adults: a randomized trial. JAMA 2003;290:2588–98.

49. Michalopoulos A, Kasiakou SK, Mastora Z, et al. Aerosolized colistin for the treatment of nosocomial pneumonia due to multidrug-resistant Gram-negative bacteria in patients without cystic fibrosis. Crit Care 2005;9:R53–9.

50. Baughman RP, Kerr MA. Ventilator-associated pneumonia patients who do not reduce bacterial from the lungs have a worse prognosis. J Intensive Care Med 2003;18(5):269–74.

Bronchiectasis: New Approaches to Diagnosis and Management

Charles Feldman, MB, BCh, DSc, PhD, FRCP, FCP(SA)

KEYWORDS

- Bronchiectasis • Corticosteroids • High-resolution CT scan
- Macrolides • Physiotherapy • Vaccination

The term bronchiectasis is derived from the Greek words *bronkia* (bronchial tubes), *ek* (out), and *tasis* (stretching), which together literally mean "the outstretching of the bronchi." The condition is generally defined as an abnormal and permanent dilatation of the cartilage-containing airways (bronchi).[1] Although bronchiectasis occurring unrelated to cystic fibrosis (CF) is a common and potentially serious condition, it has historically received little attention or research and many of the recommendations for its management, rather than being based on appropriate research, have been extrapolated from the extensive studies informing the recommendations for the management of CF.[2] More recently, this condition has been extensively reviewed and a comprehensive guideline for its management developed.[3,4]

PREVALENCE OF BRONCHIECTASIS

The true prevalence of bronchiectasis is unknown for most regions of the world. There is a commonly held belief that, with the advent of vaccination that effectively prevents many serious childhood respiratory illnesses, as well as the ready availability of potent antibiotics that rapidly treat acute respiratory tract infections, bronchiectasis is on the decline.[5] Studies have reported an incidence of bronchiectasis in Finland of 3.9 per 100,000 per year in the overall population (0.49 per 100,000 per year in those aged under 15 years) and

a prevalence in New Zealand of 3.7 per 100,000 per year in those aged under 15 years.[6] In the United States the prevalence has commonly been quoted as being 52 cases per 100,000 adults,[7,8] although Weycker and colleagues[9] reported the prevalence to be 4.2 per 100,000 persons aged between 18 and 34 years and 272 per 100,000 persons in those equal to or greater than 75 years of age. Very high prevalences have been described in certain indigenous populations, such as Alaskan Natives, New Zealand Maoris, and Australian Aborigines.[6,10]

One recent study from the United States, which sought to estimate the burden and trends of bronchiectasis-associated hospitalizations, documented the average annual age-adjusted hospitalization rate from 1993 to 2006 to be 16.5 hospitalizations per 100,00 population, which increased significantly over these years with an annual increase of 2.4% in men and 3.0% in women.[8] The highest rate of hospitalizations was in women and persons over 60 years. Because most persons with bronchiectasis are not admitted to hospital, these rates of hospitalization would significantly underestimate the prevalence of bronchiectasis in the general population. Similarly, to provide information of the burden of bronchiectasis in England and Wales, trends in mortality from non-CF bronchiectasis were analyzed.[5] Between 2001 and 2007, there was an increase in bronchiectasis deaths of approximately 3%

Financial disclosure: The author has nothing to disclose.

Division of Pulmonology, Department of Internal Medicine, Faculty of Health Sciences, Charlotte Maxeke Johannesburg Academic Hospital, University of the Witwatersrand, 7 York Road, Parktown, 2913 Johannesburg, South Africa

E-mail address: charles.feldman@wits.ac.za

chestmed.theclinics.com

per year, which were similar among men and women. As with the hospitalization rates, mortality rates will clearly underestimate the total burden of the bronchiectasis problem in the population.

CAUSES AND PATHOGENESIS

A detailed description of the pathophysiology and associated causes of bronchiectasis is beyond the scope of this article, but has been extensively reviewed elsewhere.[11–15] Bronchiectasis results from the occurrence of one of three main pathogenic mechanisms: bronchial wall injury, bronchial lumen obstruction, and traction from adjacent fibrosis.[14] The dominant feature of bronchiectasis is clearly the presence of airway inflammation, in association with bacterial infection, and, in particular, nonclearing infection.[10] This theory was put forward as the "vicious cycle hypothesis" by Professor Peter Cole[16] many years ago, which proposed that an initial airway insult, such as an infection, often on the background of genetic susceptibility, compromised host clearance mechanisms and, in particular, the mucociliary escalator mechanism, which facilitated persistent bacterial colonization and infection. This damages the airway further, both directly and indirectly. as a consequence of the initiation of a secondary host inflammatory response.[10,13]

There are many medical conditions that may lead to the development of bronchiectasis and these are detailed elsewhere.[1,2,10,13,14] **Box 1** depicts the potential causes of bronchiectasis. An important and frequent question is whether knowledge of the underlying medical cause leads to a change in management of patients with bronchiectasis. One study investigating this question in two tertiary pediatric units in the United Kingdom and Hong Kong identified the cause in 74% of cases. Furthermore, they found that immunodeficiency and intrinsic abnormalities accounted for the majority of cases of non-CF bronchiectasis and that knowledge of a specific causal agent (in 56% of children) led to a modification in management.[17] This has been confirmed in the adult setting in a study at the Brompton hospital in London, United Kingdom.[18] In that study, 165 patients were confirmed to have bronchiectasis on CT scan of the chest. An underlying cause was identified in 122 (74%) patients. Knowledge of the underlying cause directly affected management of 61 (37%) patients. All these studies suggest that investigation of the underlying causes of bronchiectasis leads to an alteration in therapy to target these specific conditions in many more cases than was previously thought, which can have significant prognostic implications.[19,20]

Box 1
Recognized causes of bronchiectasis (associated conditions in italics)

- Postinfective
  - Severe pneumonia
  - Tuberculosis
  - Pertussis
  - Measles
- Impaired mucociliary clearance
  - CF
  - Primary ciliary dyskinesia
  - Young's syndrome
- Immune deficiency
  - Common variable immune deficiency
  - Specific polysaccharide antibody deficiency
  - Secondary immunodeficiency, eg, malignancy (chronic lymphocytic leukemia) or human immunodeficiency virus infection
- Exaggerated immune response
  - Allergic bronchopulmonary aspergillosis
  - Graft versus host disease
  - *Inflammatory bowel disease (ulcerative colitis* and *Crohn's disease)*
- Congenital abnormalities of the bronchial wall
  - Mounier-Kuhn syndrome
  - Williams-Campbell syndrome
  - Marfan syndrome
- Inflammatory pneumonitis
  - Aspiration of gastric contents
  - Smoke inhalation
- Fibrosis (traction bronchiectasis)
  - Sarcoidosis
  - Idiopathic pulmonary fibrosis
- Mechanical obstruction
  - Foreign body
  - Tumor
  - Extrinsic compression (eg, lymph node)
- Miscellaneous conditions
  - Primary *Mycobacterium avium* complex infection ("Lady Windermere syndrome")
  - *Connective tissue diseases,* eg, *rheumatoid arthritis, systemic lupus erythematosus, Sjögren syndrome*
  - Pulmonary sequestration
  - Yellow nail syndrome
  - Infertility (primary ciliary dyskinesia, cystic fibrosis, Young syndrome)
  - *Diffuse panbronchiolitis*
  - α_1-Antitrypsin deficiency

Data from Zoumot Z, Wilson R. Respiratory infection in noncystic fibrosis bronchiectasis. Curr Opin Infect Dis 2010;23:165–70.

Examples of treatable conditions are common variable immunodeficiency, allergic bronchopulmonary aspergillosis, nontuberculosis mycobacterial infections, airway obstruction, inflammatory bowel disease, and several others.[20,21]

DIAGNOSIS

The diagnosis of bronchiectasis should be suspected in any individual presenting with persistent daily cough with mucopurulent sputum.[22] Interestingly, it is said that sputum volume correlates with quality of life and the lung function decline in patients with bronchiectasis.[23] Furthermore, the Leicester Cough Questionnaire (LCQ), a symptom-specific questionnaire designed to assess the impact of cough severity, has been found reliable for use in patients with non-CF bronchiectasis. It can discriminate disease severity and does respond to change in status as a consequence of treatment.[24]

A large number of additional symptoms may be present, including hemoptysis, chest pain, dyspnea, decreased effort tolerance; as well as constitutional symptoms, including fatigue, malaise, lethargy and weight loss—but these are nonspecific.[1,7,10,22] Physical findings are also nonspecific and may include clubbing of the digits and crackles and wheezing in the chest.[1,10,22]

A plain chest radiograph is said to be essential and may arouse suspicion or show the features characteristic of bronchiectasis.[2] However, it is insufficiently sensitive for the adequate diagnosis of the condition,[1,7,22] detecting fewer than 50% of cases in one study in which the presence of bronchiectasis was subsequently confirmed on bronchography.[25]

Although bronchography was previously commonly used to confirm the presence and extent of bronchiectasis, it was replaced many years ago by high-resolution CT (HRCT) scanning of the chest, which has become the gold standard for the diagnosis; standard HRCT criteria for establishing the diagnosis exist.[1,7,10,14,22] The most specific HRCT scanning findings suggestive of bronchiectasis are (1) internal diameter of the bronchus is wider than the adjacent pulmonary artery (ie, signet ring formation), (2) failure of the bronchi to taper, and (3) bronchi being visualized in the outer 1 to 2 cm of the lung fields.[10,13,22] A number of less sensitive findings are also described. In contrast to established bronchiectasis occurring in adults, some children with bronchiectasis have been shown to have resolution or considerable improvement of the changes seen on CT scanning, suggesting the possibility that the condition may be reversible in some cases.[6]

Interestingly, the extent of involvement of lungs documented on HRCT scanning has been shown to correlate with both functional changes and clinical outcomes,[22,26,27] with one study showing a correlation between HRCT score and both lung function testing and systolic pulmonary artery pressure.[28] Clearly, the improved ability to diagnose bronchiectasis with the use of HRCT scanning has contributed, at least partly, to the apparent increased prevalence of bronchiectasis noted.[8] A detailed description of the HRCT scan findings in the different conditions associated with bronchiectasis is discussed elsewhere.[14] **Fig. 1** demonstrates the presence of severe cystic bronchiectasis in the right lower lobe of an adult patient on HRCT scan of the chest.

Because of concerns about radiation exposure as a consequence of HRCT scanning, particularly in children, Montella and colleagues[29] studied the validity of 3.0T MRI scanning compared with four-slice HRCT scanning of the chest in 41 subjects aged 16 to 29 years with non-CF bronchiectasis. The researchers compared the prevalence of lung abnormalities found using each technique, the agreement between the modified Helbich scores for the two techniques, and the correlation between the modified Helbich scores and the lung function tests. They found a similar prevalence of lung abnormalities using the two imaging techniques, with a good to excellent agreement between the two modalities for all subscores and total score. Furthermore, HRCT and MRI total scores and bronchiectasis scores correlated significantly with pulmonary function tests. The investigators indicated that these results suggest that MRI is a radiation-free alternative to HRCT scanning for the follow up of non-CF

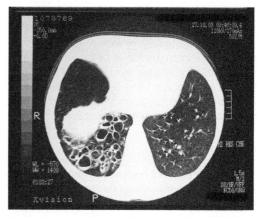

Fig. 1. Severe cystic bronchiectasis in the right lower lobe of an adult patient, demonstrated with HRCT scan of the chest.

bronchiectasis.[29] Limitations to its widespread use include limited availability and the need for respiratory gating or prolonged breath holding during the acquisition of the MRI images.

The lung function studies in patients with bronchiectasis usually show an obstructive defect and there may or may not be evidence of airway hyperreactivity.[1,7,22] Additional testing that is recommended in patients with bronchiectasis, once the presence of the condition is confirmed on HRCT scanning, includes a further diagnostic workup to reveal the underlying cause, and an evaluation of sputum microbiology.[1,2,7,13,22] Routinely recommended additional investigations in patients with bronchiectasis, together with investigations that are recommended to be reserved for selected cases, are shown in **Box 2**.

With regard to sputum examination in patients with established bronchiectasis, a large number of different pathogens have been identified in the various microbiological studies and, conversely, even in the presence of good quality and purulent sputum samples, pathogenic bacteria may fail to grow.[13] The main bacterial pathogens that are commonly isolated are *Haemophilus influenzae* (29%–70%) followed by *Pseudomonas aeruginosa* (12%–31%). It has been suggested that the microbiological flora varies with the severity of the disease, that patients with best preserved lung function may not have bacteria cultured from their sputum, and that, as lung function declines, *H influenza*, becomes dominant, followed with the presence of more severe disease by *P aeruginosa*.[13] Additional microorganisms that may be encountered include *Streptococcus pneumoniae*, *Haemophilus parainfluenzae*, *Staphylococcus aureus*, and *Moraxella catarrhalis*.[25] It is commonly recommended that sputum examination should be performed, because identification of a pathogen and characterization of its antimicrobial susceptibility pattern would aid in decisions regarding antibiotic therapy, should it become needed.

It is also important to remember that, in addition to these common bacterial pathogens, patients with bronchiectasis may have infection with tuberculosis or nontuberculosis mycobacteria, and occasionally even fungi, such as *Aspergillus* spp, warranting therapy that is more specific.[30]

MANAGEMENT

A myriad of treatment options are potentially available for the management of patients with bronchiectasis, but only a limited number of studies have investigated these options in non-CF cases. Many of them included small numbers of patients and few were randomized or blinded.[15,31,32] Many of

---

Box 2
Recommendations for the investigation of bronchiectasis

- All patients

  o Chest radiograph (posterior anterior and lateral)
  o Sinus radiographs
  o Respiratory function tests
  o Blood investigations[a]
  o Sputum microscopy eosinophils and culture
  o Sputum smear and culture for acid-fast bacilli
  o Skin tests (atopy, *Aspergillus*)
  o High-resolution, thin-section CT scan
  o Sweat test (nasal potential difference, genotyping)
  o Nasal mucociliary clearance (cilia studies if abnormal)

- Selected patients

  o Fiberoptic bronchoscopy
  o Barium swallow (video fluoroscopy)
  o Respiratory muscle function
  o Semen analysis
  o Tests for associated conditions
  o Blood tests for rarer immune deficiencies

[a] To include: differential white blood cell count; total immunoglobulin (Ig) levels of IgA, IgE, and IgG subclasses; *Aspergillus* radioallergosorbent test and precipitins; rheumatoid factor and antinuclear antibodies; α_1-antiproteinase.

Data from Wilson R. Bronchiectasis. In: Niederman MS, Sarosi G, Glassroth J, editors. Respiratory infections. 2nd edition. Philadelphia: Lippincott, Williams and Wilkins; 2001. p. 347–59.

---

the current recommendations are based on studies and recommendations in patients with CF and extrapolation from the management of other respiratory conditions, or based on expert opinion.[21] The general goals of the treatment in bronchiectasis are to limit the cycle of infection and inflammation and, therefore, the progression of the airway damage, to improve the symptoms, to reduce the number of exacerbations, and to improve the quality of life.[1,7,22]

General Supportive Therapy

General health measures such as adoption of good nutrition, nonsmoking strategy, regular exercise, and exposure to fresh air are all considered to be beneficial to patients with respiratory diseases.[15,32] Furthermore, pulmonary rehabilitation, which is of proven benefit in patients with chronic obstructive pulmonary disease (COPD) may also be of benefit to patients with bronchiectasis. Severely affected cases may benefit from long-term oxygen therapy and even noninvasive ventilation using bilevel positive airway pressure (BiPAP).[15] In general, it is recommended that patients with bronchiectasis be managed by a team of health care professionals trained in the management of this condition, including physicians, physiotherapists, nurses, occupational therapists, and psychologists.[15] In this regard, one group of investigators undertook a randomized controlled crossover trial of nurse practitioner-led versus doctor-led outpatient care of patients in a bronchiectasis clinic and concluded that nurse practitioner-led care for such patients within a chronic chest clinic was safe and as effective as doctor-led care, but may consume more resources.[33,34] The development of a management plan for patients with bronchiectasis may be beneficial and should be tailored to individual cases.[32]

Treatment of the Underlying Causative Conditions

As indicated above, there is evidence that investigation for the cause in patients with bronchiectasis may identify the underlying condition in a substantial number of cases. Furthermore, it is recommended that should an underlying treatable cause be identified, it should be appropriately managed. However, what is less clear is whether this has a clear-cut effect on the natural history of the bronchiectasis in many cases.[22]

Prevention of Secondary Infection with Vaccination

Influenza vaccination
There is no evidence for or against routine influenza vaccination in children or adults with bronchiectasis.[35] However, influenza vaccination is widely recommended for use in both groups of patients, in adults in particular because of a reduction in exacerbations in patients with COPD, many of whom have coexistent bronchiectasis.[2]

Pneumococcal vaccination
The use of pneumococcal vaccination as routine management of bronchiectasis in adults and children was evaluated in a Cochrane review.[36] One open-label, randomized study in 167 adults with chronic lung diseases, including bronchiectasis, compared 23-valent pneumococcal vaccine together with influenza vaccine to influenza vaccine alone and found a significant reduction in exacerbations in the former group, but no difference in pneumonia episodes in the two groups and no data on lung function decline.[36] The investigators also identified one small,

nonrandomized, study in children, which, although it showed eradication of S pneumoniae in sputum, had no clinical benefit.[2,36] The investigators concluded that there was limited evidence to support use of 23-valent pneumococcal vaccination in adults and circumstantial evidence to support its use of children with bronchiectasis.[36] However, there is a general recommendation for routine vaccination against pneumococcal infection in both adults and children with bronchiectasis.

Mobilization of Airway Secretions

Effective clearance of mucus from the airways is one of the most important, perhaps crucial, treatment modalities that can be instituted in patients with bronchiectasis. It may break the vicious cycle of the disease process by decreasing the stagnation of mucus and mucus plug formation with associated bacterial colonization, recurrent infection, and inflammation.[32] Chest physiotherapy has been used for many years and a number of techniques are available for mobilizing secretions, such as postural drainage, active cycle of breathing techniques (ACBT), positive expiratory pressure (PEP), oscillatory PEP devices, and high-frequency chest wall percussion.[32] One recent, small, randomized control trial using the LCQ as the primary endpoint, and multiple secondary endpoints, concluded that regular chest physiotherapy in patients with non-CF bronchiectasis had small, but significant, benefits[37] despite earlier negative systematic reviews. However, few controlled trials have evaluated the optimal technique and multiple questions still remain.[38] Eaton and colleagues[39] compared the use of a flutter (PEP) device versus ACBT, with or without postural drainage (PD). The three techniques were studied in random order over a week in 36 patients with non-CF bronchiectasis. All three techniques were well tolerated, and patient preference was 44% for the Flutter device, 22% for ACBT, and 33% for ACBT-PD. However, ACBT-PD proved most effective acutely, with total sputum production wet weight twice that of the other two techniques. Exercise and inspiratory muscle training appear to improve exercise tolerance and capacity, as well as quality of life.[32,40]

Mucolytics and inhaled hyperosmolar agents
With regard to the use of adjunctive agents to improve clearance of mucus, the latest Cochrane review indicated that there was not enough evidence to evaluate their routine use, although high-dose bromhexine coupled with antibiotics may help sputum production and clearance.[41] Some benefit was also shown in one study with

erdosteine.[7,42] Certainly recombinant human DNase has not shown to be beneficial in non-CF bronchiectasis and may be potentially harmful.[32,43]

A number of recent studies and an earlier Cochrane review suggested that inhaled mannitol improved the physical properties of mucus and increased tracheobronchial mucus clearance in patients with bronchiectasis.[44–49] Furthermore, a small study of nebulized hypertonic saline as an adjunct to physiotherapy in patients with stable bronchiectasis showed small but significant benefits; thus warranting a longer term study.[50]

Bronchodilator Therapy

Although a substantial number of patients with bronchiectasis have airflow obstruction with airway hyperreactivity and a significant bronchodilator response, for which bronchodilators are used, there are no randomized, controlled trails investigating the effects of short-acting or long-acting beta-agonists, short-acting anticholinergics, or methylxanthines in the management of patients with bronchiectasis.[1,51–55] One study evaluated the role of the long-acting anticholinergic, tiotropium in patients with chronic airway mucus hypersecretion, including three cases with bronchiectasis, and showed improved symptoms of cough, sputum, and breathlessness, warranting further investigation.[56]

Furthermore, no randomized controlled trials were identified investigating the potential role of leukotriene antagonists for the management of bronchiectasis.[57]

Antibiotic Therapy

A myriad of articles have been written regarding appropriate antibiotic management in patients with bronchiectasis. Antibiotics may be instituted for the management of acute infective exacerbations, but have also been used for maintenance therapy, and options for therapy include both short-course and prolonged antibiotic therapy, given orally and/or parenterally, as well as nebulized antibiotic therapy, such that these decisions remain a complicated issue.[32] With regard to the different classes of antibiotics, it is important to remember that different patients may be colonized and/or infected with different pathogens, there may be changes in the bacteria isolated at different stages of disease, and some patients may be colonized simultaneously with multiple pathogens.[32] It is useful to obtain sputum specimens for microbiological culture (sometimes multiple) to help identify the infecting microorganisms, which should be targeted for antibiotic therapy.[32]

Antibiotics are most commonly used for the management of acute exacerbations and the specific choice of agent would best be guided by the pathogens isolated and their antimicrobial susceptibility patterns. In general terms, in clinical practice patients appear to respond well to broad spectrum antibiotics effective against *P aeruginosa*, *H influenzae*, and *S aureus*.[43] One or two standard agents may be given orally, commonly for between 7 and 14 days. Although longer courses are sometimes used there is no clear cut evidence for their benefit.[32] Intravenous antibiotics may be given to patients who are severely ill or who are not responding to oral therapy.[32] In one study, a 14-day course of intravenous antibiotics improved systemic symptoms, sputum volume and bacterial clearance, inflammatory markers, and quality of life (but not forced expiratory volume in 1 second and forced vital capacity).[58]

There is also a substantial body of literature on the use of prolonged antibiotics in patients with bronchiectasis, most commonly in patients with severe and purulent bronchiectasis (severe bronchial sepsis), and particularly in cases not responding to conventional courses of antibiotics.[59–63] These studies have shown small benefit with regard to reduction of symptoms, improved sputum parameters, reduction in lung inflammation, and improvement in lung function.[32] It is commonly recommended that if long-term antibiotics are to be used in patients with bronchiectasis their use be confined to the subset of patients with chronic bronchial sepsis who are not responding to conventional antibiotic therapy or perhaps in cases with frequent exacerbations. There is, however, emerging evidence for the use of long-term macrolide therapy in patients with bronchiectasis (see later discussion).

Similarly, there are also a large number of publications describing the use of inhaled antibiotics (in particular tobramycin[64–66] and gentamicin,[67] as well as other antibiotics[68,69]) in patients with bronchiectasis and particularly in the setting of *P aeruginosa* infection. Although some benefits have been documented in these studies, including a decrease in bacterial density, the benefits appear to be less than in CF cases and adverse events, such as bronchospasm, appear to be more common in adults with non-CF bronchiectasis than reported in the CF population.[70]

Antiinflammatory Therapy

The two agents that may be considered for use because of their antiinflammatory properties are corticosteroids and the macrolides. **Table 1** is a summary of studies on the use of inhaled

Table 1
Summary of clinical trials of ICS and macrolides in bronchiectasis

Study (Year)	No. of Pts	Study Design	Therapy (Daily Dose) and Duration	Findings
ICS				
Elborn et al,[75] 1992	20	Randomized, double-blind, crossover, placebo-controlled	Beclomethasone (1500 µg) 6 wk	↓Daily sputum, minor changes in PEFR and FEV_1
Tsang et al,[76] 1998	24	Randomized, double-blind, placebo-controlled	Fluticasone propionate (500 µg) 52 wk	↓Sputum markers (IL-1, IL-8, LTB4)
Tsang et al,[71] 2005	73	Randomized, double-blind, placebo-controlled	Fluticasone propionate (1000 µg) 52 wk	↓Sputum volume in subgroups
Martinez-Garcia et al,[72] 2006	86	Randomized	Fluticasone propionate (50 and 1000 µg) 6 mo	↓Sputum volume and cough, ↑quality of life
Macrolides				
Koh et al,[88] 1997	25	Randomized, double-blind, placebo-controlled	Roxithromycin (8 mg/kg) 12 wk	↓Airway reactivity (methacholine challenge)
Tsang et al,[81] 1999	21	Randomized, double-blind, placebo-controlled	Erythromycin (1000 mg) 8 wk	↑FEV_1 and FVC, ↓sputum volume
Davies and Wilson,[89] 2004	39	Prospective study	Azithromycin (dose varied) 4 mo	↓Symptoms and sputum, ↑spirometry (D_{LCO})
Cymbala et al,[83] 2005	11	Randomized, open-label, crossover	Azithromycin (1000 mg) 6 mo	↓Sputum volume
Yalcin et al,[84] 2006	34	Randomized, placebo-controlled	Clarithromycin (15 mg/kg) 3 mo	↓Sputum volume, ↓sputum markers

Abbreviations: D_{LCO}, pulmonary diffusion capacity for carbon monoxide; FEV_1, forced expiratory volume in 1 second; FVC, forced vital capacity; ICS, inhaled corticosteroids; IL, interleukin; LT, leukotriene; PEFR, peak expiratory flow rate; pts, patients; ↑, increased; ↓, decreased.

Data from King P. Is there a role for inhaled corticosteroids and macrolide therapy in bronchiectasis? Drugs 2007;67:965–74.

corticosteroids and macrolides in patients with bronchiectasis.

Corticosteroids

Corticosteroids may be indicated for use in patients with bronchiectasis for associated asthma, COPD, or airway hyperreactivity. However, there has been an interest in the use of corticosteroids for the management of patients with bronchiectasis, per se, both in the stable state and during exacerbations, because of the inflammatory nature of the

condition, and a number of studies have been published.[71–76] Although some benefits were demonstrated, particularly in short-term trials (generally <6 months) of high-dose inhaled corticosteroids (ICS), a Cochrane review concluded that there was insufficient evidence to recommend the routine use of ICS in adults with stable-state bronchiectasis, but that a trial of this form of therapy may be justified in adults with difficult to control symptoms and in certain subgroups of cases, which needed to be balanced against potential risks of high dose ICS.[73] Furthermore, the review indicated that no recommendations could be made with regard to ICS in adults during exacerbations or in children. Interestingly, a recent study indicated that a significant proportion of patients with bronchiectasis have evidence of adrenal suppression, particularly when ICS are also used, and that impaired cortisol response to stimulation is associated with poor health status.[77] These findings need to be investigated further.

The latest Cochrane review of oral corticosteroids in patients with bronchiectasis indicated that there were no randomized controlled trails on which to make a recommendation regarding oral corticosteroid use in either acute or stable bronchiectasis.[78]

Nonsteroidal antiinflammatory therapy

A Cochrane review published in 2010 indicated that there was insufficient evidence to support or refute the use of inhaled nonsteroidal antiinflammatory drugs (NSAIDs) in either adults or children with bronchiectasis, although one small study reported a reduction in sputum production and improved dyspnea in adults with chronic lung disease treated with inhaled indomethacin, suggesting the need for further studies.[79] A Cochrane review of oral NSAIDs for children and adults with bronchiectasis failed to identify any randomized controlled trials, but the investigators concluded that, based on some benefit shown by inhaled NSAIDs in bronchiectasis, randomized, controlled trails need to be performed in this area.[80]

Macrolides

Likewise, there is a substantial body of literature describing the use of macrolides (a range of 14- and 15-membered ring macrolides) in the management of patients with bronchiectasis, including adults and children.[42,74,81–89] An overview of these studies suggests that these agents appear to be very promising in the management of bronchiectasis and have the capacity to improve clinical status and lung function, while reducing lung inflammatory markers and volume of sputum in patients. One investigator's practice is to try the use of macrolides in selected patients with bronchiectasis for a 3 to 6 month period and discontinue therapy if there is no evidence of benefit with regard to quality of life and/or frequency of exacerbations.[42]

As is the case with many other therapies investigated for this condition, most studies with macrolides were performed on relatively small patient cohorts, with varying length of treatment and follow-up.[74,86] Furthermore, their long-term use needs to be balanced against the potential side effects with these agents, including gastrointestinal and cardiac, and the potential for selection of antimicrobial resistance among respiratory pathogens.[90] Caution also needs to be exercised if the possibility of Mycobacterium avium (MAC) infection exists in a patient for whom macrolide therapy is being contemplated because macrolide monotherapy increases the likelihood of emergence of macrolide resistance in MAC, which would be extremely problematic to treat.[42] In such cases, the presence of MAC infection should be excluded with at least two negative, good-quality sputum specimens before macrolide therapy is commenced.[42]

The mechanisms by which macrolides exert their beneficial effect in patients with bronchiectasis and other chronic inflammatory conditions of the airway is most likely multifactorial and extends beyond their antimicrobial activity. The 14- and 15-membered ring macrolides have been documented to have a number of useful properties, in addition to their antibacterial effects. They have significant effects on the mucociliary clearance mechanism through effects on ciliated airway epithelium and on mucus production and quality. They also have effects on the hosts' immune system and on the quorum sensing activity of bacteria, including pathogens important in patients with bronchiectasis, such as P aeruginosa, that are otherwise totally resistant to these antibiotics.[74,91]

Surgery

Aggressive medical therapy is recommended before surgery is contemplated.[11] Specific surgical indications include (1) life-threatening conditions, such as hemoptysis, (2) localized disease causing severe symptoms, which are nonresponsive to medical therapy, (3) resectable disease causing persistent focal infection, and (4) localized resectable disease with failure to thrive.[11] Although there are a large number of studies published describing the clinical experience with various surgical techniques in the management of bronchiectasis from individual thoracic surgery units, including several recent ones,[92–99] the latest Cochrane review indicated that there were no randomized or controlled trials comparing surgery with nonsurgical treatment for bronchiectasis such that it was not possible to provide an unbiased estimate of the benefit of surgery compared with conservative treatment.[100]

PROGNOSIS

In the pre-antibiotic era, the mortality rate in patients with bronchiectasis was estimated to be greater than 25%, but this has undoubtedly improved with the advent of antibiotics, although it still remains significant and further investigations are clearly required to better define the natural history of the condition.[101] Bronchiectasis morality appears to be up to 13% over a 5-year follow-up period and patients of older age with chronic hypoxia, hypercapnia, and greater radiological extent of the disease appear to be most vulnerable.[1,97]

SUMMARY

The purpose of this article is to review the subject of bronchiectasis with the emphasis on new aspects of diagnosis and management. A summary of the main findings in this regard are as follows:

- Thin-slice HRCT of the chest is considered to be the gold standard for the diagnosis of bronchiectasis
- Because of concerns of the level of radiation exposure with HRCT, particularly in children, MRI has been studied more recently for the diagnosis of bronchiectasis and been found to be a potentially suitable radiation-free alternative to HRCT
- It is important to investigate patients with bronchiectasis for an underlying medical cause, because identification of such a cause frequently leads to a change in medical management in adults and children, and may have significant prognostic implications
- Patients are best managed by a team of health care professionals experienced in the management of bronchiectasis
- As part of management, routine influenza and pneumococcal vaccination is recommended for adults and children
- Effective clearance of mucus from the airways is one of the most important treatment modalities that can be instituted in patients with bronchiectasis
- Chest physiotherapy has been shown to have small, but significant, benefit and should include ACBT and/or use of PEP devices or techniques, with or without postural drainage. There is emerging evidence that inhalation of hypertonic agents such as mannitol and saline, as an adjunct to physiotherapy, may assist in improving tracheobronchial mucus clearance. Exercise and inspiratory muscle training improve exercise tolerance and capacity, and quality of life
- Bronchodilators are recommended for the treatment of airway hyperreactivity, if

present, and/or for the management of associated asthma or COPD
- Antibiotic therapy is recommended for use primarily for acute infective exacerbations, given as a short course either orally or parenterally depending on the severity of illness. Prolonged antibiotic therapy and/or nebulized antibiotics are recommended only in certain circumstances, such as severe and purulent bronchiectasis (chronic bronchial sepsis) and recurrent exacerbations, particularly in cases not responding to conventional courses of antibiotics
- There is a definite emerging role for the use of antiinflammatory therapies, such as inhaled corticosteroids and especially macrolides, which needs to be more clearly defined by additional studies
- Surgery is reserved for selected cases in which sufficient improvement has not been achieved with aggressive medical management.

REFERENCES

1. Pappalettera M, Aliberti S, Castellotti P, et al. Bronchiectasis: an update. Clin Respir J 2009;3: 1752–6981.
2. Stafler P, Carr SB. Non-cystic fibrosis bronchiectasis: its diagnosis and management. Arch Dis Child Educ Pract Ed 2010;95:73–82.
3. Leikin JB. Bronchiectasis. Dis Mon 2008;54:514–64.
4. Pasteur MC, Bilton D, Hill AT, et al. British Thoracic Society guideline for non-CF bronchiectasis. Thorax 2010;65:i1–58.
5. Roberts HJ, Hubbard R. Trends in bronchiectasis mortality in England and Wales. Respir Med 2010;104:981–5.
6. Al Subie H, Fitzgerald DA. Non-cystic fibrosis bronchiectasis. J Paediatr Child Health 2010. DOI:10.1111/j.1365-2230.2010.03857.x.
7. Goeminne P, Dupont L. Non-cystic fibrosis bronchiectasis: diagnosis and management in 21st century. Postgrad Med J 2010;86:493–501.
8. Seitz AE, Olivier KN, Steiner CA, et al. Trends and burden of bronchiectasis-associated hospitalizations in the United States, 1993–2006. Chest 2010;138(4):944–9.
9. Weycker D, Edelsberg J, Oster G, et al. Prevalence and economic burden of bronchiectasis. Clin Pulm Med 2005;12:205–9.
10. King PT, Daviskas E. Pathogenesis and diagnosis of bronchiectasis. Breathe 2010;6:343–51.
11. Dagli E. Non cystic fibrosis bronchiectasis. Paediatr Respir Rev 2000;1:64–70.
12. Fuschilllo S, De Felice A, Balzano G. Mucosal inflammation in idiopathic bronchiectasis: cellular

and molecular mechanisms. Eur Respir J 2008;31: 396–406.

13. King PT. The pathophysiology of bronchiectasis. Int J Chron Obstruct Pulmon Dis 2009;4:411–9.

14. Javidan-Nejad C, Bhalla S. Bronchiectasis. Radiol Clin North Am 2009;47:289–306.

15. Tsang KW, Bilton D. Clinical challenges in managing bronchiectasis. Respirology 2009;14: 637–50.

16. Cole PJ. Inflammation: a two-edged sword—the model of bronchiectasis. Eur J Respir Dis Suppl 1986;147:6–15.

17. Li AM, Sonnappa S, Lex C, et al. Non-CF bronchiectasis: does knowing the aetiology lead to changes in management? Eur Respir J 2005;26:8–14.

18. Shoemark A, Ozerovitch L, Wilson R. Aetiology in adult patients with bronchiectasis. Respir Med 2007;101:1163–70.

19. Rosen MJ. Chronic cough due to bronchiectasis. Chest 2006;129(Suppl):122S–31S.

20. Zoumot Z, Wilson R. Respiratory infection in non-cystic fibrosis bronchiectasis. Curr Opin Infect Dis 2010;23:165–70.

21. Loebinger MR, Wilson R. Pharmacotherapy for bronchiectasis. Expert Opin Pharmacother 2007; 8(18):3183–93.

22. O'Donnell AE. Bronchiectasis. Chest 2008;134: 815–23.

23. Martinez-Garcia MA, Perpina-Tordera M, Roman-Sanchez P, et al. Quality-of-life determinants in patients with clinically stable bronchiectasis. Chest 2005;128:739–45.

24. Murray MP, Turnbull K, MacQuarrie S, et al. Validation of the Leicester Cough Questionnaire in non-cystic fibrosis bronchiectasis. Eur Respir J 2009; 34(1):125–31.

25. Wilson R. Bronchiectasis. In: Niederman MS, Sarosi G, Glassroth J, editors. Respiratory infections. 2nd edition. Philadelphia: Lippincott, Williams and Wilkins; 2001. p. 47–359.

26. Sheehan RE, Wells AU, Copley SJ, et al. A comparison of serial computed tomography and functional change in bronchiectasis. Eur Respir J 2002;20:581–7.

27. Eshed I, Minski I, Katz R, et al. Bronchiectasis: correlation of high resolution CT findings with health-related quality of life. Clin Radiol 2007;62:152–9.

28. Alzeer AH. HRCT score in bronchiectasis: correlation with pulmonary function tests and pulmonary artery pressure. Ann Thorac Med 2008;3:82–6.

29. Montella S, Santamaria F, Salvatore M, et al. Assessment of chest high-field magnetic resonance imaging in children and young adults with noncystic fibrosis chronic lung disease: comparison to high-resolution computed tomography and correlation with pulmonary function. Invest Radiol 2009;44:532–8.

30. Ilowite J, Spiegler P, Kessler H. Pharmacological treatment options for bronchiectasis. Focus on anti-microbial and anti-inflammatory agents. Drugs 2009;69(4):407–19.

31. Ten Hacken N, Kerstjens H, Postma D. Bronchiectasis. Clin Evid (Online) 2008;2008:1507.

32. King PT, Daviskas E. Management of bronchiectasis. Breathe 2010;6:353–64.

33. Sharples LD, Edmunds J, Bilton D, et al. A randomized controlled crossover trial of nurse practitioner versus doctor led outpatient care in a bronchiectasis clinic. Thorax 2002;57:661–6.

34. French J, Bilton D, Campbell F. Nurse specialist care for bronchiectasis. Cochrane Database Syst Rev 2003;3:CD004319.

35. Chang CC, Morris PS, Chang AB. Influenza vaccine for children and adults with bronchiectasis. Cochrane Database Syst Rev 2007;3:CD006218.

36. Chang CC, Singleton RJ, Morris PS, et al. Pneumococcal vaccine for children and adults with bronchiectasis. Cochrane Database Syst Rev 2009;2:CD006316.

37. Murray MP, Pentland JL, Hill AT. A randomized crossover trial of chest physiotherapy in non-cystic fibrosis bronchiectasis. Eur Respir J 2009; 34:1086–92.

38. Martinez-Garcia MA, Soriano JB. Physiotherapy in bronchiectasis: we have more patients, we need more evidence. Eur Respir J 2009;34:1011–2.

39. Eaton T, Young P, Zeng I, et al. A randomized evaluation of the acute efficacy, acceptability and tolerability of flutter and active cycle of breathing with and without postural drainage in non-cystic fibrosis bronchiectasis. Chron Respir Dis 2007;4:23–30.

40. Bradley J, Moran F, Greenstone M. Physical training for bronchiectasis. Cochrane Database Syst Rev 2002;3:CD002166.

41. Crockett AJ, Cranston JM, Latimer KM, et al. Mucolytics for bronchiectasis. Cochrane Database Syst Rev 2000;2:CD001289.

42. Metersky ML. New treatment options for bronchiectasis. Ther Adv Respir Dis 2010;4:93–9.

43. Chang AB, Bilton D. Exacerbations in cystic fibrosis: 4—Non-cystic fibrosis bronchiectasis. Thorax 2008;63:269–76.

44. Daviskas E, Anderson SD, Eberl S, et al. Inhalation of dry powder mannitol improves clearance of mucus in patients with bronchiectasis. Am J Respir Crit Care Med 1999;159(6):1843–8.

45. Daviskas E, Anderson SD, Eberl S, et al. The 24-h effect of mannitol on the clearance of mucus in patients with bronchiectasis. Chest 2001;119: 414–21.

46. Daviskas E, Anderson SD, Gomes K, et al. Inhaled mannitol for the treatment of mucociliary dysfunction in patients with bronchiectasis: effect on lung

function, health status and sputum. Respirology 2005;10(1):46–56.

47. Daviskas E, Anderson SD, Eberl S, et al. Effect of increasing doses of mannitol on mucus clearance in patients with bronchiectasis. Eur Respir J 2008; 31:765–72.

48. Daviskas E, Anderson SD, Young IH. Effect of mannitol and repetitive coughing on the sputum properties in bronchiectasis. Respir Med 2010;104:371–7.

49. Wills P, Greenstone M. Inhaled hyperosmolar agents for bronchiectasis. Cochrane Database Syst Rev 2006;2:CD002996.

50. Kellett F, Redfern J, Niven RM. Evaluation of nebulised hypertonic saline (7%) as an adjunct to physiotherapy in patients with stable bronchiectasis. Respir Med 2005;99(1):27–31.

51. Hassan JA, Saadiah S, Roslan H, et al. Bronchodilator response to inhaled beta-2 agonist and anticholinergic drugs in patients with bronchiectasis. Respirology 1999;4:423–6.

52. Sheikh A, Nolan D, Greenstone M. Long-acting beta-2-agonists for bronchiectasis. Cochrane Database Syst Rev 2001;4:CD002155.

53. Lasserson T, Holt K, Evans D, et al. Anticholinergic therapy for bronchiectasis. Cochrane Database Syst Rev 2001;4:CD002163.

54. Steele K, Greenstone M, Lasserson JA. Oral methyl-xanthines for bronchiectasis. Cochrane Database Syst Rev 2001;1:CD002734.

55. Franco F, Sheikh A, Greenstone M. Short acting beta-2 agonists for bronchiectasis. Cochrane Database Syst Rev 2003;3:CD003572.

56. Saito Y, Azuma A, Morimoto T, et al. Tiotropium ameliorates symptoms in patients with chronic airway mucus hypersecretion which is resistant to macrolide therapy. Intern Med 2008;47:585–91.

57. Corless JA, Warburton CJ. Leukotriene receptor antagonists for non-cystic fibrosis. Cochrane Database Syst Rev 2000;4:CD002174.

58. Murray MP, Turnbull K, MacQuarrie S, et al. Assessing response to treatment of exacerbations of bronchiectasis in adults. Eur Respir J 2009;33:312–7.

59. Hill SL, Burnett D, Hewetson KA, et al. The response of patients with purulent bronchiectasis to antibiotics for four months. Q J Med 1988; 66(250):163–73.

60. Currie DC, Garbett ND, Chan KL, et al. Double-blind randomized study of prolonged higher-dose oral amoxicillin in purulent bronchiectasis. Q J Med 1990;76(280):799–816.

61. Rayner CF, Tillotson G, Cole PJ, et al. Efficacy and safety of long-term ciprofloxacin in the management of severe bronchiectasis. J Antimicrob Chemother 1994;34(1):149–56.

62. Evans DJ, Greenstone M. Long-term antibiotics in the management of non-CF bronchiectasis—do they improve outcome? Respir Med 2003;97:851–8.

63. Evans DJ, Bara A, Greenstone M. Prolonged antibiotics for purulent bronchiectasis in children and adults. Cochrane Database Syst Rev 2007;2:CD001392.

64. Drobnic ME, Sune P, Montoro JB, et al. Inhaled tobramycin in non-cystic fibrosis patients with bronchiectasis and chronic bronchial infection with *Pseudomonas aeruginosa*. Ann Pharmacother 2005;39(1):39–44.

65. Scheinberg P, Shore E, on behalf of the PC-TNDS-008 Study Group. A pilot study of the safety and efficacy of tobramycin solution for inhalation in patients with severe bronchiectasis. Chest 2005; 127:1420–6.

66. Bilton D, Henig N, Morrissey B, et al. Addition of inhaled tobramycin to ciprofloxacin for acute exacerbations of *Pseudomonas aeruginosa* infection in adult bronchiectasis. Chest 2006;130:1503–10.

67. Murray MP, Govan JR, Doherty CJ, et al. A randomized controlled trial of nebulised gentamicin in non-cystic fibrosis bronchiectasis. Am J Respir Crit Care Med 2011;183(4):491–9.

68. Orriols R, Rolg J, Ferrer J, et al. Inhaled antibiotic therapy in non-cystic fibrosis patients with bronchiectasis and chronic bronchial infection by *Pseudomonas aeruginosa*. Respir Med 1999; 93(7):476–80.

69. Macleod DL, Barker LM, Sutherland JL, et al. Antibacterial activities of a fosfomycin/tobramycin combination: a novel inhaled antibiotic for bronchiectasis. J Antimicrob Chemother 2009;64(4):829–36.

70. Rubin BK. Aerosolized antibiotics for non-cystic fibrosis bronchiectasis. J Aerosol Med Pulm Drug Deliv 2008;21(1):71–6.

71. Tsang KW, Tan KC, Ho PL, et al. Inhaled fluticasone in bronchiectasis: a 12 month study. Thorax 2005; 60(3):239–43.

72. Martinez-Garcia MA, Perpina-Tordera M, Roman-Sanchez P, et al. Inhaled steroids improve quality of life in patients with steady-state bronchiectasis. Respir Med 2006;100:1623–32.

73. Kapur N, Bell S, Kolbe J, et al. Inhaled steroids for bronchiectasis. Cochrane Database Syst Rev 2009;1:CD000996.

74. King P. Is there a role for inhaled corticosteroids and macrolide therapy in bronchiectasis? Drugs 2007;67:965–74.

75. Elborn JS, Johnston B, allen F, et al. Inhaled steroids in patients with bronchiectasis. Respir Med 1992;86:121–4.

76. Tsang KW, Ho PL, Lam WK, et al. Inhaled fluticasone reduces sputum inflammatory indices in severe bronchiectasis. Am J Respir Crit Care Med 1998;158:723–7.

77. Holme J, Tomlinson JW, Stockley RA, et al. Adrenal suppression in bronchiectasis and the impact of inhaled corticosteroids. Eur Respir J 2008;32: 1047–52.

78. Lasserson T, Holt K, Greenstone M. Oral steroids for bronchiectasis (stable and acute exacerbations). Cochrane Database Syst Rev 2001;4:CD002162.

79. Pizzutto SJ, Upham JW, Yerkovich ST, et al. Inhaled non-steroid anti-inflammatories for children and adults with bronchiectasis (review). Cochrane Database Syst Rev 2010;4:CD007525.

80. Kapur N, Chang AB. Oral non steroid anti-inflammatories for children and adults with bronchiectasis. Cochrane Database Syst Rev 2007;4: CD006427.

81. Tsang KW, Ho PI, Chan KN, et al. A pilot study of low-dose erythromycin in bronchiectasis. Eur Respir J 1999;13:361–4.

82. Tagaya E, Tamaoki J, Kondo M, et al. Effect of a short course of clarithromycin therapy on sputum production in patients with chronic airway hypersecretion. Chest 2002;122(1):213–8.

83. Cymbala AA, Edmonds LC, Bauer MA, et al. The disease-modifying effects of twice-weekly oral azithromycin in patients with bronchiectasis. Treat Respir Med 2005;4(2):117–22.

84. Yalcin E, Kiper N, Ozcelik U, et al. Effects of clarithromycin on inflammatory parameters and clinical conditions in children with bronchiectasis. J Clin Pharm Ther 2006;31:49–55.

85. Anwar GA, Bourke SC, Afolabi G, et al. Effects of long-term low-dose azithromycin in patients with non-CF bronchiectasis. Respir Med 2008;102:1494–6.

86. Crosbie PAJ, Woodhead MA. Long-term macrolide therapy in chronic inflammatory airway disease. Eur Respir J 2009;33:171–81.

87. Friedlander AL, Albert RK. Chronic macrolide therapy in inflammatory airways diseases. Chest 2010;138(5):1202–12.

88. Koh YY, Lee MH, Sun YH, et al. Effect of roxithromycin on airway responsiveness in children with bronchiectasis: a double-blind, placebo-controlled study. Eur Respir J 1997;10:994–9.

89. Davies G, Wilson R. Prophylactic antibiotic treatment of bronchiectasis with azithromycin. Thorax 2004;59:540–1.

90. Altenburg J, de Graaff CS, van der Werf TS, et al. Immunomodulatory effects of macrolide antibiotics—part 2: advantages and disadvantages of long-term, low-dose macrolide therapy. Respiration 2011;81(1):75–87.

91. Giamarellos-Bourboulis EJ. Macrolides beyond the conventional antimicrobials: a class of potent immunomodulators. Int J Antimicrob Agents 2008; 31:12–20.

92. Fujimoto T, Hillejan L, Stamatis G. Current strategy for surgical management of bronchiectasis. Ann Thorac Surg 2001;72:1711–5.

93. Balkanli K, Genc O, Dakak M, et al. Surgical management of bronchiectasis: analysis and short-term results in 238 patients. Eur J Cardiothorac Surg 2003;24:699–702.

94. Giovannetti R, Alifano M, Stefani A, et al. Surgical treatment of bronchiectasis: early and long-term results. Interact Cardiovasc Thorac Surg 2008;7: 609–12.

95. Titman A, Rogers CA, Bonser RS, et al. Disease-specific survival benefit of lung transplantation in adults: a national cohort study. Am J Transplant 2009;9:1640–9.

96. Bagheri R, Haghi SZ, Fattahi Masoum SH, et al. Surgical management of bronchiectasis: analysis of 277 patients. Thorac Cardiovasc Surg 2010; 58(5):291–4.

97. Gursoy S, Ozturk AA, Ucvet A, et al. Surgical management of bronchiectasis: the indications and outcomes. Surg Today 2010;40:26–30.

98. Hayes D, Meyer KC. Lung transplantation for advanced bronchiectasis. Semin Respir Crit Care Med 2010;31(2):123–38.

99. Zhang P, Jiang G, Ding J, et al. Surgical treatment of bronchiectasis: a retrospective analysis of 790 patients. Ann Thorac Surg 2010;90:246–51.

100. Corless JA, Warburton CJ. Surgery vs non-surgical treatment for bronchiectasis. Cochrane Database Syst Rev 2000;4:CD002180.

101. Prasad M, Tino G. Bronchiectasis, part 2: management. J Respir Dis 2008;29(1):20–5.

Diagnosis of Ventilator-Associated Respiratory Infections (VARI): Microbiologic Clues for Tracheobronchitis (VAT) and Pneumonia (VAP)

Donald E. Craven, MD[a,b],*, Jana Hudcova, MD[b,c],
Yuxiu Lei, PhD[a]

KEYWORDS

- Ventilator-associated pneumonia
- Ventilator-associated tracheobronchitis
- Ventilator-associated respiratory infection
- Microbiologic criteria for diagnosis • Endotracheal aspirates
- Bronchoalveolar lavage antibiotics
- Multidrug-resistant bacteria

Ventilator-associated respiratory infections (VARIs) may be manifested as tracheobronchitis (VAT) and ventilator-associated pneumonia (VAP).[1–6] VARI is usually caused by bacteria colonizing the patient's oropharynx or stomach that enter the lower respiratory tract around the endotracheal tube cuff or through the lumen.[1,3,4] Initial antibiotic management of VARI is complicated by delays in identification and antibiotic sensitivity data for a wide spectrum of potential pathogens that are increasingly multidrug-resistant (MDR).[4]

Placement of an endotracheal tube facilitates bacterial entry into the lower respiratory tract, impairs bacterial clearance by host defenses, and increases the risk of VAP 6-fold to 20-fold.[1] The differentiation between VARI and colonization is initially based on the presence of clinical signs and symptoms suggesting infection, such as fever, purulent sputum, and elevated peripheral leukocyte counts. Microbiologic data are also critical, but specific criteria vary with the sampling method and type of sample. For example, endotracheal aspirates (EAs) are readily available in intubated patients and bronchoalveolar lavage (BAL) or protected specimen brush (PSB) technique.[1,4,7–10] Gram-stained EA might assist diagnosis of VARI and is employed in many hospitals and intensive care units. The presence of polymorphonuclear leukocytes (PMNL) indicates possible inflammation or infection, whereas information about bacterial morphology may suggest likely pathogens. Culture of the EA either by a quantitative (Q-EA) or semiquantitative methods (SQ-EA) is used to distinguish colonization from VARI.[2,4,7] Identification and sensitivity data are usually available within 48 to 72 hours.

Lack of standardized definitions for the diagnosis of VAT and VAP based on EA samples has created confusion for clinicians using either Q-EA or SQ-EA methods versus bronchoscopic

[a] Center for Infectious Disease & Prevention, Lahey Clinic Medical Center, 41 Mall Road, Burlington, MA 01805, USA
[b] Tufts University School of Medicine, 136 Harrison Avenue, Boston, MA 02110, USA
[c] Department of Critical Care & Surgery, Lahey Clinic Medical Center, 41 Mall Road, Burlington, MA 01805, USA
* Corresponding author. Centers for Infectious Diseases & Prevention, Lahey Clinic Medical Center, 41 Mall Road, Burlington, MA 01805.
E-mail address: donald.e.craven@lahey.org

Clin Chest Med 32 (2011) 547–557
doi:10.1016/j.ccm.2011.06.001

(B) or nonbronchoscopic (NB) BAL or PSB samples.[3,10,11] The purpose of this article is to highlight the epidemiology, pathogenesis, diagnosis, and management strategies for VARI. The authors' primary aim is to clarify current diagnostic criteria to diagnose VAT and VAP versus tracheal colonization and to underscore specific clinical and microbiologic clues that could lead to earlier, appropriate antibiotic treatment of VARI.[3,7,8,12]

EPIDEMIOLOGY

VAT and VAP are defined as infections that occur more than 48 hours after intubation.[1,3,4,7] Early VAP occurs within the first 5 days of intubation. Late-onset VAP occurs after 5 days, is more commonly caused by MDR pathogens, and carries higher morbidity and mortality (**Table 1**). The reported crude mortality rate for VAP ranges from 20% to 50%, and health care costs are estimated to be $15,000 to $40,000 per episode.[1,4,13] In a recent study of outcomes of 126 intensive care unit (ICU) patients who received long-term ventilation in 5 ICUs at Duke University, the survival rate at 1 year was 56%, and only 9% of the patients were not in dependent care. Many patients had multiple admissions to a spectrum of transitional care facilities, with an estimated cost of $3.4 million dollars per patient.[14]

Medical and surgical patients diagnosed with VAT also experience a significantly longer length of ICU stay and duration of mechanical ventilation with possible progression to VAP.[2] The incidence of VAT in Europe has ranged from 2.7% to 10%, depending on the population studied.[3] A recent study in the United States, using a different model and definitions, reported an incidence of VAT of 1.4%, compared with a 4.0% incidence of VAP.[6] However, 32% of patients with VAT progressed to VAP.

BACTERIAL PATHOGENS

The most frequent pathogens isolated from patients with VAT and VAP are shown in **Table 1**. Over the past 20 years, there has been an increased incidence of infections due to MDR gram-negative pathogens, such as *Pseudomonas aeruginosa, Acinetobacter baumannii, Stenotrophomonas maltophilia,* or *Enterobacteriaceae,* such as *Escherichia coli* and *Klebsiella pneumonia.*[4] In addition, there has also been a dramatic increase in infections due to methicillin-resistant *Staphylococcus aureus* (MRSA) that is likely to continue.[3,4,15]

VARI may rarely be caused by pathogens that are not regularly identified by routine EA and BAL cultures or Gram stains, such as *Legionella pneumophila,* anaerobic bacteria, coagulase-negative staphylococci; viruses such as influenza A and B, respiratory syncytial virus, herpes simplex virus, coronavirus, or cytomegalovirus. Reactivation of *Mycobacterium tuberculosis* is rare, as are fungal pathogens such as *Cryptococcus neoformans, Aspergillus fumigatus,* and *Candida* species, which occur rarely, except in immunocompromised patients.

PATHOGENESIS

Understanding the pathogenesis of VAT and VAP is essential for establishing principles and strategies for therapy and prevention (**Fig. 1**).[1,4,7] Intubation with mechanical ventilation increases the risk of bacterial pneumonia sixfold to 20-fold.[1,4] The endotracheal tube (ETT) and oro/nasogastric tube (OG/NT) facilitate bacterial entry into the lower respiratory tract and tracheal colonization, which may progress in some intubated patients to VAT or VAP (**Fig. 2**).[1,2,4,7] Bacteria usually enter the lower respiratory tract by leakage around the ETT cuff or via the ETT lumen.[1,7,16] The inflated ETT cuff prevents the exit of bacteria and secretions from the lower airway, which increases the need for manual tracheabronchial suctioning of infected secretions. Furthermore, ETT biofilm-encased bacteria may also contribute to lower airway infection from biofilm emboli.[17,18]

Table 1	
Pathogens associated with ventilator-associated respiratory infection	
Antibiotic-Sensitive Pathogens	**Multidrug-Resistant (MDR) Pathogens**
Gram-Positive Cocci: *Streptococcus pneumoniae (pneumococcus)* Methicillin-sensitive *Staphyloccus aureus (MSSA)*	Gram-Positive Cocci: Methicillin-resistant *Staphylococcus aureus* (MRSA)
Gram-Negative Bacilli (GNB): *Haemophilus influenzae* *Escherichia coli* *Klebsiella pneumoniae* *Enterobacter aerogenes* *Proteus species*	GNB: *Pseudomonas aeruginosa* *E coli*[a] *K pneumoniae*[a,b] *Enterobacter species*[a,b] *Acinetobacter species* *Stenotrophomonas maltophilia*

[a] ESBL-positive (extended-spectrum β-lactamase).
[b] CRE (carbapenemase-resistant *Enterobacteriacaea*).

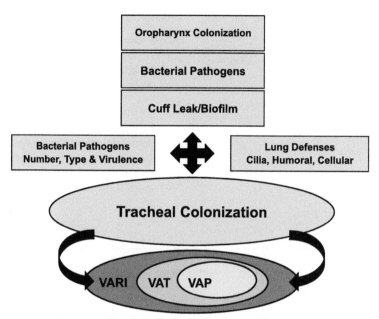

Fig. 1. Pathogenesis of ventilator-associated respiration infections (VARI). Bacteria enter the lower respiratory tract from the oropharynx by leakage around the endotracheal tube (ETT) cuff or from intraluminal biofilm. The black arrows represent the battle between the entering bacterial pathogen(s) and host defenses. The circles correspond to either colonization or VARI, manifest as either tracheobronchitis (VAT), pneumonia (VAP), or both.

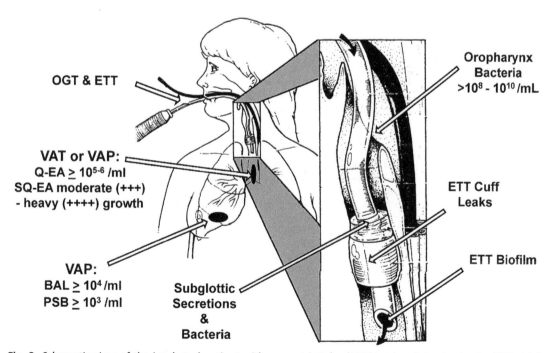

Fig. 2. Schematic view of the intubated patient with orogastric tube (OGT) and endotracheal tube (ETT). High levels of bacteria are present in the oropharyngeal secretions that may collect in the subglottic space above the ETT cuff. Bacteria-encased biofilm in the ETT lumen may colonize or embolize into the distal airways. Ventilator-associated respiratory infection (VARI) includes tracheobronchitis (VAT) or pneumonia (VAP) or both. Endotracheal aspirates (EA) examined by quantitative methods (Q-EA) or semiquantitative methods (SQ-EA) are used to distinguish infection versus colonization, and bronchoalveolar lavage (BAL) and protected specimen brush (PSB) are used to define VAP versus VAT or colonization.

The numbers, type, and virulence of bacterial pathogen(s) entering the trachea, as well as host defenses, are important factors in disease progression. In addition to a wide spectrum of potential pathogens, bacterial virulence may vary within the same bacterial species.[19,20] Mechanical host defenses (mucus and cilia), polymorphonuclear leukocyts (PMNLs), and macrophages with their respective cytokines, work in conjunction with humoral antibodies (eg, immunoglobulin M [IgM], IgG, and IgA) and complement to prevent progression of colonization to VAT or VAP.[4,21]

DIAGNOSIS AND DEFINITIONS

Similarities and differences in diagnostic criteria for VAT and VAP are summarized in **Table 2** and **Fig. 3**. Note that there is a considerable overlap in clinical definitions in terms of fever, leukocytosis, purulent sputum, and change in oxygenation.[22] Some clinicians and investigators have relied on a combination of these factors that are included in the clinical pulmonary infection score (CPIS).[23–26] A score of at least 6 has been suggested as a marker of VAP. Clinical differentiation between VAT and VAP can be difficult due to current

Table 2
Diagnostic criteria used for the diagnosis of ventilator-associated respiratory infection that includes pneumonia and tracheobronchitis

	VAP	VAT
Clinical Signs and Symptoms	At least one of these Temperature (>38°C or 100.4° F) Or Leukocyte count >12,000/mm^3 or leukopenia <4000/mm^3 Plus One of these New onset of purulent secretions or change in suctioning requirements Or Worsening oxygen requirements (increasing FIO$_2$) or PaO$_2$/FIO$_2$ ratio) Or CPIS Score ≥6	
Radiologic Signs	Chest radiograph or CT scan: New or persistent infiltrate, consolidation or cavitation	Chest radiograph or CT scan: No new infiltrate Findings consistent with diagnosis of atelectasis, ARDS, CHF
Microbiologic Criteria Smear Cultures	Endotracheal aspirate (EA) Gram stain: Many polymorphonuclear leukocytes (PMNL) Many bacteria (morphology: cocci vs bacilli) Bacterial culture: SQ-EA = many/++++ growth correlates with Q-EA = 10^6 cfu/mL Or SQ-EA = moderate/+++ growth correlates with Q-EA = 10^5 cfu/mL Bronchoscopic B-BAL/PSB Cytospin: many PMNL & bacteria B-BAL≥10^4 cfu/mL Or PSB≥10^3 cfu/mL Or Nonbronchoscopic N-BAL: Cytospin: many PMNL & bacteria N-BAL≥10^3 cfu/mL	Bronchoscopic B-BAL/PSB: Cytospin: few PMNL, no bacteria B-BAL<10^4 cfu/mL Or PSB<10^3 cfu/mL Or Nonbronchoscopic N-BAL: Cytospin: few PMNL, no bacteria N-BAL<10^3 cfu/mL

Note the overlapping microbiologic criteria when endotracheal aspirates are used for diagnosis in contrast to different criteria when bronchoalveolar lavage or protected specimen brush are used.

Abbreviations: ARDS, acute respiratory distress syndrome; BAL, bronchoalveolar lavage; CHF, congestive heart failure; CT, computerized tomography; FiO$_2$, inspired oxygen concentration; PaO$_2$, partial pressure of oxygen in arterial blood; PMNL, polymorphonuclear leukocytes; PSB, protected specimen brush; VAP, ventilator-associated pneumonia; VARI, ventilator-associated respiratory infection; VAT, ventilator-associated tracheobronchitis.

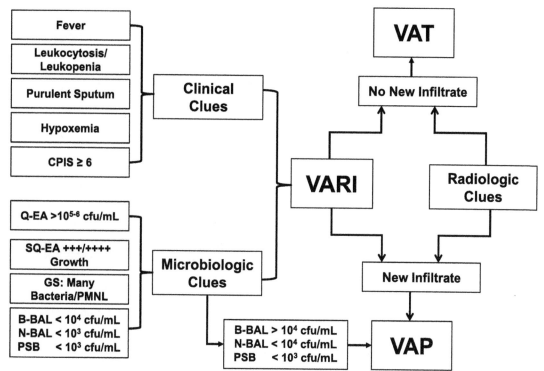

Fig. 3. Clues for diagnosis of ventilator-associated respiratory infection (VARI), which includes tracheobronchitis (VAT), pneumonia (VAP), or both. Clinical clues are common to all (VARI, VAT, VAP). Radiology clues may help to discriminate VAP from VAT based on the presence or absence of a new pulmonary infiltrate. By comparison, microbiology clues differ depending on the diagnostic methodology employed. Note that the significant growth of pathogen on bronchoscopic–bronchoalveolar lavage (B-BAL$\geq 10^4$ cfu/mL), nonbronchoscopic BAL (N-BAL>10^4 cfu/mL), or protected specimen brush (PSB$\geq 10^3$ cfu/mL) is diagnostic for VAP. Absence of significant growth (B-BAL<10^4 cfu/mL, N-BAL<10^4 cfu/mL, PSB<10^3 cfu/mL) is consistent with VAT or colonization. When endotracheal aspirates (EAs) are used for diagnosis, it is difficult to discriminate between VAT and VAP, but they are helpful for distinguishing between colonization and infection (VARI).

definitions and overlap between these infections when EAs are used for the microbiologic diagnosis.[7]

In contrast to VAT, VAP requires radiographic evidence of a new infiltrate, which may be difficult to assess, especially in patients with preexisting infiltrates, severe congestive heart failure, or acute respiratory distress syndrome (ARDS) (**Fig. 4**).[4,27–29] Unfortunately, portable chest radiographs are often of poor quality that can reduce sensitivity, and there are concerns about specificity as well, particularly in patients with pre-existing pulmonary infiltrates due to non-infectious causes.[27,28] Nseir and colleagues[10] reported that 38% of their ventilated study patients had an abnormal chest radiograph at the time of admission to the ICU. Similar problems with chest radiograph interpretation and specificity have been noted by others.[27,30,31] Data suggest that computerized tomography (CT) lung scans provide better resolution, but also have limitations,

and are not readily available in many ICUs. Interpretation of chest infiltrates in critically ill patients could be improved with the use of CT lung scans, but this may be impractical for many ICU patients. In addition, the dose of radiation exposure is high and is equivalent to greater than100 portable chest radiographs.[32,33] Based on these clinical and radiological reservations, microbiologic criteria become the cornerstone for the diagnosis of VAT or VAP due to aerobic bacterial pathogens (see **Table 2**).

QUANTITATIVE MICROBIOLOGY

Standardized criteria for the microbiological diagnosis of VAP exist for B-BAL (>10^4 cfu/mL) and NB-BAL (>10^3 cfu/mL), as well as B-PSB (>10^3 cfu/mL) techniques (see **Fig. 3**, **Table 2**; **Table 3**). Smears from EAs and cytospins of BAL or PSB specimens can be examined for PMNL and bacteria. Many PMNLs, along with bacteria,

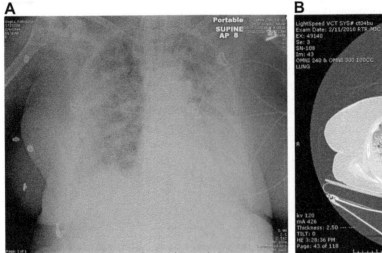
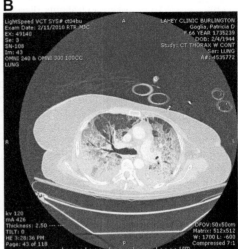

Fig. 4. Chest radiograph and computerized tomographic (CT) scan of patient with acute respiratory failure and diffuse bilateral infiltrates. Radiographic findings demonstrating diffuse airspace disease are also consistent with diagnosis of acute respiratory distress syndrome (ARDS) or congestive heart failure with or without infection. Patient also displayed clinical clues of ventilator-associated respiratory infection (VARI). Due to pre-existing changes on chest radiograph, no new infiltrate could be detected to confirm a diagnosis of ventilator-associated pneumonia (VAP). The quantitative endotracheal aspirate had greater than 10^6 colony forming units (cfu)/mL indicating ventilator-associated tracheobronchitis (VAT) or pneumonia (VAP). Bronchoalveolar lavage (BAL) could not be performed due to the severity of her ARDS.

suggest infection and the presence of bacteria on Gram stain of EA corresponds to a bacterial colony count of greater than 10^5 colony forming units (cfu)/mL. Gram stain provides clues about bacterial morphology (cocci or bacilli), morphologic arrangement (clusters vs pairs or chains) and whether the bacteria belong to the gram-positive or gram-negative group. Absence of PMNL reduces the likelihood of bacterial infection, and the presence of many is suggestive of VARI. No bacteria on the smear, in the absence of recent treatment with antibiotics, suggests noninfectious or nonbacterial causes.

There has been more confusion and less standardization for quantitative culture assessment of EA samples. Many microbiology laboratories use SQ-EA methods, and report the growth of the bacterial pathogen(s) isolated as: rare (+), few (++), moderate (+++), or many (++++), as shown in **Fig. 5**. Cultures with + or ++ growth usually represent colonization, and the presence of +++ or ++++ growth is more consistent with VARI (VAT or VAP). Other laboratories have used Q-EA and report results as a number of cfu/mL of specimen. There is no clear-cut value for diagnosis of VARI, and different providers use different thresholds (eg, 10^5 vs 10^6 cfu/mL). Quantitative cultures less than these values suggest colonization.

Several combinations of clinical and microbiologic criteria exist for the diagnosis of VAT and VAP, which vary considerably, and the merits of each have been debated for decades.[1,3,4,7,12,27,31,34,35] For the diagnosis of VAT and VAP, Q-EA$\geq 10^6$ cfu/mL has been proposed by French investigators, which corresponds well with moderate or many (++++) growth by SQ-EA and many bacteria on Gram stain. Dallas and colleagues[6] have suggested a threshold of Q-EA greater than or equal to 10^5 cfu/mL. SQ-EA with moderate (+++) or many (++++) growth also correlated with few-to-moderate bacteria present on Gram-stained smears of EA.[7,10,35] El-Ebiary and colleagues[8] reported that although Q-EA at greater than 10^5 cfu/mL had good sensitivity and specificity, Q-EA was less specific than PSB and BAL for diagnosing VAP. Nseir used a Q-EA result of greater than 10^6 cfu/mL for the diagnosis of VAT, because it had better specificity than 10^5 cfu/mL.[12]

The lack of accepted universal definitions and microbiological benchmarks for assessing Q-EA and SQ-EA is unfortunate as it is often based on the sensitivity and specificity of the criteria compared with a gold standard that remains elusive. Specific definitions are critical, not only for patient care, but also for surveillance, assessing the efficacy of prevention strategies, public

Table 3
Microbiologic clues for the diagnosis and management of VAT, VAP or VARI

EA	Clues & Interpretation
Gram stain smear	
Polymorphonuclear leukocytes (PMNL/LPF)	
Rare: <1	No infection
Few: 1–10	Unlikely infection
Moderate: 10–25	Suggests infection
Many: >25	Suggests infection
Bacteria–gram stain color	
Blue	Gram positive (G+)
Red	Gram negative (G−)
Bacteria–morphology	
Round	G+ cocci in chains: streptococci or clusters: staphylococci
Rods	G− bacilli: eg, *Escherichia coli* or *Pseudomonas aeruginosa*
Number of bacteria	
None or rare	Colonization
Moderate to many	Suggests infection, consider therapy
Culture data	
Semiquantitative culture (SQ-EA):	
Rare (+), few (++) colonies	Colonization, observe
Moderate (+++), many (++++) colonies	Possible infection, consider therapy
Quantitative (Q-EA):	
<10^5 cfu/mL	Colonization, observe
≥10^{5-6} cfu/mL	Infection, consider therapy

Note differences in Gram stain and culture criteria for EA sputum samples examined by quantitative (Q-EA) and semi-quantitative (SQ-EA) methods and diagnostic criteria for samples obtained by bronchoscopic (B) and non-bronchoscopic (N) bronchoalveolar lavage (BAL) and protected specimen brush (PSB).

Abbreviations: cfu, colony forming units; Ea, endotracheal aspirate; HPF, high power field of microscope; LPF, Low power field of microscope; VAP, ventilator-associated pneumonia; VARI, ventilator-associated respiratory infection; VAT, ventilator-associated tracheobronchitis.

reporting, improving patient outcomes, and reducing health care cost.

SURVEILLANCE CULTURES

Serial EAs have been used for microbiologic surveillance to identify the likely pathogen(s) and antibiotic sensitivities before the development of VARI.[36–40] The EA Gram-stain and culture data could also be a predictor of patients at risk for VAT or VAP. Positive surveillance EA cultures will enable distinction between colonization and infection, facilitate earlier appropriate antibiotic therapy, and improve patient outcome (**Fig. 6**).

Three studies have examined the use of serial, respiratory surveillance cultures collected at different times. Michel and colleagues[36] obtained Q-EA twice weekly in an intubated cohort, and when compared with a culture from BAL performed at the time of VAP, the causative organism was identified by prior Q-EA in 83% of study patients. VAP was most commonly late-onset, and the offending organism was *P aeruginosa.* Deputdt and colleagues[37] used weekly Q-EA to detect VAP due to MDR pathogens, and found that VAP was due to MDR pathogens in 69% of the episodes. Surveillance cultures led to the appropriate antibiotic therapy in 96% of the patients. In a similar study with BAL confirmed VAP, Hayon and colleagues reported that Q-EA surveillance cultures identified at least one of the pathogens isolated by BAL, with the highest predictive value of cultures obtained within 72 hours of the VAP diagnosis.[38,39] Finally, Yang and colleagues[38] used daily Q-EA cultures to identify patients with MDR *P aeruginosa*, and reported that colonized patients were more likely to develop VAP. Further studies are clearly needed to expand and confirm these results in different patient populations. There is also a need to look for optimal intervals between surveillance cultures to provide appropriate and timely therapy and improve patient outcome (see **Fig. 6**).

RATIONALE FOR TREATING VAT

VAT may be a precursor to or overlap with VAP.[3,6,11,40] Treatment provides an opportunity for earlier intervention and targeted rather than empiric antibiotic therapy. Several observation and randomized VAT studies have been published and are summarized.

A'Court and colleagues[40] studied tracheal colonization in 150 mechanically ventilated patients, using serial quantitative, nonbronchoscopic BAL samples and reported increases in lower respiratory tract colonization over time that appeared to peak about 2 days before the onset of clinical signs of VAP. In a prospective, observational cohort of medical and surgical patients by Nseir and colleagues,[3] VAT was associated with increased length of ICU stay, more mechanical ventilator days, and higher mortality in medical but not surgical ICU patients. In a later study of

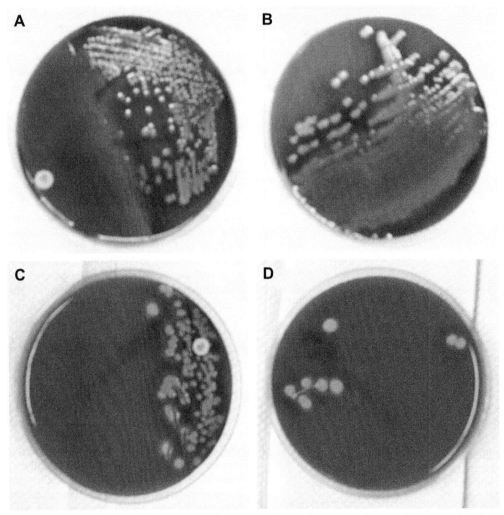

Fig. 5. Patient "MJ" had clinical signs (fever, leukocytosis and purulent sputum) of ventilator-associated respiratory infection (VARI). Her semiquantitative endotracheal aspirate (SQ-EA) showed many/++++ bacterial growth (*A*), and a simultaneous Q-EA demonstrated >10^6 cfu/mL of *Pseudomonas aeruginosa* on blood agar plates (*B*), consistent with the diagnosis of ventilator-associated tracheobronchitis (VAT) or pneumonia (VAP). Patient "YL" had clinical signs of VARI; an SQ-EA showed few/++ bacterial growth (*C*) and Q-EA<10^4 cfu/mL of *Escherichia coli* (*D*), consistent with endotracheal colonization.

patients with chronic obstructive pulmonary disease (COPD), the same authors reported that patients with VAT, when compared with matched controls, had significantly lower median days of mechanical ventilation and more ICU days, but antibiotic therapy did not appear to protect against VAP.[41] In a later prospective, observational case–control study of patients with VAT, patients who were treated with antibiotics had significantly fewer days of mechanical ventilation and ICU stay, but no difference was noted in mortality rates.[42]

Two randomized studies of antibiotic therapy for VAT have recently been conducted, but the study populations, definitions of VAT, and interventions were different. Nseir and colleagues[12] reported results from a controlled, unblinded trial of 58 patients with a clinical diagnosis of VAT. VAT was defined by a Q-EA greater than 10^6 cfu/mL and no infiltrate on chest radiograph. Patients were randomized to receive targeted intravenous antibiotic therapy versus no or delayed therapy. The antibiotic-treated group displayed better outcomes: more mechanical ventilation-free days (median 12 vs 2 days, *P*<.001), a lower ICU mortality (18% vs 47%, *P*<.05), and a significant decrease in VAP (47% vs 14%, *P*<.02). The same bacterial pathogens were identified in each study group, supporting the concept that VAT appeared to progress to VAP in some patients.

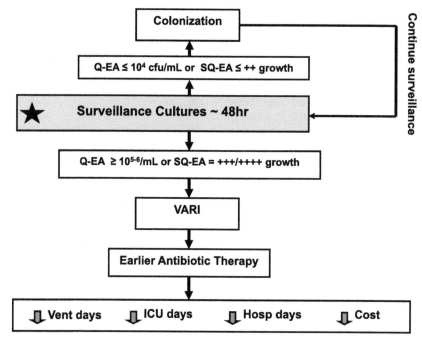

Fig. 6. Model for the use of quantitative (Q) and semiquantitative (SQ) endotracheal aspirates (EAs) to initiate "argeted rather than empiric antibiotic therapy. Ventilator-associated respiratory infections (VARIs) include tracheobronchitiis (VAT) and pneumonia (VAP). The goal is early targeted appropriate antibiotic therapy to improve patient outcomes in terms of reduced mortality, morbidity, and health care costs.

Important limitations of this study included low numbers of patients, an imbalance in the numbers of patients randomized to each group, and lack of an independent, blinded evaluation of endpoints such as interpretation of chest radiographs to exclude early VAP.

Palmer and colleagues[43] performed a double-blind, randomized, placebo-controlled study of medical ICU (MICU) and surgical ICU (SICU) patients, comparing aerosolized antibiotic treatment (gentamicin every 8 hours if gram-negative bacilli were present, vancomycin every 8 hours if gram-positive bacteria were detected, or both for those with mixed infections) for 14 days or until extubation (n = 19) versus a saline placebo (n = 24). VAT was defined as the production of at least 2 mL of purulent EA over a 4-hour period with a Gram stain demonstrating bacteria. Systemic antibiotics were given at the discretion of treating physician and frequently prescribed in both groups. Compared with the placebo group, the aerosolized antibiotic group had significantly better outcomes, manifested as lower rates of clinical signs and symptoms of VAP, faster weaning of the ventilator, reduced numbers of MDR pathogens, and lower use of systemic antibiotic, with all endpoints, $P<.05$. Notable limitations of this study included the definition of VAT, lack of Q-EA, high numbers of patients who had prior VAP,

lack of data on radiographic signs of VAP, small numbers of study patients, and potential confounding effect by the use of systemic antibiotics.

Different results were reported by Dallas and colleagues[6] in a retrospective study of VAT and VAP in medical and surgical ICU patients. Dalllas and colleagues reported that VAT occurs less commonly than VAP when using an EA cutoff of 10^5 cfu/mL. Most patients had MDR pathogens; patients diagnosed with VAT frequently progressed to VAP and VAT, and VAP patients had similar mortality (19% vs 21%). These conclusions may have been related to the definitions used for VAT and VAP, the well-known limitations of portable chest radiograph interpretation to define VAP, lack of surveillance cultures, and retrospective chart review.

VARI: A NEW PARADIGM FOR CLINICAL MANAGEMENT

Diagnosis of VAT or VAP by B-BAL/N-BAL/PSB has been clearly delineated. However, when EAs are used for diagnosis, discrimination between VAP and VAT is almost impossible, because of low sensitivity and specificity of clinical and radiologic findings and overlapping microbiologic criteria. However, quantitative and semiquantitative EAs can discriminate between colonization and infection.[4] VARI is a term that clearly discriminates between colonization and infection due to VAT, VAP, or both.

Due to the limited availability of B-BAL/N-BAL/PSB in many ICUs, EAs are commonly used for the diagnosis VAP. The authors emphasize the importance of quantitative and semiquantitative EA criteria for assessing for VARI and as a trigger point to consider initiating early, appropriate antibiotic therapy. For example + or ++ growth of *Klebsiella* species on SQ-EA or Q-EA less than 10^5 most likely represents colonization that likely does not require treatment with antibiotics. However, at least 3 caveats apply to these recommendations:

The patient is not critically ill (eg, shock)
No cultures have been performed within 24 to 48 hours
Patients have not received antibiotics within 24 hours before the cultures were obtained.

In addition, these recommendations pertain to the bacterial pathogens associated with VARI that are summarized in **Table 1**.

Early, appropriate antibiotic therapy, as emphasized in the 2005 American Thoracic Society/Infectious Diseases Society of America guidelines, is associated with improved patient outcomes.[4] These guidelines recommend broad-spectrum, empiric antibiotic therapy until culture and antibiotic sensitivity data are available, and then de-escalation of antibiotics based on the microbiologic data. However, for intubated patients, the use surveillance EA may provide earlier information on colonization with MDR pathogens that could be used for targeted antibiotic therapy. This approach could reduce inappropriate antibiotic therapy, reduce overuse of antibiotics that can result in selection of MDR pathogens, improve clinical outcomes, and reduce health care costs.

SUMMARY

The clinical definitions for the diagnosis of VAT and VAP lack specificity, and differentiating between them may be difficult. These definitions are important to guide clinicians on when antibiotic treatment should be initiated and which antibiotics should be used. VARI is a term that indicates infection that deserves consideration for antibiotic therapy. Surveillance cultures will identify pathogens and help clinicians to initiate earlier targeted antibiotic therapy. The purpose of this communication is to highlight the importance of microbiologic clues to aid clinicians in distinguishing between infection and colonization. The authors' goal is to drive down rates of VARI and to

emphasize prevention strategies to decrease rates or VAT or VAP. Strategies to improve outcomes include early identification of infection, avoiding intubation, removing endotracheal tubes as soon as possible, use of sedation vacation, treating infections early, and limiting inappropriate antibiotic use.

REFERENCES

1. Chastre J, Fagon JY. Ventilator-associated pneumonia. Am J Respir Crit Care Med 2002;165:867–903.
2. Nseir S, Ader F, Marquette CH. Nosocomial tracheobronchitis. Curr Opin Infect Dis 2009;22:148–53.
3. Nseir S, Di Pompeo C, Pronnier P, et al. Nosocomial tracheobronchitis in mechanically ventilated patients: incidence, aetiology, and outcome. Eur Respir J 2002;20:1483–9.
4. Niederman MS, Craven DE, Bonten MJ, et al. Guidelines for the management of adults with hospital-acquired, ventilator-associated, and healthcare-associated pneumonia. Am J Respir Crit Care Med 2005;171:388–416.
5. Craven DE, Hjalmarson KI. Ventilator-associated tracheobronchitis and pneumonia: thinking outside the box. Clin Infect Dis 2010;51(Suppl 1):S59–66.
6. Dallas J, Skrupky L, Abebe N, et al. Ventilator-associated tracheobronchitis (VAT) in a mixed surgical and medical ICU population. Chest 2011;139(3):513–8.
7. Craven DE, Chroneou A, Zias N, et al. Ventilator-associated tracheobronchitis: the impact of targeted antibiotic therapy on patient outcomes. Chest 2009;135:521–8.
8. el-Ebiary M, Soler N, Monton C, et al. Markers of ventilator-associated pneumonia. Clin Intensive Care 1995;6:121–6.
9. Marquette CH, Copin MC, Wallet F, et al. Diagnostic tests for pneumonia in ventilated patients: prospective evaluation of diagnostic accuracy using histology as a diagnostic gold standard. Am J Respir Crit Care Med 1995;151:1878–88.
10. Nseir S, Deplanque X, Di Pompeo C, et al. Risk factors for relapse of ventilator-associated pneumonia related to nonfermenting Gram-negative bacilli: a case–control study. J Infect 2008;56:319–25.
11. Craven DE. Ventilator-associated tracheobronchitis (VAT): questions, answers, and a new paradigm? Crit Care 2008;12:157.
12. Nseir S, Favory R, Jozefowicz E, et al. Antimicrobial treatment for ventilator-associated tracheobronchitis: a randomized, controlled, multicenter study. Crit Care 2008;12:R62.
13. Rello J, Lorente C, Bodi M, et al. Why do physicians not follow evidence-based guidelines for preventing ventilator-associated pneumonia? a survey based on the opinions of an international panel of intensivists. Chest 2002;122:656–61.

14. Unroe M, Kahn JM, Carson SS, et al. One-year trajectories of care and resource utilization for recipients of prolonged mechanical ventilation: a cohort study. Ann Intern Med 2010;153:167–75.

15. Lam AP, Wunderink RG. Methicillin-resistant *S aureus* ventilator-associated pneumonia: strategies to prevent and treat. Semin Respir Crit Care Med 2006;27:92–103.

16. Kollef MH, Afessa B, Anzueto A, et al. Silver-coated endotracheal tubes and incidence of ventilator-associated pneumonia: the NASCENT randomized trial. JAMA 2008;300:805–13.

17. Bauer TT, Torres A, Ferrer R, et al. Biofilm formation in endotracheal tubes. Association between pneumonia and the persistence of pathogens. Monaldi Arch Chest Dis 2002;57:84–7.

18. Inglis TJ, Millar MR, Jones JG, et al. Tracheal tube biofilm as a source of bacterial colonization of the lung. J Clin Microbiol 1989;27:2014–8.

19. El Solh AA, Akinnusi ME, Wiener-Kronish JP, et al. Persistent infection with *Pseudomonas aeruginosa* in ventilator-associated pneumonia. Am J Respir Crit Care Med 2008;178:513–9.

20. Alcon A, Fabregas N, Torres A. Pathophysiology of pneumonia. Clin Chest Med 2005;26:39–46.

21. Craven DE. Preventing ventilator-associated pneumonia in adults: sowing seeds of change. Chest 2006;130:251–60.

22. Barreiro B, Dorca J, Manresa F, et al. Protected bronchoalveolar lavage in the diagnosis of ventilator-associated pneumonia. Eur Respir J 1996;9:1500–7.

23. Pugin J. Clinical signs and scores for the diagnosis of ventilator-associated pneumonia. Minerva Anestesiol 2002;68:261–5.

24. Pelosi P, Barassi A, Severgnini P, et al. Prognostic role of clinical and laboratory criteria to identify early ventilator-associated pneumonia in brain injury. Chest 2008;134:101–8.

25. Luna CM, Blanzaco D, Niederman MS, et al. Resolution of ventilator-associated pneumonia: prospective evaluation of the clinical pulmonary infection score as an early clinical predictor of outcome. Crit Care Med 2003;31:676–82.

26. Luyt CE, Chastre J, Fagon JY. Value of the clinical pulmonary infection score for the identification and management of ventilator-associated pneumonia. Intensive Care Med 2004;30:844–52.

27. Klompas M. Does this patient have ventilator-associated pneumonia? JAMA 2007;297:1583–93.

28. Klompas M, Kulldorff M, Platt R. Risk of misleading ventilator-associated pneumonia rates with use of standard clinical and microbiological criteria. Clin Infect Dis 2008;46:1443–6.

29. Wunderink RG. Clinical criteria in the diagnosis of ventilator-associated pneumonia. Chest 2000;117: 191S–4S.

30. Graat ME, Choi G, Wolthuis EK, et al. The clinical value of daily routine chest radiographs in a mixed medical–surgical intensive care unit is low. Crit Care 2006;10:R11.

31. Klompas M, Kleinman K, Platt R. Development of an algorithm for surveillance of ventilator-associated pneumonia with electronic data and comparison of algorithm results with clinician diagnoses. Infect Control Hosp Epidemiol 2008;29:31–7.

32. Syrjala H, Broas M, Suramo I, et al. High-resolution computed tomography for the diagnosis of community-acquired pneumonia. Clin Infect Dis 1998;27:358–63.

33. Winer-Muram HT, Rubin SA, Ellis JV, et al. Pneumonia and ARDS in patients receiving mechanical ventilation: diagnostic accuracy of chest radiography. Radiology 1993;188:479–85.

34. Torres A. Implementation of guidelines on hospital-acquired pneumonia: is there a clinical impact on outcome? Chest 2005;128:1900–2802.

35. Nseir S, Di Pompeo C, Soubrier S, et al. Impact of ventilator-associated pneumonia on outcome in patients with COPD. Chest 2005;128:1650–6.

36. Michel F, Franceschini B, Berger P, et al. Early antibiotic treatment for BAL-confirmed ventilator-associated pneumonia: a role for routine endotracheal aspirate cultures. Chest 2005;127:589–97.

37. Depuydt PO, Vandijck DM, Bekaert MA, et al. Determinants and impact of multidrug antibiotic resistance in pathogens causing ventilator-associated-pneumonia. Crit Care 2008;12:R142.

38. Yang K, Zhuo H, Guglielmo BJ, et al. Multidrug-resistant *Pseudomonas aeruginosa* ventilator-associated pneumonia: the role of endotracheal aspirate surveillance cultures. Ann Pharmacother 2009;43: 28–35.

39. Hayon J, Figliolini C, Combes A, et al. Role of serial routine microbiologic culture results in the initial management of ventilator-associated pneumonia. Am J Respir Crit Care Med 2002;165:41–6.

40. A'Court CH, Garrard CS, Crook D, et al. Microbiological lung surveillance in mechanically ventilated patients, using nondirected bronchial lavage and quantitative culture. Q J Med 1993;86:635–48.

41. Nseir S, Di Pompeo C, Soubrier S, et al. Outcomes of ventilated COPD patients with nosocomial tracheobronchitis: a case–control study. Infection 2004;32: 210–6.

42. Nseir S, Di Pompeo C, Soubrier S, et al. Effect of ventilator-associated tracheobronchitis on outcome in patients without chronic respiratory failure: a case-control study. Crit Care 2005;9:R238–45.

43. Palmer LB, Smaldone GC, Chen JJ, et al. Aerosolized antibiotics and ventilator-associated tracheobronchitis in the intensive care unit. Crit Care Med 2008;36:2008–13.

Aerosolized Antibiotics in the Intensive Care Unit

Lucy B. Palmer, MD

KEYWORDS

- Aerosolized antibiotics
- Ventilator-associated tracheobronchitis
- Ventilator-associated pneumonia • Bacterial resistance

Ventilator-associated pneumonia (VAP) is the leading cause of death related to infection in critically ill patients and accounts for more than 50% of the antibiotic use in the intensive care unit (ICU).[1–8] The morbidity and mortality related to respiratory infections remain significant. In a 2010 review of clinical outcomes of health care–related infection in European ICUs, 4457 patients were identified with VAP caused by *Pseudomonas aeruginosa*, *Acinetobacter baumannii*, *Escherichia coli*, or *Staphylococcus aureus*.[9] The excess risk of death from VAP (hazard ratio) was 1.7 (95% confidence interval [CI], 1.4–1.9) for drug-sensitive *S aureus* and 3.5 (95% CI, 2.9–4.2) for ceftazidime-resistant *Pseudomonas*. Increasing microbial resistance in the ICU is a major challenge for physicians because it is driven primarily by systemic antibiotic use. Rates of resistance correlate directly with amounts of antibiotic used.[6,10–12] The increasing difficulty of treatment of multidrug-resistant organisms (MDROs) is occurring at a time when there is a dearth of new systemic antibiotics available. Furthermore, few new antibiotics are in development in the pipelines of the pharmaceutical industry. In the past 40 years, there have been only 2 new classes of antibiotics introduced, oxazolidinones (linezolid) and the cyclic lipopeptides (daptomycin). Both these antibiotics are used for the treatment of gram-positive organisms, leaving options for resistant gram-negative organisms even more limited.[13–15] This shrinking armamentarium of systemic antibiotics in a battlefield of rising minimum inhibitory concentrations (MICs) compels us to examine the current data on the efficacy of aerosolized antibiotics. At present, the American Thoracic Society (ATS) guidelines suggest, "adjunctive therapy with an inhaled aminoglycoside or polymyxin for MDR Gram-negative pneumonia should be considered, especially in patients who are not improving on systemic therapy"[1] and cite 1 nonrandomized trial[16] because these guidelines were written in 2005. In this article, the author reviews the literature with emphasis on the most recent data concerning the following questions:

1. What is the evidence that aerosolized antibiotics result in improved outcome in the treatment of respiratory tract infection in mechanically ventilated patients in the ICU?
2. What should be the indication for aerosolized antibiotics?
3. Are there data available that suggest this method of delivery decreases or increases the emergence of MDROs?

The earliest studies of topical antibiotic therapy were driven by the same clinical problem that plagues us more than 40 years later.[17–21] Resistant gram-negative organisms, in particular *Pseudomonas* species, were causing respiratory infections in intubated patients and patients with tracheostomy, and clinical response to intravenous (IV) therapy was poor. At that time, aminoglycosides given intravenously were the primary

Disclosure: Dr Lucy B Palmer and her associate Dr Gerald Smaldone have a patent with the Research Foundation of SUNY Stony Brook for the use endobronchial antibiotics, which is licensed to Nektar Therapeutics.
Pulmonary, Critical Care and Sleep Division, SUNY at Stony Brook, HSC T17-040, Stony Brook, NY 11794-8172, USA
E-mail address: lbpalmer@notes.cc.sunysb.edu

Clin Chest Med 32 (2011) 559–574
doi:10.1016/j.ccm.2011.05.012
0272-5231/11/$ – see front matter © 2011 Elsevier Inc. All rights reserved.

treatment of gram-negative organisms, and treatment failure occurred in up to 60% of patients.[19–21] These poor outcomes were thought primarily to be caused by poor penetration of the aminoglycosides into the lung, so the methods of increasing the concentration in the lung were studied.

Early investigations used endotracheal instillation of the antibiotic. The concentrations of the aminoglycoside in the bronchial secretions were shown to be 1000-fold higher than the serum concentrations of patients receiving IV therapy, and bactericidal activity was more than 30-fold greater than that in serum.[20] These investigators had also demonstrated the clinical benefit from the instillation of aminoglycosides for the treatment of bronchial infections in intubated patients, which is now called ventilator-associated tracheobronchitis (VAT), as well as in bronchopneumonia.[19,20] At that time the investigators wrote, "endotracheal administration might thus represent the ideal adjunct to systemic antimicrobial therapy for bronchopneumonina." Despite these initial positive studies in the 1970s, there have been no large multisite clinical randomized trials of aerosolized antimicrobials for the treatment of respiratory infection in mechanically ventilated patients.

Why have advances in antibiotic delivery to the lung in ventilated patients progressed so slowly? There have been several drugs approved for patients with cystic fibrosis, but almost all aerosol treatments of VAT or VAP have been off label. There has been only one phase 2 randomized controlled trial (RCT) in ventilated patients for VAP.[22] This delay of research and development in aerosolized antibiotics for the ventilated patient was primarily driven by the negative results of an investigation of topical antibiotics used for the prevention of pneumonia in critically ill patients in the 1970s.[23,24] It is worthwhile reviewing this work because the data teach the importance of methods of delivery and the duration of prophylactic or treatment protocols.

Two seminal studies came out in 1975 using polymyxin B, a potent cationic cyclic polypeptide antibiotic against gram-negative organisms.[23,24] In a preliminary observational study, all patients in the ICU, whether intubated or not, were given prophylactic polymyxin B. The polymyxin B was administered via an atomizer to the oropharynx or, if the patients were intubated, for 2-month cycles with both atomizer and instillation, alternating with 2-month cycles with no polymyxin B. A total of 744 patients were enrolled.[23] The results were encouraging because both colonization rates with Pseudomonas and the incidence of VAP were decreased. The same investigators then published a follow-up study,[24] which gave the same regimen

in a 7-month trial to 292 patients, but now the antibiotic was given continuously to all the patients without any 2-month cycles off the antibiotic. This study had markedly different results. There was an increase in the incidence of VAP with organisms resistant to polymyxin, including Flavobacterium, Serratia, and Streptococcus species, and the mortality from VAP was 64% (7 of the 11 patients who acquired pneumonia during the study died). The investigators stated that continuous topical antibiotics were a dangerous form of therapy. These results led to reluctance to further study topical therapy, and there were no significant advances in aerosolized antibiotic treatment trials for nearly 30 years. In retrospect, analysis of the design of this trial predicts the development of resistant organisms. As the investigators themselves noted, it was the continuous use of polymyxin given to all patients, all the time, whether intubated or not, that was problematic. Also, dose and deposition site were not well defined with the use of an atomizer and instillation. All these factors may have contributed to the emergence of resistant organisms.

Now that the treatment of MDRO has become increasingly problematic, targeted therapy to the lung is being revisited. The first RCTs in targeted delivery to the lung were treatment protocols in spontaneously breathing patients with cystic fibrosis. In these patients with chronic airway infection, aerosolized antibiotics are a mainstay of therapy, and investigations have shown decreased hospitalizations and preservation of lung function.[25,26] These studies have led to 2 Food and Drug Administration (FDA)-approved aerosolized antibiotics with defined delivery devices.

Mechanically ventilated patients' airways and respiratory infections share many attributes of those of patients with cystic fibrosis once VAT is present. Both groups present an airway epithelium that is injured and inflamed with poor mucociliary clearance, and, in addition, it is well known now that the endotracheal tube develops a biofilm similar to that found in the airways of patients with cystic fibrosis.[27,28] Biofilm may also be present in ventilated patients' airways (Fig. 1). Furthermore, increasingly resistant Pseudomonas species and S aureus are important pathogens in both groups. These similarities suggest that the aerosolized delivery of antimicrobial therapy should be of benefit for mechanically ventilated patients as well. The off-label, FDA-approved, and phase 2 trial drugs used for these 2 groups of patients are shown in Box 1. Toxicities associated with the use of these antibiotics are shown in Box 2.

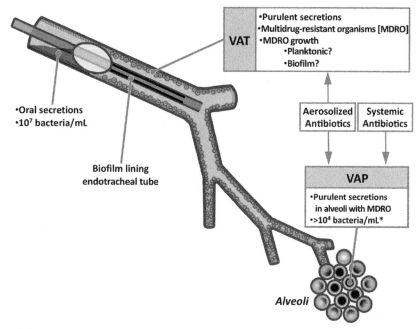

Fig. 1. The multifactorial process that leads to VAT and VAP. Subglottic secretions, disturbed mucociliary clearance, damaged mucosa, and bacterial biofilm may all play a role in the pathogenesis of proximal and distal infections. Within a few days of ICU admission, the bacteria frequently become MDROs. * The cutoff of 10^4 colony-forming units per milliliter for the microbiological diagnosis of VAP may not pertain to patients with prolonged mechanical ventilation.

RATIONALE FOR AEROSOLIZED ANTIBIOTIC THERAPY IN THE ICU

The theoretical reasons for using targeted antimicrobial therapy in mechanically ventilated patients are compelling. With proper delivery, the drug is delivered directly to the site of infection, concentrations in the lung are high, and systemic toxicity is minimized.[22,29–31] Furthermore, the microflora of the gut is not altered, thus reducing the emergence of MDRO and infection with *Clostridium difficile*. The high antibiotic concentrations achieved with targeted therapy far exceed the MIC and result in a large ratio of maximum concentration to MIC, an index shown to be important for eradication of these organisms in the milieu of thick purulent secretions, biofilm, and diminished mucociliary clearance.[32] Conversely, if only IV therapy is used and concentrations are not bactericidal, biofilm formation may be induced, making the infections even harder to eradicate.[33] There is some evidence that the use of these aerosolized agents with systemic antibiotics may reduce the need for additional systemic antibiotic added for poor response to initial treatment.[34,35] Although untested, it is also possible that the use of aerosolized antibiotics could shorten the duration of systemic antibiotic use for respiratory tract infections and thus reduce the selection pressure for MDRO.

WHAT ARE THE CURRENT UNCERTAINTIES ABOUT AEROSOLIZED THERAPY

Devices used for aerosolized delivery have never been held to the same rigorous FDA regulations to which medications are subject. Medications given intravenously with appropriate attention to dosing are not subject to large variability of concentrations in the blood stream. Unlike IV therapy, whereby dose is primarily related to concentration in the blood and the blood flow within the infected organ, aerosolized delivery depends on all the factors listed in **Box 3**. In addition to all these important factors, delivery devices and mechanical ventilators are designed with increasingly complex interactive technology that may alter drug deposition. Devices have evolved from a simple syringe or atomizer to jet and ultrasonic nebulizers, vibrating mesh technology, and, in animal studies, magnetic field–guided aerosols with superparamagnetic iron oxide nanoparticles in the solutions to be aerosolized.[36] Despite all these variables that may influence lung dose and site of deposition, there are no specific standards for aerosolized drug delivery in intubated patients.

Because of the complexity of all these variables, currently available proprietary drugs are sold as a combination drug and device product to optimize the delivery of the antimicrobial. This review

of 2 antibiotics, imipenem and tobramycin. Bronchial and serum concentrations of both were compared.

One and 2 hours after the administration of the second dose, instilled imipenem/cilastatin produced imipenem concentrations of 4695 ± 3580 mg/L and 4278 ± 3104 mg/L, respectively, whereas concentrations after nebulization were 72 ± 76.1 mg/L after

does not focus on these technological aspects of delivery because the data are well summarized in several excellent reviews.[37–44]

ANTIBIOTIC DELIVERY: WHAT IS KNOWN ABOUT CENTRAL AND DISTAL CONCENTRATIONS OF ANTIBIOTIC DELIVERED VIA AEROSOL
Instillation

The earliest data about proximal concentrations of drug are from the trials in the 1960s to 1970s of instillation of aminoglycosides through the endotracheal tube or tracheostomy. As mentioned previously, tracheal aspirate concentrations were found to be 1000 times more than those of serum concentrations.[20] More recently, Badia and colleagues,[45] in a prospective, randomized, open-label trial in critically ill mechanically ventilated patients, compared instillation with aerosolization

1 hour and 120.9 ± 181.2 mg/L after 2 hours (P = .022 and P = .0029, respectively). These differences in concentration were striking. Instilled concentrations of imipenem were well above the MIC for *P aeruginosa* even 8 hours after administration (86% of *P aeruginosa* isolates [MIC of 4 mg/L]). Antibiotic concentrations greater than the MIC were also attained with nebulized imipenem, but concentrations from instillation were 60-fold greater.

Unlike imipenem, tobramycin concentrations were similar after either methods of delivery (nebulized: 102 ± 61 mg/L after 2 hours, instilled: 142 ± 125 mg/L 2 hours after dose; P>.05). These data confirm that the dose and deposition site of molecule/solvent delivered via different devices or methods can never be assumed without in vivo testing.

Jet Nebulizer Delivery

The data concerning the concentration of aerosolized antibiotics delivered via jet nebulizer in the airways consistently demonstrate that secretion (tracheal aspirates) levels may be 20- to 100-fold greater than the in vitro MIC of the organisms being treated. Palmer and colleagues,[29] in a study of chronically ventilated patients, administered 80 mg of gentamicin placed in a jet nebulizer (AeroTech II; CIS-US, Bedford, MA, USA) every 8 hours. Mean sputum concentrations ranged from 289 ± 41.4 mg/mL to 1179 ± 394.5 mg/mL, trough and peak, respectively, after 5 days of treatment. Serum concentrations were undetectable, except for 1 patient who had renal failure. Deposition studies of using the jet nebulizer suggest that central deposition was greater than peripheral.[46]

Miller and colleagues[31] in their investigation of drug delivery compared bench model testing of drug delivery with in vivo studies to determine key factors in drug delivery. The antibiotic treatment regimen consisted of aerosolized antibiotics given every 8 hours given for 24 hours. When delivery was optimized (humidification off during treatment and breath-actuated nebulization), sputum concentrations ranged from 550 mg/mL to 5790 mg/mL for amikacin and 200 to 790 mg/mL for gentamicin and 2352 mg/mL for a subject who received vancomycin.

Sputum concentrations of aerosolized vancomycin have also been studied in parallel with serum concentrations in patients who were also receiving IV vancomycin. Zarilli and colleagues[47] aerosolized 120 mg of vancomycin every 8 hours via jet nebulizer (AeroTech) to 10 mechanically ventilated patients with suspected infection with methicillin-resistant *S aureus* (MRSA). Concentrations of vancomycin were compared in patients treated with IV vancomycin alone and after aerosolized therapy. The concentration in those receiving only IV therapy was 10.8 ± 1.3 mg/mL, whereas those receiving aerosol had concentrations that were 20-fold greater than this.

Vibrating Mesh Technology

In a recent study using vibrating mesh technology, Niederman and colleagues[22] randomized 69 mechanically ventilated patients with gram-negative VAP to receive proprietary aerosolized amikacin or placebo. Aerosolized amikacin was given, 400 mg every 12 hours or once daily, followed by placebo 12 hours later in conjunction with IV antimicrobials. The investigators found that the nebulized drug was well distributed in the lung parenchyma with high tracheal levels (6.9 mg/mL for once daily and 16.2 mg/mL for twice daily). Serum concentrations were low and less than renal toxic concentrations.

Luyt and colleagues[30] administered aerosolized amikacin (400 mg twice a day) to the lungs of 28 mechanically ventilated patients with gram-negative pneumonia for 7 to 14 days, adjunctive to IV therapy administered by the responsible clinician according to the ATS guidelines. On the third day of treatment, 30 minutes after completing aerosol delivery, all the patients underwent bronchoalveolar lavage in the infection-involved area, and the amikacin concentration was determined in epithelial lining fluid (ELF). The same day, amikacin concentrations were determined in sera, starting the morning of amikacin aerosolization delivery. The median (range) ELF amikacin level was 976.1 μg/mL (135.7–16,127.6 μg/mL), whereas the maximum serum amikacin concentration was 0.9 μg/mL (0.62–1.73 μg/mL). ELF concentrations were greater than the MIC for amikacin for common gram-negative pathogens for VAP. These data suggest that high concentrations may be possible in the deep lung with vibrating mesh nebulizers, although variability in concentration in this investigation was significant. Further studies are needed to assess deep lung concentrations with this delivery method and should be done for each different design of delivery device and molecule to be delivered.

CLINICAL EFFECTS OF AEROSOLIZED ANTIBIOTICS

Aerosolized antibiotics have been used in trials to prevent VAP and in treatment protocols. The author focuses primarily on the treatment protocols but briefly summarizes the VAP prophylactic trials.

Prophylaxis Trials

The use of aerosolized antibiotics as prophylaxis for VAP is not well supported at this time. The polymyxin B data from the 1970s have been discussed previously. A recent meta-analysis by Falagas and colleagues[48] reviewed the literature from 1950 to 2005. Of the 12 prophylactic trials, there were only 8 investigations[22,49–55] that were either RCTs or prospective comparative trials (5 RCTs and 3 nonrandomized prospective comparative trials). Aerosolized gentamicin was used in 3 trials, polymyxin in 2, tobramycin in 1, and ceftazidime in 1. There were 1877 patients included in the meta-analysis. Primary outcomes were incidence of VAP and mortality. Secondary outcome was colonization with P aeruginosa.

Analysis of the 5 RCTs demonstrated a reduction in VAP in the treated patients with an odds ratio (OR) of 0.49 (95% CI, 0.32–0.76). However, there was no effect on mortality, and there were insufficient data to assess the effect on bacterial colonization. Addition of the 2 nonrandomized trials to their meta-analysis yielded similar results for VAP; however, in this analysis, there was a reduction in VAP in patients colonized with P aeruginosa in the group that received prophylaxis compared with the group of patients that received no prophylaxis (OR, 0.51; 95% CI, 0.30–0.86). Although these data are of interest, current guidelines from both the Centers for Disease Control and Prevention and the ATS do not recommend this therapy.[1,3] These older prophylactic studies used a variety of delivery devices, often have no data on concentrations of the antibiotic in the lung, and represent pathogens that have currently evolved to be more resistant. RCTs with standardized delivery methods; appropriate new end points, such as ventilator-free days; reduction in the use of systemic antibiotics; and effects on bacterial resistance are necessary for preventive protocols to be reconsidered.

ARE AEROSOLIZED ANTIBIOTICS USEFUL IN TREATING VAT AND/OR VAP

At present, there are no large multisite investigations examining the effect of aerosolized antibiotics on VAP. Ioannidou and colleagues[56] recently performed a meta-analysis on small RCTs done from 1950 to 2007 that compared topical administration (aerosolization or instillation) with or without concurrent usage of systemic antibiotics for the treatment of VAP. Of the 685 potential relevant articles, there were only 5 RCTs[20,57–60] with a combined total of 176 patients suitable for analysis. This meta-analysis demonstrated that patients receiving aerosolized or instilled antibiotics had less VAP (clinical diagnosis) in the intention-to-treat group (fixed effect model: OR, 2.39; 95% CI, 1.29–4.44 and random effect model: OR, 2.75; 95% CI, 1.06–7.17) and clinically evaluable group (fixed effect model: OR, 3.14; 95% CI, 1.48–6.70 and random effects model: OR, 3.07; 95% CI, 1.15–8.19). There were no statistically significant differences between the therapeutic regimens for mortality, microbiological success, and toxicity.

Aerosolized Colistin for VAP

The increasing prevalence of VAP caused by highly resistant P aeruginosa and Acinetobacter has led to the reintroduction of colistin (polymyxin E) in an aerosolized form and the IV form. Colistin was used extensively in the 1960s and 1970s. The mechanism of colistin's bactericidal activity is destabilization of the lipopolysaccharide (LPS) of the outer membrane, and, in addition, it neutralizes the LPS, thereby decreasing antiendotoxin activitites.[48] The use of colistin was discontinued because of multiple reports of neurologic and renal toxicity when used parenterally.[48,60–63]

Recently, there have been multiple small nonrandomized clinical trials, and one review focused on aerosolized colistin treatment of multidrug-resistant (MDR) Pseudomonas and Acinetobacter species.[48,64–73] Both these bacteria produce extended-spectrum β-lactamases and metallolactamases. Acinetobacter is often sensitive only to polymyxin B or colistin (polymyxin E), and there are now reports of colistin resistance as well.[74,75]

Included in the meta-analysis by Ioannidou and colleagues[56] mentioned earlier were 2 nonrandomized prospective trials of aerosolized colistin that included patients infected by these organisms. Kwa and colleagues[65] treated 21 patients with respiratory tract infections with Acinetobacter and Pseudomonas species. Patients who received systemic antibiotics and aerosolized colistin had a good clinical response with a reduction in signs/symptoms of infection. Hamer[16] treated MDR Pseudomonas with aerosolized colistin in a small case series of 3 mechanically ventilated patients with VAP who also showed an improvement in signs of infection.

In an open-label noncontrolled prospective investigation, Michalopoulos and colleagues[66] treated 60 critically ill patients with a mean Acute Physiology and Chronic Health Evaluation (APACHE) II score of 16.7. Patients received aerosolized colistin for the treatment of VAP caused by MDR pathogens. Among the 60 patients, A baumannii was present in 37 patients, P aeruginosa in 12, and Klebsiella pneumoniae in 11. Half of these pathogens were susceptible only to colistin. Of the 60 patients, 57 received concomitant IV treatment with colistin or other antimicrobial agents. Bacteriologic and clinical response of VAP was observed in 83% of their patients.

Berlana and colleagues[64] described the microbiological outcomes in an investigation including 71 courses of aerosolized colistin used to treat 60 respiratory infections with A baumannii and 11 with P aeruginosa. The mean duration of the therapy was 12 ± 8 days. The Acinetobacter was eradicated in all the end-of-treatment cultures that were available; however, Pseudomonas was eradicated only in 57%.

Most recently, Kofteridis and colleagues[72] in a retrospective matched case-control study compared the effect of IV colistin alone with that of IV colistin and aerosolized colistin. Each group had 43 patients. A baumannii was the most common pathogen (77% of isolates), followed by K. pneumoniae (14%) and P aeruginosa (9.3%). The patients in the aerosolized and IV colistin group had a higher rate of clinical cure than patients in the IV colistin group, 23 (54%) of the 43 patients versus 14 (32.5%) of the 43 patients ($P = .05$). No significant differences in eradication of pathogens ($P = .679$) or mortality ($P = .289$) between the 2 groups were observed. Overall, the mortality rate in the ICU was 42% (18 of 43 patients) in the IV colistin alone group compared with 24% (10 of 43 patients) in the aerosol and IV colistin group ($P = .066$). This study, unlike all others described, found IV therapy no different from IV and aerosolized colistin in bacterial eradication. The reasons for this less-robust microbiological response are not clear. Methods of aerosolization are not described, so comparison of methods of drug delivery with those of other studies cannot be made.

Korbila and colleagues,[73] in a similar retrospective cohort study, compared IV colistin alone (43 patients) with IV colistin plus aerosolized colistin (78 patients) and demonstrated a significant improvement in clinical outcome (resolution of signs and symptoms of infection) in 62 of 78 (79.5%) patients who received IV plus inhaled colistin versus 26 of 43 (60.5%) patients who received IV colistin alone ($P = .025$). The use of inhaled colistin was independently associated with the cure of VAP in a multivariable analysis (OR, 2.53; 95% CI, 1.11–5.76). No significant differences were observed in the 2 groups, inhaled colistin plus IV colistin and IV colistin alone, respectively, for all-cause ICU mortality (28 of 78 patients [35.9%] vs 17 of 43 [39.5%], respectively; $P = .92$) and oral-cause in-hospital mortality (31 of 78 patients [39.7%] vs 19 of 43 patients [44.2%], respectively; $P = .63$).

RCTS OF AEROSOLIZED ANTIBIOTICS FOR VAT OR VAP

There have only been 4 randomized placebo-controlled studies with important positive clinical outcomes. A double-blind placebo-controlled phase 2 study of aerosolized amikacin delivered via vibrating mesh technology was given to 67 patients as adjunctive therapy in ventilated patients with gram-negative pneumonia. Systemic antibiotic therapy was given by the responsible clinician following ATS guidelines.[34] Randomization was to aerosolized amikacin 400 mg daily with placebo (normal saline) 12 hours later or 400 mg twice daily or placebo twice daily. The mean number of IV antibiotics at the end of the study (mean 7 days) was 2 times greater with placebo than with twice-daily amikacin ($P<.02$).

Palmer and colleagues[35] in a double-blind placebo-controlled trial randomized 43 critically ill intubated patients with VAT (defined as the production of 2 mL of purulent secretions for longer than 4 hours) to aerosolized (AeroTech II nebulizer) gentamicin (80 mg every 8 hours) and/or vancomycin treatment (120 mg every 8 hours) dictated by Gram stain at the time of randomization. Systemic antibiotics were administered by the clinician responsible for the patient. Both the placebo and active treatment groups received similar amounts of appropriate systemic antibiotics at randomization. Treatment with aerosolized antibiotics resulted in decreased signs and symptoms of VAP, decreased Clinical Pulmonary Infection Score (CPIS), facilitated weaning, and reduction in the use of systemic antibiotics (**Table 1**) compared with the placebo patients. **Fig. 2** shows the effect of treatment on bacterial growth in tracheal aspirates by the semiquantitative technique at the time of randomization, week 1, and week 2 of treatment. Patients treated with aerosolized antibiotics had marked reduction in bacterial growth. Gram stains of cultures with zero growth revealed that in the aerosolized antibiotic group, 7 of 12 (58%) during week 1 and 6 of 8 (75%) during week 2 had no organisms on Gram stain. In placebo, only 3 of 14 cultures (21%) during week 1 and 4 of 18 (22%) during week 2 had Gram stains with no organisms.

This investigation also provided the first promising data for the treatment of MRSA via aerosolized vancomycin in ventilated patients. Three placebo patients who had VAT secondary to MRSA as well as VAP at the time of randomization had no improvement during the study despite being on appropriate systemic antibiotics. Three patients with MRSA and VAT received aerosolized vancomycin. Two of these patients did not have

Table 1
Effect of aerosolized antibiotics on systemic antibiotic use

Group	Number of Subjects on Systemic Antibiotics at Time of Randomization	P	Number of Subjects on Systemic Antibiotics at End of Treatment	P
Aerosolized Antibiotics	17 (89%)	.44[a]	8	.042[a]
Placebo	19 (79%)		17	

[a] P values for differences in systemic antibiotic use between aerosolized antibiotic group and placebo group.

VAP at randomization and remained free of VAP at the end of the treatment. The one patient who had MRSA and VAP had clinical resolution at the end of aerosolized vancomycin treatment as well as eradication of the MRSA.

In another randomized and placebo-controlled study done by this same group, 4 of 5 patients with MRSA as their cause of VAT had the organisms eradicated while on aerosolized vancomycin.[76] Furthermore, the Gram stains of the tracheal aspirates showed no organisms present after treatment, suggesting true eradication rather than an in vitro phenomenon due to high drug concentration. Although these numbers are small and need to be confirmed in much larger trials, they suggest that aerosolized therapy for MRSA may be useful.

The most recent randomized controlled study compared the effects of normal saline with those of aerosolized colistimethate (CMS), a prodrug

that is converted in the lung to active colistin, on VAP.[77] All patients were on systemic antibiotics chosen by the responsible physicians. The baseline characteristics of the patients were similar, and mean APACHE scores of both groups were 18.5 and 19.1 for the placebo and CMS groups, respectively. Conventional systemic antibiotic therapy for VAP in both groups was comparable. Most cases of VAP were caused by MDR, A baumannii, and/or P aeruginosa. All isolates of gram-negative bacteria were susceptible to colistin. Favorable clinical outcome was 51.0% in the aerosol CMS plus systemic antibiotic group and 53.1% in the placebo plus systemic antibiotic group (P = .84). Patients in the CMS group had significantly more favorable microbiological outcome (defined as eradication or presumed eradication) when compared with patients in the control group (60.9% vs 38.2%, P = .03). This

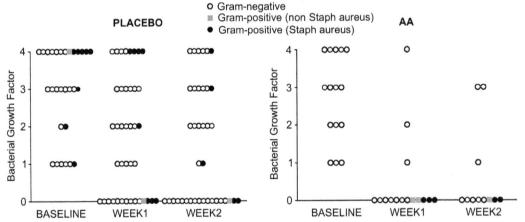

Fig. 2. Bacterial growth from tracheal aspirate cultures obtained at time of randomization (baseline) and after the first and second weeks of treatment. The quantity of growth is assessed on a graded scale of 0 to 4 from semi-quantitative cultures. Each filled circle represents S aureus, each shaded circle represents other gram-positive organisms, and open circles represent gram-negative organisms. Some patients had multiple isolates. Most patients were on systemic antibiotics. At week 1, all the isolates with zero growth represent organisms detected at baseline that did not grow in isolates sampled at week 1. At week 2, the isolates with zero growth represent organisms detected at baseline or at week 1 that did not grow in samples obtained at week 2. There was a clear difference in the pattern of bacterial growth between the aerosolized antibiotic (AA) group and placebo. In addition, most of the zero growth cultures of the AA group were free of organisms on Gram stain. (Modified from Palmer LB, Smaldone GC, Chen JJ, et al. Aerosolized antibiotics and ventilator-associated tracheobronchitis in the intensive care unit. Crit Care Med 2008;36:2011; with permission.)

Table 2
Microbiological response to aerosolized antibiotics

Authors	Year	Setting	Design	Indication	Method of Aerosolization; Drug	Number of Patients	Number of Patients on Systemic Antibiotic Use	Number of Organisms in Patients	Number of Patients with Eradication of Causative Organism	Number of Patients with Resistant Organisms
Michalopoulos et al[66]	2005	ICU, Greece	Retrospective chart review	VAP for 6 patients, HAP for 2 patients	Aerosolized via Siemens Servo Ventilator; colistin	8	7/8	7, *Acinetobacter*; 1, *Pseudomonas*	4/5	None
Kwa et al[65]	2005	ICU, Singapore	Retrospective chart review	VAP	Aerosolized colistin; no data on method	21	Yes, but not active against causative organism	17, *Acinetobacter*; 4, *Pseudomonas*	11/11 available cultures	Not described
Berlana et al[64]	2005	ICU, Spain	Retrospective chart review	Pulmonary infection	Aerosolized with various compressors; colistin	71	78% of patients	60, *Acinetobacter*; 11, *Pseudomonas*	*Acinetobacter* (33/33); *Pseudomonas* (4/7)	Not described
Michalopoulos et al[68]	2008	ICU, Greece	Prospective	VAP	Aerosolized via Siemens Servo Ventilator; colistin	60	57	37, *Acinetobacter*; 12, *Pseudomonas*; 11, *Klebsiella*	50/60	Not described
Palmer et al[35]	2008	ICU, United States	Randomized, double blind, placebo controlled	VAT≥2-mL sputum/4 h and organism on Gram stain	AeroTech jet nebulizer; vancomycin and/or gentamicin	24, placebo; 19, AA	32/43	Multiple species of gram-negative and gram-positive organisms	See Table 1	Placebo (8/24), AA (0/19)
Kofteridis et al[72]	2010	ICU, Greece	Retrospective review, matched case control	VAP	Aerosolized colistin; no details on method	43 IV & aerosolized colistin; 43 IV colistin	All patients	66, *Acinetobacter*; 12, *Klebsiella*; 8, *Pseudomonas*	Placebo, 17 (50%); aerosolized 19 (45%)	Not described
Korbila et al[73]	2010	ICU, Greece	Retrospective review, matched case control	VAP	Aerosolized via Siemens Servo Ventilator; colistin	43 IV colistin 78 aerosolized colistin + IV	All patients	MDR gram-negative organisms	Placebo, 26 (60.5%); aerosolized, 62 (79.5%)	Not described

Abbreviations: AA, aerosolized antibiotic; HAP, hospital-acquired pneumonia.

investigation differs from all others described because CMS was used, which is thought to be less potent than colistin. The concentration of the active drug in the lung is not as predictable as that in those studies using colistin and may explain the less-favorable clinical outcome compared with the other RCT's.

HOW DO AEROSOLIZED ANTIBIOTICS AFFECT THE EMERGENCE OF BACTERIAL RESISTANCE COMPARED WITH SYSTEMIC ANTIBIOTICS

Increased bacterial resistance in the ICU has been shown to have a direct relationship to the amount of systemic antibiotics used.[6] However, there have been little data in the recent literature analyzing the impact of aerosolized antibiotics on the emergence of resistance.

Prophylactic Trials

In the meta-analysis of prophylactic trials (1950–2005) mentioned previously,[48] of the 8 studies worthy of analysis (5 RCTs and 3 prospective comparative studies), 6 noted that there was no significant increase in resistant organisms described, but there are little actual culture and susceptibility data presented in these investigations. Any future clinical trials for prophylaxis of VAP should include microbiological outcomes, including not only respiratory tract organisms but also multisite surveillance cultures, to determine effects on ICU microbial resistance patterns.

Treatment Trials

The emergence of resistance in aerosolized antibiotic treatment protocols was reviewed in the meta-analysis described previously by Ioanoudiu.[56] In the 5 RCT investigations from 1972 to 2007, of the 46 participants with susceptible organisms at randomization, only 3 (6.5%) who received an endotracheal regimen of aminoglycoside with an initially susceptible pathogen had a resistant one after the completion of the treatment.

Palmer and colleagues[35] demonstrated that 8 of 24 placebo participants acquired resistant organisms during treatment compared with 0 of 19 patients administered aerosolized antibiotics (P = .0056). In the placebo group, 4 participants had initially sensitive bacteria (3 *P aeruginosa* and 1 *K pneumoniae*) that developed resistance on treatment. Two participants acquired a resistant *Acinetobacter* and 2 acquired MRSA. One of the 19 aerosolized antibiotic participants transiently acquired a resistant organism, a resistant *Acinetobacter* that resolved during therapy. All patients who acquired resistant organisms received systemic antibiotics.

Table 2 shows the currently available data on the eradication of pathogens and the emergence of resistance for studies published between 2005 and 2010.[35,64–67,72,73] The amount of data is limited. Only 2 trials report any data on the emergence of resistance. In these 2 trials, no new resistance was detected. These investigations suggest that aerosolized therapy provides concentrations that can eradicate pathogens and, in 1 investigation, that placebo and systemic antibiotics are associated with the emergence of newly resistant organisms, whereas aerosolized antibiotics with systemic antibiotics are not.[35] Multisite RCTs confirming these data are needed.

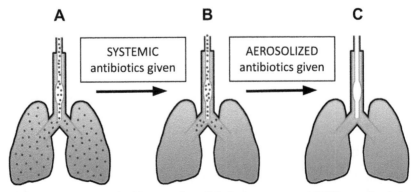

Fig. 3. Model of how VAP (A), treated with systemic antibiotics, may not treat VAT in proximal airway effectively (B). Aerosolized antibiotics with primarily central deposition eliminate VAT effectively (C). VAT could be targeted alone before VAP and/or as an adjuvant with systemic antibiotics in VAP. (*Modified from* Palmer. Aerosolized antibiotics in critically ill ventilated patients. Current Opinion in Critical Care 2009;15:414; with permission.)

INDICATIONS FOR AEROSOLIZED ANTIBIOTICS

There are no new consensus guidelines on the appropriate indications for aerosolized antibiotics since 2005. The current guidelines from the ATS state that "aerosolized antibiotics may also be useful to treat microorganisms that, on the basis of high minimum inhibitory concentration values, are 'resistant' to systemic therapy" but further studies are needed.[1] So should adjunctive therapy remain the only indication or should the indication be extended to VAT? If VAT should be included, what definition should be used?

Currently available data suggest that VAT may be a useful trigger for therapy.[29,35,76,78–84] Early treatment protocols in the 1970s by Klastersky and colleagues[19] targeted tracheobronchitis, which is now called VAT. These intubated or tracheostomized patients treated with airway instillation of antibiotics showed clinical improvement, lessening of secretions, and eradication of bacteria. Palmer and colleagues[29] treated VAT in a group of chronically ventilated patients and found a reduction in the volume of secretion and eradication of pathogens. A recent study by Nseir[82] randomized patients with VAT defined as

---

Box 4
Definitions of VAT

The Centers for Disease Control and Prevention diagnosis of tracheobronchitis[81,a]

    Two of the following signs or symptoms with no other cause

        New or increased purulent secretions

        Fever greater than 38°C

        Cough

        Rhonchi or wheezing

    One of the following

        Tracheal aspirate with positive culture result

        Positive antigen test result on respiratory secretions

        No infiltrate on chest radiography

Nseir and colleagues[82]

    Purulent sputum production

    Fever greater than 38°C with no other recognizable cause

    Endotracheal aspirate with 10^6 or more colony-forming units (CFUs) per milliliter

    No infiltrate on chest radiography

Craven and colleagues[83]

    Temperature (>38°C) or leukocytosis (>12,000/mL) or leukopenia (<4000/mL) (at least 1 of these) plus new onset of purulent endotracheal secretions or change in sputum

    Endotracheal aspirate; Gram stain with polymorphonuclear leukocytes with/without bacteria (note morphology and color); semiquantitative

    Endotracheal aspirate (moderate to heavy growth) or quantitative endotracheal aspirate, 10^5 to 10^6 CFUs/mL. Bronchoalveolar lavage, if done, must exclude VAP

    No infiltrate

Palmer and colleagues[35]

    Production of 2 mL or more of purulent secretions for 4 hours

    Gram stain shows organisms

    No radiographic requirement

[a] This diagnosis was established for nonventilator patients, and the presence of the endotracheal tube makes the symptoms of cough and abnormal breath sounds very nonspecific.

Data from Palmer LB. Ventilator-associated tracheobronchitis. Current Respiratory Medicine Reviews 2010;6:58–64.

greater than 10^6 bacteria in endotracheal aspirate associated with fever and no infiltrate on chest radiography to IV antibiotics versus a group that received no therapy. The treated group had a significantly less VAP ($P<.02$), increased ventilator-free days ($P<.001$), and lower mortality ($P<.05$). The data are promising, but the mortality effects need further study because of the small number of patients and some weakness in design and statistical analysis.

In a recent investigation in critically ill patients by Palmer and colleagues,[35] VAT was used as the trigger for randomization to aerosolized antibiotics. As mentioned previously, the definition of VAT for this study did not include any systemic signs of infection. VAT was defined simply as a volume of purulent secretions greater or equal to 2 mL per 4 hours and Gram stain showing organisms. Many of these patients with VAT had VAP as well. There were significant improvements in clinical and microbiological outcomes in the aerosolized treatment group compared with placebo. In addition, the 5 patients who had VAT with no evidence of VAP who received aerosolized antibiotics had a decrease in their CPIS and bacterial eradication, and none progressed to VAP. These data suggest that treatment of VAT, with or without concomitant VAP, may be beneficial. **Fig. 3** depicts how high concentrations in the proximal airway may be able to eradicate bacteria that are not eliminated by systemic antibiotics because of insufficient concentrations in this area of diminished capillary interface and thick mucoid secretions.

Clearly, well-designed multisite studies are needed to confirm the data summarized in this review. These protocols need objective criteria for the diagnostic criteria for VAT, or they share the nonspecificity of current diagnostic criteria for VAP. **Box 4** shows the current diagnostic criteria for VAT as defined by different investigators.[35,82–84]

Recently, an argument has been made for doing serial endotracheal cultures as a surveillance method for VAT using a cutoff of 10^5 to 10^6, which would lead to treatment before the onset of deep lung infections in the presence of fever and elevation of WBC.[83] This method, although attractive, shares the problem of VAP diagnosed by bronchoalveolar lavage when patients are already on systemic antibiotics. False-negative results cannot be excluded in this setting. The importance of standard criteria is most evident in **Box 5**.[35,78,84–86] Dramatic differences of VAT incidence are seen with different criteria and duration of mechanical ventilation.

The question if it is possible that the appropriate use of aerosolized antibiotics for the treatment of

---

Box 5
Incidence of VAT

- German multicenter study; 515 patients in the ICU: 2.7%[85]
- Single-center study in Spain: 5.5%[86]
- Patients in the ICU in France: 10%[82]
- Multicenter study; cardiac surgery patients requiring longer than 72 hours on vent; United States: 10.6%[87]
- Single-center study; ICU and surgical ICU; United States: 70% by day 7 on ventilator[35]

VAT could lead to (1) decreased incidence of VAP, (2) a reduced use of systemic antibiotics as seen in the 2 prior studies, and (3) decreased development of MDRO arises. Points (1) and (2) already have early supportive data.[34,35] Point (3) is potentially the most powerful end point, but, as seen in **Table 2**, none of the current publications have been designed to specifically answer this question.

SUMMARY

After 40 years of off-label use of aerosolized antibiotic in mechanically ventilated patients, with many promising results, there is neither consensus on the use of aerosolized antibiotics for VAT or VAP beyond the 2005 ATS guidelines nor any FDA-approved product for these diagnoses. There is, however, a growing body of data that suggest aerosolized antibiotics may have a role in the treatment of respiratory infection in the ICU. Three recent RCTs have shown positive clinical outcomes, with reduction in CPIS, facilitation of weaning, and/or a reduction in the use of systemic antibiotics when aerosolized antibiotics were used as an adjunctive therapy for VAT and/or VAT with VAP. Furthermore, those patients receiving active treatment had a decrease in the emergence of resistance in 2 RCTs compared with placebo.

In view of the threat of increasingly resistant organisms present in the ICU, including both MDR gram-negative organisms and MRSAs, large multicenter trials targeting antimicrobial therapy to the lung are needed. By targeting VAT, there is the potential for a significant reduction in the use of systemic antibiotics. Trials must be designed to assess clinical end points, such as resolution of signs and symptoms of respiratory infection, and data should be acquired for new primary outcomes, such as effects on the amounts, types, and duration of systemic antibiotic used while also documenting antimicrobial resistance in the ICU and incidence of nosocomial infections such as *Clostridium difficile.*

It is clear that bacterial growth and the emergence of resistance in the ICU are a moving target. Intensivists are responsible for the evolution of MDRO because they prescribe the drugs that are driving the problem. Future investigations are needed to determine not only if treatment of VAT and/or VAP with aerosolized antibiotics is clinically effective but also its effects on selective pressure for MDRO. Contrary to the data on topical therapy from the 1970s,[24] it is now worth exploring whether targeted therapy may become one of the new tools combating antimicrobial resistance.

REFERENCES

1. American Thoracic Society, Infectious Diseases Society of America. Guidelines for the management of adults with hospital-acquired, ventilator-associated, and healthcare-associated pneumonia. Am J Respir Crit Care Med 2005;171(4):388–416.
2. Chastre J, Fagon JY. Ventilator-associated pneumonia. Am J Respir Crit Care Med 2002;165(7): 867–903.
3. Richards MJ, Edwards JR, Culver DH, et al. Nosocomial infections in medical intensive care units in the United States. National Nosocomial Infections Surveillance System. Crit Care Med 1999;27(5): 887–92.
4. Masterton RG, Galloway A, French G, et al. Guidelines for the management of hospital-acquired pneumonia in the UK: report of the working party on hospital-acquired pneumonia of the British Society for Antimicrobial Chemotherapy. J Antimicrob Chemother 2008;62(1):5–34.
5. Kollef MH, Morrow LE, Niederman MS, et al. Clinical characteristics and treatment patterns among patients with ventilator-associated pneumonia. Chest 2006;129(5):1210–8.
6. Chastre J, Luyt CE. Optimising the duration of antibiotic therapy for ventilator-associated pneumonia. Eur Respir Rev 2007;16(103):40–4.
7. Chastre J, Wolff M, Fagon JY, et al. Comparison of 8 vs 15 days of antibiotic therapy for ventilator-associated pneumonia in adults: a randomized trial. JAMA 2003;290(19):2588–98.
8. Safdar N, Dezfulian C, Collard HR, et al. Clinical and economic consequences of ventilator-associated pneumonia: a systematic review. Crit Care Med 2005;33(10):2184–93.
9. Lambert ML, Suetens C, Savey A, et al. Clinical outcomes of health-care-associated infections and antimicrobial resistance in patients admitted to European intensive-care units: a cohort study. Lancet Infect Dis 2011;11(1):30–8.

10. Neuhauser MM, Weinstein RA, Rydman R, et al. Antibiotic resistance among gram-negative bacilli in US intensive care units: implications for fluoroquinolone use. JAMA 2003;289(7):885–8.
11. Landman D, Quale JM, Mayorga D, et al. Citywide clonal outbreak of multiresistant Acinetobacter baumannii and Pseudomonas aeruginosa in Brooklyn, NY: the preantibiotic era has returned. Arch Intern Med 2002;162(13):1515–20.
12. Arias CA, Murray BE. Antibiotic-resistant bugs in the 21st century—a clinical super-challenge. N Engl J Med 2009;360(5):439–43.
13. Wenzel RP. The antibiotic pipeline—challenges, costs, and values. N Engl J Med 2004;351(6):523–6.
14. Peterson LR. Bad bugs, no drugs: no ESCAPE revisited. Clin Infect Dis 2009;49(6):992–3.
15. Spellberg B, Guidos R, Gilbert D, et al. The epidemic of antibiotic-resistant infections: a call to action for the medical community from the Infectious Diseases Society of America. Clin Infect Dis 2008; 46(2):155–64.
16. Hamer DH. Treatment of nosocomial pneumonia and tracheobronchitis caused by multidrug-resistant Pseudomonas aeruginosa with aerosolized colistin. Am J Respir Crit Care Med 2000;162(1):328–30.
17. Pino G, Conterno G, Colongo PG. Clinical observations on the activity of aerosol colimycin and of endobronchial instillations of colimycin in patients with pulmonary suppurations. Minerva Med 1963; 54:2117–22 [in Italian].
18. Pines A, Raafat H, Plucinski K. Gentamicin and colistin in chronic purulent bronchial infections. Br Med J 1967;2(5551):543–5.
19. Klastersky J, Geuning C, Mouawad E, et al. Endotracheal gentamicin in bronchial infections in patients with tracheostomy. Chest 1972;61(2):117–20.
20. Klastersky J, Carpentier-Meunier F, Kahan-Coppens L, et al. Endotracheally administered antibiotics for gram-negative bronchopneumonia. Chest 1979;75(5): 586–91.
21. Smith CR, Baughman KL, Edwards CQ, et al. Controlled comparison of amikacin and gentamicin. N Engl J Med 1977;296(7):349–53.
22. Niederman MS, Sanchez M, Corkery K, et al. Amikacin aerosol achieves high tracheal aspirate concentrations in intubated mechanically ventilated patients with Gram-negative pneumonia: a pharmacokinetic study. Am J Respir Crit Care Med 2007; 175:A326.
23. Klick JM, du Moulin GC, Hedley-Whyte J, et al. Prevention of gram-negative bacillary pneumonia using polymyxin aerosol as prophylaxis. II. Effect on the incidence of pneumonia in seriously ill patients. J Clin Invest 1975;55(3):514–9.
24. Feeley TW, Du Moulin GC, Hedley-Whyte J, et al. Aerosol polymyxin and pneumonia in seriously ill patients. N Engl J Med 1975;293(10):471–5.

25. Ramsey BW, Dorkin HL, Eisenberg JD, et al. Efficacy of aerosolized tobramycin in patients with cystic fibrosis. N Engl J Med 1993;328(24):1740–6.

26. Ramsey BW, Pepe MS, Quan JM, et al. Intermittent administration of inhaled tobramycin in patients with cystic fibrosis. Cystic Fibrosis Inhaled Tobramycin Study Group. N Engl J Med 1999;340(1):23–30.

27. Singh PK, Schaefer AL, Parsek MR, et al. Quorum-sensing signals indicate that cystic fibrosis lungs are infected with bacterial biofilms. Nature 2000; 407(6805):762–4.

28. Inglis TJ, Lim TM, Ng ML, et al. Structural features of tracheal tube biofilm formed during prolonged mechanical ventilation. Chest 1995;108(4):1049–52.

29. Palmer LB, Smaldone GC, Simon SR, et al. Aerosolized antibiotics in mechanically ventilated patients: delivery and response. Crit Care Med 1998;26(1):31–9.

30. Luyt CE, Clavel M, Guntupalli K, et al. Pharmacokinetics and lung delivery of PDDS-aerosolized amikacin (NKTR-061) in intubated and mechanically ventilated patients with nosocomial pneumonia. Crit Care 2009;13:R200.

31. Miller DD, Amin MM, Palmer LB, et al. Aerosol delivery and modern mechanical ventilation: in vitro/in vivo evaluation. Am J Respir Crit Care Med 2003; 168:1205.

32. Palmer LB, Spitzer E, Monteforte M, et al. Methicillin-resistant Staphylococcus aureus (MRSA) minimum inhibitory concentration for amikacin: can aerosolized amikacin treat MRSA in the airway? Am J Respir Crit Care Med 2011;183:A3933.

33. Marr AK, Overhage J, Bains M, et al. The Lon protease of Pseudomonas aeruginosa is induced by aminoglycosides and is involved in biofilm formation and motility. Microbiology 2007;153:474.

34. Niederman MS, Chastre J, Corkery K, et al. Inhaled amikacin reduces IV antibiotic use in intubated mechanically ventilated patients [abstract]. Am J Respir Crit Care Med 2007;175:A326.

35. Palmer LB, Smaldone GC, Chen JJ, et al. Aerosolized antibiotics and ventilator-associated tracheobronchitis in the intensive care unit. Crit Care Med 2008;36:2008–13.

36. Coates AL. Guiding aerosol deposition in the lung. N Engl J Med 2008;358:304.

37. O'Riordan TG, Palmer LB, Smaldone GC. Aerosol deposition in mechanically ventilated patients. Optimizing nebulizer delivery. Am J Respir Crit Care Med 1994;149:214.

38. Smaldone GC. Aerosolized antibiotics in mechanically ventilated patients. Respir Care 2004;49:635.

39. Dhand R. Aerosol delivery during mechanical ventilation: from basic techniques to new devices. J Aerosol Med Pulm Drug Deliv 2008;21:45.

40. Dhand R, Guntur VP. How best to deliver aerosol medications to mechanically ventilated patients. Clin Chest Med 2008;29:277.

41. Dhand R, Mercier E. Effective inhaled drug administration to mechanically ventilated patients. Expert Opin Drug Deliv 2007;4:47.

42. Dhand R, Sohal H. Pulmonary drug delivery system for inhalation therapy in mechanically ventilated patients. Expert Rev Med Devices 2008;5:9.

43. Hess DR. Nebulizers: principles and performance. Respir Care 2000;45:609.

44. Hess D, Fisher D, Williams P, et al. Medication nebulizer performance. Effects of diluent volume, nebulizer flow, and nebulizer brand. Chest 1996;110:498.

45. Badia JR, Soy D, Adrover M, et al. Disposition of instilled versus nebulized tobramycin and imipenem in ventilated intensive care unit (ICU) patients. J Antimicrob Chemother 2004;54:508.

46. Smaldone GC, Palmer LB. Aerosolized antibiotics: current and future. Respir Care 2000;45:667.

47. Zarrilli GM, Monteforte M, Baram D, et al. Systemic versus aerosolized delivery of vancomycin for MRSA: concentrations in lungs and serum [abstract]. Am J Respir Crit Care Med 2008;177: A286.

48. Falagas ME, Siempos II, Bliziotis IA, et al. Administration of antibiotics via the respiratory tract for the prevention of ICU-acquired pneumonia: a meta-analysis of comparative trials. Crit Care 2006;10: R123.

49. Greenfield S, Teres D, Bushnell LS, et al. Prevention of gram-negative bacillary pneumonia using aerosol polymyxin as prophylaxis. I. Effect on the colonization pattern of the upper respiratory tract of seriously ill patients. J Clin Invest 1973;52:2935.

50. Klastersky J, Huysmans E, Weerts D, et al. Endotracheally administered gentamicin for the prevention of infections of the respiratory tract in patients with tracheostomy: a double-blind study. Chest 1974; 65:650.

51. Lode H, Hoffken G, Kemmerich B, et al. Systemic and endotracheal antibiotic prophylaxis of nosocomial pneumonia in ICU. Intensive Care Med 1992; 18(Suppl 1):S24.

52. Rathgeber J, Zielmann S, Panzer C, et al. Prevention of pneumonia by endotracheal micronebulization of tobramycin. Anasthesiol Intensivmed Notfallmed Schmerzther 1993;28:23 [in German].

53. Rouby JJ, Poete P, Martin de Lassale E, et al. Prevention of gram negative nosocomial bronchopneumonia by intratracheal colistin in critically ill patients. Histologic and bacteriologic study. Intensive Care Med 1994;20:187.

54. Vogel F, Werner H, Exner M, et al. Prophylaxis and treatment of respiratory tract infection in ventilated patients by endotracheal administration of aminoglycosides (author's transl). Dtsch Med Wochenschr 1981;106:898 [in German].

55. Wood GC, Boucher BA, Croce MA, et al. Aerosolized ceftazidime for prevention of ventilator-associated

pneumonia and drug effects on the proinflammatory response in critically ill trauma patients. Pharmacotherapy 2002;22:972.

56. Ioannidou E, Siempos II, Falagas ME. Administration of antimicrobials via the respiratory tract for the treatment of patients with nosocomial pneumonia: a meta-analysis. J Antimicrob Chemother 2007;60: 1216.

57. Hallal A, Cohn SM, Namias N, et al. Aerosolized tobramycin in the treatment of ventilator-associated pneumonia: a pilot study. Surg Infect (Larchmt) 2007;8:73.

58. Le Conte P, Potel G, Clementi E, et al. Administration of tobramycin aerosols in patients with nosocomial pneumonia: a preliminary study. Presse Med 2000; 29:76 [in French].

59. Brown RB, Kruse JA, Counts GW, et al. Double-blind study of endotracheal tobramycin in the treatment of gram-negative bacterial pneumonia. The Endotracheal Tobramycin Study Group. Antimicrob Agents Chemother 1990;34:269.

60. Falagas ME, Kasiakou SK, Tsiodras S, et al. The use of intravenous and aerosolized polymyxins for the treatment of infections in critically ill patients: a review of the recent literature. Clin Med Res 2006;4:138.

61. Tallgren LG, Liewendahl K, Kuhlbaeck B. The therapeutic success and nephrotoxicity of colistin in acute and chronic nephropathies with impaired renal function. Acta Med Scand 1965;177:717.

62. Duncan DA. Colistin toxicity. Neuromuscular and renal manifestations. Two cases treated by hemodialysis. Minn Med 1973;56:31.

63. Elwood CM, Lucas GD, Muehrcke RC. Acute renal failure associated with sodium colistimethate treatment. Arch Intern Med 1966;118:326.

64. Berlana D, Llop JM, Fort E, et al. Use of colistin in the treatment of multiple-drug-resistant gram-negative infections. Am J Health Syst Pharm 2005;62:39.

65. Kwa AL, Loh C, Low JG, et al. Nebulized colistin in the treatment of pneumonia due to multidrug-resistant Acinetobacter baumannii and Pseudomonas aeruginosa. Clin Infect Dis 2005;41:754.

66. Michalopoulos A, Kasiakou SK, Mastora Z, et al. Aerosolized colistan for the treatment of nosocomial pneumonia due to multidrug-resistant Gram-negative bacteria in patients without cystic fibrosis. Crit Care 2005;9:R53–9. DOI:10.1186/cc3020.

67. Falagas ME, Kasiakou SK. Colistin: the revival of polymyxins for the management of multidrug-resistant gram-negative bacterial infections. Clin Infect Dis 2005;40:1333.

68. Michalopoulos A, Fotakis D, Virtzili S, et al. Aerosolized colistin as adjunctive treatment of ventilator-associated pneumonia due to multidrug-resistant Gram-negative bacteria: a prospective study. Respir Med 2008;102:407.

69. Karageorgopoulos DE, Falagas ME. Current control and treatment of multidrug-resistant Acinetobacter baumannii infections. Lancet Infect Dis 2008;8:751.

70. Rios FG, Luna CM, Maskin B, et al. Ventilator-associated pneumonia due to colistin susceptible-only microorganisms. Eur Respir J 2007;30:307.

71. Li J, Nation RL, Milne RW, et al. Evaluation of colistin as an agent against multi-resistant Gram-negative bacteria. Int J Antimicrob Agents 2005;25:11.

72. Kofteridis DP, Alexopoulou C, Valachis A, et al. Aerosolized plus intravenous colistin versus intravenous colistin alone for the treatment of ventilator-associated pneumonia: a matched case-control study. Clin Infect Dis 2010;51:1238.

73. Korbila IP, Michalopoulos A, Rafailidis PI, et al. Inhaled colistin as adjunctive therapy to intravenous colistin for the treatment of microbiologically documented ventilator-associated pneumonia: a comparative cohort study. Clin Microbiol Infect 2010;16: 1230.

74. Munoz-Price LS, Weinstein RA. Acinetobacter infection. N Engl J Med 2008;358:1271.

75. Moffatt JH, Harper M, Harrison P, et al. Colistin resistance in Acinetobacter baumannii is mediated by complete loss of lipopolysaccharide production. Antimicrob Agents Chemother 2010;54:4971.

76. Palmer LB, Baram D, Gunther MS, et al. Aerosolized vancomycin for treatment of Gram-positive respiratory infection in mechanically ventilated patients. Am J Respir Crit Care Med 2003;167(7):A604.

77. Rattanaumpawan PLJ, Ungprasert P, Angkasekwinai N, et al. Randomized controlled trial of nebulized colistimethate sodium as adjunctive therapy of ventilator-associated pneumonia caused by Gram-negative bacteria. J Antimicrob Chemother 2010; 65(12):2645–9.

78. Nseir S, Di Pompeo C, Pronnier P, et al. Nosocomial tracheobronchitis in mechanically ventilated patients: incidence, aetiology and outcome. Eur Respir J 2002;20(6):1483–9.

79. Nseir S, Di Pompeo C, Soubrier S, et al. Outcomes of ventilated COPD patients with nosocomial tracheobronchitis: a case-control study. Infection 2004; 32(4):210–6.

80. Nseir S, Di Pompeo C, Soubrier S, et al. Effect of ventilator-associated tracheobronchitis on outcome in patients without chronic respiratory failure: a case-control study. Crit Care 2005;9(3):R238–45.

81. Garner JS, Jarvis WR, Emori TG, et al. CDC definitions for nosocomial infections, 1988. Am J Infect Control 1988;16(3):128–40.

82. Nseir S, Favory R, Jozefowicz E, et al. Antimicrobial treatment for ventilator-associated tracheobronchitis: a randomized, controlled multicenter study. Crit Care 2008;12:R62 doi:1186/cc6890.

83. Craven DE, Chroneou A, Zias N, et al. Ventilator-associated tracheobronchitis: the impact of targeted

antibiotic therapy on patient outcomes. Chest 2009; 135(2):521–8.

84. Nseir S, Ader F, Marquette CH. Nosocomial tracheobronchitis. Curr Opin Infect Dis 2009;22(2):148–53.

85. Kampf G, Wischnewski N, Schulgen G, et al. Prevalence and risk factors for nosocomial lower respiratory tract infections in German hospitals. J Clin Epidemiol 1998;51(6):495–502.

86. Rello J, Ausina V, Castella J, et al. Nosocomial respiratory tract infections in multiple trauma patients. Influence of level of consciousness with implications for therapy. Chest 1992;102(2):525–9.

87. Hortal J, Munoz P, Cuerpo G, et al. Ventilator-associated pneumonia in patients undergoing major heart surgery: an incidence study in Europe. Crit Care 2009;13(3):R80.

Should Management of Pneumonia be an Indicator of Quality of Care?

Mark L. Metersky, MD

KEYWORDS

- Pneumonia, Bacterial • Community-acquired pneumonia
- Performance measurement • Public reporting
- Quality improvement • Guideline
- Quality indicators, Health care • Guideline adherence

There is overwhelming evidence that the quality of medical care provided in the United States is frequently not optimal.[1] This realization has prompted extensive efforts by regulatory agencies, payers, and purchasers to encourage quality improvement through the use of financial incentives, disincentives, and public reporting programs.[2] Adherence by the provider to measureable indices of quality of care generally serves as the basis for these efforts. For several reasons that are discussed in detail, the care provided to patients hospitalized with pneumonia has been one of the most frequent components of hospital performance measurement programs. In this article, the rationale for targeting pneumonia care is examined. The strengths and weaknesses of the evidence base in support of specific performance measurement are also critically reviewed. Because community-acquired pneumonia (CAP) in the hospital has been the target of performance measurement programs more frequently than ventilator-associated pneumonia, this article is limited to CAP (**Table 1** lists Center for Medicare & Medicaid Services [CMS] CAP performance measures). However, the article should provide a useful framework for evaluating the appropriateness of performance measurement programs directed at other types of pneumonia, such as ventilator-associated pneumonia or outpatient-treated CAP.

QUALITY OF CARE AND PNEUMONIA

There are several factors to consider when determining whether it is useful to measure quality of care for a given disease process. The first that must be considered is whether the disease is important enough to spend time and resources assessing quality of care. On a population basis, is the disease common enough and does it cause enough morbidity, mortality, or cost such that it is an appropriate use of resources to measure and report quality of care?

There can be little debate that pneumonia is a condition that has a great societal impact. More than 5 million cases occur each year in the United States, of which approximately 1.2 million result in admission to the hospital.[3] The in-hospital mortality was 4.7% during 2003 to 2005, whereas the 30-day mortality of admitted Medicare patients is 12%.[4] Furthermore, an abundance of literature shows that patients who survive an episode of pneumonia have increased risk of

Disclosures: Dr Metersky has served as a consultant to the Centers for Medicare & Medicaid Services and to Qualidigm (Connecticut's Medicare Quality Improvement Organization) on various quality improvement and patient safety initiatives. His employer has received remuneration for some of these activities.
Funding source: None.
Division of Pulmonary and Critical Care Medicine, University of Connecticut Health Center, 263 Farmington Avenue, Farmington, CT 06030-1321, USA
E-mail address: Metersky@nso.uchc.edu

Clin Chest Med 32 (2011) 575–589
doi:10.1016/j.ccm.2011.05.005
0272-5231/11/$ – see front matter © 2011 Elsevier Inc. All rights reserved.

Table 1
CMS CAP measures

Measure	Status
PN-1 Oxygenation assessment	Discontinued
PN-2 Pneumococcal vaccination	Likely to be discontinued[a]
PN-3a Blood cultures performed within 24 h for patients admitted to ICU	Active
PN-3b Blood cultures (if performed) collected before antibiotics collected before initial antibiotic received in hospital	Active
PN-4 Smoking cessation counseling	Likely to be discontinued[b]
PN-5 Antibiotic timing (median)	Active
PN-5a Initial antibiotic within 8 h of hospital arrival	Discontinued
PN-5b Initial antibiotic within 4 h of hospital arrival	Discontinued
PN-5c Initial antibiotic within 6 h of hospital arrival	Active
PN-6 Initial antibiotic selection for CAP in immunocompetent patients	Active
PN-6a Initial antibiotic selection for CAP in immunocompetent patients: ICU patients	Active
PN-6b Initial antibiotic selection for CAP in immunocompetent patients: non-ICU patients	Active
PN-7 Influenza vaccination	Likely to be discontinued[a]

[a] Will probably be replaced by a measure encompassing all appropriate hospitalized patients.
[b] Endorsement withdrawn by the National Quality Forum.

mortality for many months compared with patients with similar levels of comorbidities without pneumonia.[5] The direct cost of caring for patients with pneumonia in the United States is approximately $17 billion, of which about half is related to the few patients who are admitted to the hospital.[3]

Pneumonia Guideline Adherence

Despite the great cost to society, it is only useful to measure and report the quality of pneumonia care if there is credible evidence that there is a gap between the best possible care and how care is actually delivered. The definition of optimum care evolves as knowledge is gained. However, if we assume that adherence to evidence-based guidelines is a reasonable surrogate for optimum quality of care, there is ample evidence that pneumonia care often is not concordant with guideline recommendations.

In 1 study, patients admitted to 5 community hospitals with CAP in the winter of 1999 to 2000 received guideline-concordant antibiotic therapy in only 57% of cases.[6] In 2004, Mortensen and colleagues[7] reported that among 420 patients admitted with CAP to 2 tertiary teaching hospitals, only 323 (77%) received guideline-concordant antibiotic therapy. Similar low rates of guideline-concordant antibiotic use have been measured in a study encompassing hospitals in Europe, Asia, the United States, and South America.[8] Adherence to the pneumonia CMS/Joint Commission core measure for the use of a guideline-concordant antibiotic regimen was 83% as recently as 2005, but had improved to approximately 90% in 2010 (Dale Bratzler, DO, MPH, Medicare National Pneumonia Project, personal communication, 2011).

Other studies have shown frequent lack of adherence to additional guideline-recommended processes of care. In 1994 to 1995, when blood cultures were recommended for all patients admitted to the hospital with pneumonia, Meehan and colleagues[9] found that only 69% of Medicare patients had blood cultures performed. Although the usefulness of performing blood cultures on all patients with pneumonia has been questioned,[10] guidelines still recommend blood cultures for all patients sick enough to go to the intensive care unit (ICU).[11] Recent data show that even for ICU patients, approximately 10% of patients did not have blood cultures performed within 24 hours of arrival (Dale Bratzler, DO, MPH, Medicare National Pneumonia Project, personal communication, 2011).

Although there has been great controversy regarding the appropriateness of the 4-hour rule for the timing of initial antibiotics, few would argue that patients who receive antibiotics after a delay of longer than 8 hours have received good care. Yet, in 1994 to 1995, 25% of patients did not receive their first dose of antibiotics within 8 hours of presentation.[9] Although there has since been improvement, even in 2004, more than 10% of patients did not receive antibiotics within 8 hours of presentation to the hospital (Dale Bratzler, DO, MPH, Medicare National Pneumonia Project, personal communication, 2011).

Is There a Link Between Processes of Care and Outcomes of Pneumonia?

Before it can be asserted that measuring quality of care for a specific condition can drive improvements in outcomes, there needs to be evidence that deviations from the recommended processes of care result in worsened outcomes. In this section, the evidence in favor of a link between pneumonia care in general and patient outcomes is reviewed. Evidence for each specific process of care is discussed subsequently.

Several lines of evidence suggest that the quality of care provided to patients hospitalized with pneumonia influences patient outcomes. After adjustment for baseline comorbidities and severity of illness, among Medicare patients, hospital-specific risk-adjusted 30-day CAP mortality varies widely, from 6.7% to 20.9%.[12] Although some of these differences are presumably related to the presence of unknown confounders, it seems likely that given the wide range in mortality, some of this variation is related to quality of care.

In addition, several observational studies have reported worsened outcomes in patients with CAP who did not receive guideline-concordant care. In a multinational study, adherence to Infectious Diseases Society of America/American Thoracic Society (IDSA/ATS) guidelines[11] for antibiotic regimen was associated with a lower mortality (8% vs 17%).[13] In the United States, guideline-nonconcordant antibiotic therapy was associated with increased propensity-adjusted 30-day mortality (odds ratio 5.7).[6] Among more than 54,000 patients hospitalized with pneumonia in Canada, guideline-concordant antibiotic therapy was associated with an adjusted mortality with a 30% lower risk.[14] Several other observational studies have shown a similar association between the use of guideline-adherent antibiotics and improved outcomes.[15–17] These observational studies all share the same limitation that the observed differences might be the result of unmeasured patient-related or provider-related factors not included in the multivariate analysis.[18] For example, patients with unusual presentations, and those at risk for aspiration pneumonia, may be at higher risk of mortality and might be more likely to be treated with a nonadherent antibiotic regimen. Randomized controlled studies are rare in the quality improvement literature, with pneumonia being no exception. However, several pre-post time series interventions have investigated the effect of guideline implementation interventions on patient outcomes.

Dean and colleagues[19,20] measured 30-day mortality among patients in Utah admitted to the hospital with pneumonia before and after initiation of a pneumonia guideline at Intermountain Healthcare. Whereas the mortality before the implementation of the guideline was similar for patients treated by physicians who were and were not affiliated with Intermountain Healthcare (13.4% vs 13.2%), after implementation of the guidelines, mortality fell to 11.0% among Intermountain Healthcare-affiliated physicians and increased to 14.2% for nonaffiliated physicians. Capelastegui and colleagues[21] performed a pre-post analysis after implementation of a pneumonia practice guideline and compared outcomes with those at 4 other hospitals. Guideline implementation resulted in a shorter hospital length of stay and improved adjusted in-hospital and 30-day mortality, whereas there were insignificant changes at the control hospitals. Although these studies provide stronger evidence than purely observational studies, they suffer from weaknesses such as lack of adequate correction for potential background temporal trends in patient outcomes, and the possibility that other systems or process changes unrelated to the guidelines influenced the observed outcomes. This finding could account for the results seen by Yealy and colleagues,[22] who randomized 32 hospital emergency departments in Connecticut and Pennsylvania to receive 1 of 3 different intensities of pneumonia guideline implementation. Although higher adherence to 4 pneumonia process of care recommendations were seen in the high-intensity hospitals, this did not translate into improved outcomes for either outpatients or inpatients. More low-risk patients at the high-intensity hospitals were appropriately treated as outpatients, likely representing a significant cost savings.

Although patient outcomes must be the primary determinant of appropriate care, there is no doubt that cost is an important factor to consider. There are wide variations between hospitals in pneumonia length of stay and cost[23] that are not explained by differences in severity of illness. The cost related to the admission to the hospital of patients who could safely be cared for as outpatients is likely even greater. The CAPITAL study[24] randomized hospitals in Canada to receive usual care in the emergency department or decision support using the pneumonia severity index (PSI).[25] Eighteen percent fewer low-risk patients were admitted to the intervention hospitals, without any worsening in outcomes. Similar results were seen in the study by Yealy and colleagues[22] mentioned earlier, in which approximately 24% fewer low-risk patients were admitted to the hospitals randomized to high-intensity and moderate-intensity guideline implementation, compared with low intensity. Given the tremendous costs associated with pneumonia care, there are extensive ongoing efforts in the United States to define efficiency or value standards for the care of patients with pneumonia, when these terms are defined as quality of care adjusted for cost.

In summary, there is a large body of literature showing wide variations in the quality of care provided to patients hospitalized with pneumonia, and there is evidence that these variations can be diminished, with resulting improved outcomes. This evidence has been summarized by Martinez and colleagues[26] in a recent review. Clearly, pneumonia is responsible for a large burden of disease, with resulting morbidity and mortality and tremendous expense to society. However, one must accept that measuring and reporting quality of care can help to drive improvement, before affirming that it is important to expend resources doing so which brings us back to the question asked by the title of this article, "Should management of pneumonia be an indicator of quality of care?"

Although a thorough review of quality improvement literature is beyond the scope of this article, a brief summary is appropriate. A central tenet of quality improvement, whether in industry or medicine, is that you cannot improve what you cannot measure. Without measurement, one may not convince stakeholders that there is need for improvement. In addition, without measurement, it is impossible to determine if a quality improvement intervention has truly resulted in an improvement, either as determined by improvement in the processes of care, or in improved outcomes. Thus, the need for measuring the effectiveness of how we care for patients is difficult to refute. More controversial are the issues of what should be measured, who is doing the measuring, to whom the results are disseminated, and what rewards or disincentives are based on the measurement results. There is ample evidence that internally measuring performance, feeding back the results, and implementing systems changes can be a highly effective method of improving quality.[27] Recently, there has been increasing use of performance measurement by external groups such as payers and regulatory agencies, with public reporting of the results using benchmarking data. It is hoped that doing so will drive improved quality by helping patients to identify and seek out the higher-quality providers. The theory is that increasing the volume at higher-quality providers improves the overall quality on a population basis.

In addition, lower-performing providers would be spurred to improve quality, to avoid losing market share. However, at this time there is little evidence that large numbers of patients access the websites that provide quality data, and even less evidence that patients act on those results to choose their provider. On the other hand, there has been marked improvement in the rate of performance by hospitals of the pneumonia core measures since public reporting of these measures began in the late 1990s (**Table 2**). It is unclear how much of this improvement was driven by the fact that these measures were being reported, and how much was driven by the fear that in the near future, reimbursement by Medicare would be based in part on performance. Significant improvements in pneumonia outcomes can also be seen during this period, (see **Table 2**) although it is impossible to determine which, if any, of these process improvements are driving the improved outcomes.

A cogent argument can be made for measuring and reporting to providers information regarding the quality of their pneumonia care. The controversy lies in what aspects of care are reported, the potential for unintended negative consequences of performance measurement, whether public reporting is an effective tool for improving quality, and the appropriateness of financial incentives and disincentives based on the pneumonia measures. At some level, the discussion is moot, because tremendous economic and societal forces are behind the increased use of performance measurement. Thus, performance measurement is here to stay. However, it is hoped that discussion of the attributes of specific performance measures can provide guidance regarding how performance measures for pneumonia can be most effectively used.

Outcomes Measures or Process Measures?

There is ongoing debate as to whether it is more useful to use outcomes measures or process measures to assess quality of care.[28] There are advantages and disadvantages to each. Outcomes measures have the advantage of assessing what we care about most, how the patient fared as a result of interaction with the medical system. Outcomes such as mortality or readmission rates have obvious importance. The other advantage is that the use of outcomes measures allows a provider to achieve a good result in the manner that best fits their system. For example, there is no penalty for using the wrong antibiotic, if the antibiotic is used in pathogen-directed therapy and leads to good outcomes. In addition, a hospital

Table 2
Trends in pneumonia process measure performance and outcomes[a]

	1998	2000	2002	2004	2006	2008
Outcomes						
Length of stay (d)	6.7	6.6	6.4	6.2	6.1	—
In-hospital mortality (%)	9.2	9.5	10.2	7.1	5.5	—
30-day mortality (%)	15.3	16.3	15.7	12.9	11.4	—
30-day readmission (%)	15.5	18.9	18.3	16.3	16.8	—
Process Measure Adherence (%)						
Antibiotic dose within 4 h	57	59	64	70	82	—
Antibiotic dose within 6 h	—	—	—	—	—	95
Antibiotic dose within 8 h	83	84	88	90	—	—
Antibiotic selection according to guidelines	—	59	71	76	85	89
Blood culture within 24 h (ICU patients only, starting in 2006)	61	62	60	73	91	93
Oxygenation assessment	92	94	98	99	100	—
Pneumococcal vaccine	8	15	28	50	78	91
Influenza vaccine	10	12	29	47	68	90

[a] For data from 1998 to 2004, the charts were abstracted by CMS clinical data abstraction centers, quarter 4, 2006 and 2008 data are hospital self-collected.
  Dale Bratzler, DO, MPH, Medicare National Pneumonia Project, personal communication, 2011.

where outcomes are being measured will be encouraged to address important aspects of care that are not addressed in the common performance measures, for example issues related to care transitions. The other advantage of outcomes measurements is that they are often amenable to calculation through the use of administrative datasets, preventing the need for costly and time-consuming chart review.

The major disadvantage of outcomes measures is the need for risk adjustment. Most outcomes are greatly affected by underlying patient characteristics that may differ greatly from hospital to hospital. Furthermore, without risk adjustment, perverse incentives can be created, with resulting negative unintended consequences. For example, without credible risk adjustment, providers would have an incentive to avoid sicker patients or patients with lower socioeconomic status. However, risk adjustment is not perfect, and the methodology is generally not reproducible by providers, so there may be less acceptance of the results of risk-adjusted outcomes measures compared with process measures.

Process measures have the advantages of simplicity and transparency. A measured low rate of adherence to appropriate antibiotic usage is immediately understandable and credible to the provider. In contrast to outcomes measure, they are generally actionable. A hospital confronted with a high risk-standardized 30-day mortality may not be able to readily identify and fix the problems leading to this poor performance. On the other hand, a hospital finding a low rate of use of guideline-concordant antibiotics can easily fix the problem. However, many process measures have been criticized because they have been implemented without a firm evidence base. Studies in pneumonia and other disease states have shown that adherence to some common process measures explains only a small amount of the variation in outcomes such as mortality.[29] Another disadvantage of process measures is that many require chart review and are therefore expensive.

PERFORMANCE MEASUREMENT CRITERIA

Before being adopted for use, a performance measure should meet a set of standards to make sure that the measure yields accurate, useful data. Four criteria used by the National Quality Forum (NQF), the independent organization that reviews and approves performance measures in the United States, provide an excellent framework for assessing performance measures. After a brief review of the NQF measure criteria, specific pneumonia measures are reviewed, using the framework provided by the NQF criteria.[30] **Table 3** shows the attributes of the CAP measures, based on the NQF framework.

Table 3
Attributes of the CAP performance measures, based on the NQF measurement criteria and potential for producing unintended negative consequences

Performance Measure	Importance	Scientific Acceptability	Usability	Feasibility	Unintended Negative Consequences
Assessment of oxygenation[a]	Limited evidence of process-outcome link, minimal opportunity for improvement	No significant issues	Limited, because performance is already near 100%	Minimal burden of extraction, especially with EHR	Minimal risk
Blood cultures for ICU patients	Limited evidence of process-outcome link	No significant issues	Results easily usable to guide process improvement	Minimal burden of extraction, especially with EHR	Overuse may lead to prolonged length of stay and increased vancomycin use (because of false-positive results)
Blood cultures before antibiotics	Strong evidence of increased yield, limited evidence of process-outcome link	No significant issues	Results easily usable to guide process improvement	Minimal burden of extraction, especially with EHR	Could theoretically result in delayed antibiotic treatment
Antibiotics within 6 h of presentation	Several observational studies support process-outcome link for antibiotic timing, controversial because of potential role of confounders	No significant issues	Results easily usable to guide process improvement	Minimal burden of extraction, especially with EHR	Less with 6 h than 4 h, but still theoretical potential for antibiotic overuse in patients without proven pneumonia
Antibiotic according to guidelines	Many observational studies support a process-outcome link, limited amount of prospective, randomized data	No significant issues	Results easily usable to guide process improvement	Minimal burden of extraction, especially with EHR or pharmacy database	Minimal risk

Prevention[a] Tobacco counseling Influenza vaccination Pneumococcal vaccination	Limited for tobacco cessation counseling and pneumococcal vaccination, given the weak evidence of impact on patient outcomes	No significant issues	Results easily usable to guide process improvement	Minimal burden of extraction, especially with EHR	Overuse because of inappropriate repeat vaccination
30-day risk-standardized mortality	High	Potential concern about adequacy of a risk-adjustment model that does not include data regarding severity of acute illness	Does not identify specific processes needing improvement	No issues, calculated by CMS	Potential that hospitals could inappropriately transfer out high-risk patients
30-day risk-standardized readmission rate	High	Potential concern about adequacy of a risk-adjustment model that does not include data regarding severity of acute illness	Does not identify specific processes needing improvement	No issues, calculated by CMS	Potential that hospitals could inappropriately transfer out high-risk patients

Abbreviation: EHR, electronic health record.
[a] These measures either have been or are likely to be discontinued.

Importance

Is the disease important enough to justify the resources required to measure and report quality of care? Specifically, is the disease common enough and associated with enough morbidity, mortality, or resource use such that poor quality care results in a significant negative impact on society? For process measures, the extent to which lack of adherence to the recommended process of care results in worsened outcomes must be considered. If there is little evidence that a recommended process of care affects outcomes, there is little justification for measuring its performance. This has been a particular issue with the pneumonia measures. In contrast to cardiac measures, there are few large randomized studies that provide evidence about pneumonia care. A recent systematic review accompanied by meta-analyses of the pneumonia measures showed that although there was evidence in support of all of the pneumonia measures except for hospital-based tobacco cessation counseling, the evidence was generally of low quality.[31] The investigators felt that only influenza vaccination and guideline-concordant antibiotic therapy had a robust enough evidence base to support their use as performance measures.

No matter how important a disease or a process of care is, it is useful to systematically measure and report quality of care only if there is evidence that there are gaps in quality. If the overall performance rate of process of care is high, there is limited benefit in measuring and reporting that process. An example of this is the assessment of oxygenation status in patients with pneumonia. This criterion was dropped as a pneumonia core measure when the overall performance rate reached more than 99%.

Scientific Acceptability of the Measure Properties

The measurement must produce results that are reliable, valid, and credible. This has generally not been a problem for the pneumonia process measures, although the potential for such problems exists. For example, a measure designed to assess the appropriateness of care of patients diagnosed with pneumonia in the outpatient setting initially relied on the diagnosis of pneumonia from claims data.[32] The investigators initially found that a high percentage of patients did not receive antibiotics. Only then was it determined that many patients were being seen for follow-up of a previous episode of pneumonia. In addition, exceptions must be considered and dealt with appropriately. For example, a measure of

appropriate antibiotic use must have a built-in allowance for penicillin allergy. There has also been concern regarding the scientific acceptability of outcomes measures, because even the best risk adjustment does not explain all variation.

Usability

The results must be understandable and must provide information that can be used to improve quality or cost of care. Can a provider use the results to improve their own quality of care? Can a patient or payer use the results to preferentially seek out physicians who provide higher quality of care? For example, in a year when influenza vaccine is in short supply, a measure of vaccination rates will likely provide data that, although accurate, will not be useful.

Feasibility

Can the data elements required for the measure be attained without undue burden? The ideal measure requires only data elements that can be collected without the need for manual chart review, for example data for an antibiotic appropriateness measure might be available from an electronic pharmacy database, minimizing the burden of data collection. However, there is often a trade-off between acceptability/accuracy of the results and simplifying data collection through the use of administrative data or automated electronic health record searches.

Unintended Negative Consequences of Performance Measurement

In addition to the above 4 NQF measure evaluation criteria, it is important to assess the potential for unintended negative consequences related to the implementation of any performance measure. This issue has received much attention related to the concern that measuring the promptness of antibiotic delivery to patients with CAP has resulted in excessive use of antibiotics in patients ultimately not diagnosed with pneumonia (see later discussion).[33]

SPECIFIC CAP MEASURES
Process Measures: Assessment and Diagnosis

Measurement of oxygenation status
Although it makes intuitive sense that detecting unrecognized hypoxemia is an important thing to do, there is limited evidence that significant patient harm results from the failure to measure oxygenation. One might theorize that in the more severely ill patients, physicians rarely neglect to determine oxygenation, so that increasing the

rate of performance for this process measure only increases the measurement of oxygenation status in patients who are unlikely to be hypoxic. For several years, in the United States, the average performance rate for this measure has been approximately 99%, diminishing the importance of measurement. For this reason, assessment of oxygenation status is no longer a performance measure tracked by CMS or the Joint Commission.

Performance of blood cultures

For many years, guidelines recommended that all patients admitted to the hospital with CAP have blood cultures performed.[34] There was limited evidence that such a practice improved outcomes. Although 1 study did report an approximately 10% lower mortality associated with blood culture performance,[9] this finding was believed to be a result of confounding. Because the rate of bacteremia in patients with CAP is less than 10% in most studies, it seems implausible that the performance of blood cultures could lead to such a large improvement in mortality. More likely, physicians who performed blood cultures routinely followed other recommended processes, accounting for the findings.

The routine performance of blood cultures on all patients admitted to the hospital was called into question by several studies that revealed extremely low yields of blood cultures in low-risk patients and questioned the cost effectiveness of routine blood culture performance.[10,35] Subsequently, a study by Metersky and colleagues[36] of more than 13,000 Medicare patients hospitalized with pneumonia found several predictors of bacteremia that were corroborated in a similar sized validation cohort. Because age was not an independent predictor of bacteremia, but has a large impact on the PSI, the PSI did not perform so well in predicting the risk of bacteremia. Furthermore, the percentage of patients with false-positive blood cultures (5.0%) was higher than the rate of true-positive blood cultures in patients with none of the noted predictors (2.5%). Adding to the concern about the negative consequences of routine blood culture performance, patients with false-positive blood cultures had a rate of vancomycin usage approximately 3 times greater and a risk-adjusted length of stay 1 day higher than patients with negative blood cultures. Based on these data, the most recent CAP guidelines[11] consider blood cultures optional unless the patient is seriously ill or has certain other risk factors for bacteremia or an unusual infection. In addition, because previous antibiotics decrease the yield of blood cultures by approximately 50%, the guidelines recommend that if

blood cultures are going to be performed, they be drawn before antibiotics are provided. Reflecting these changes in the guidelines, the current CMS performance measure regarding blood cultures is the percentage of blood cultures drawn before antibiotics are started. The Joint Commission also uses this measure, and in addition assesses the percentage of patients admitted to the ICU within 24 hours of presentation in whom at least 1 blood culture is performed. Although the performance of blood cultures makes intuitive sense, even in severely ill patients there is no convincing evidence that the performance of blood cultures improves patient outcomes. Rather, the current measures are based on expert opinion that in some cases identifying the pathogen may lead to more accurate antibiotic therapy. Given the weak evidence base, these measures are also designed to minimize the potential harm caused by the indiscriminate use of blood cultures.

Process Measures: Treatment

Timing of initial antibiotics

Perhaps no quality indicator in all of medicine has created as much controversy as the antibiotic timing measure for patients with CAP.[33,37,38] In 1997, Meehan and colleagues[9] reported a significantly increased 30-day mortality in Medicare patients admitted to the hospital with pneumonia in whom antibiotic therapy did not start until after at least 8 hours from the time of hospital presentation. After Houck and colleagues[39] reported significantly lower mortality in patients who received antibiotics within 4 hours in a similarly designed study, CMS and the Joint Commission in 2003 adopted a 4-hour target for the performance measure regarding the timing of antibiotics. There has been great concern about the use of antibiotic timing as a publicly reported performance metric for several reasons. It has been argued that the association between delayed antibiotics and mortality may be a result of confounding. For example, patients with an abnormal mental status are at higher risk of mortality, and receive antibiotics later, likely because of increased difficulty in obtaining an adequate history and physical examination.[40] It has been suggested that the increased risk of mortality in patients who received their antibiotics after 4 hours may be a result of a higher rate of delirium in these patients. After the institution of the 4-hour timing measure, retrospective studies documented an increased percentage of patients admitted with a diagnosis of pneumonia whose discharge diagnosis was not pneumonia.[41,42] The implication was that patients were being given a diagnosis of pneumonia prematurely to avoid a late diagnosis and a failure on the antibiotic timing measure. Another report suggested that an outbreak of *Clostridium difficile* colitis at 1 hospital may have been in part related to inappropriate antibiotic use as a result of the antibiotic timing measure.[43] None of the other reports related to this issue found evidence of patient harm related to the antibiotic timing measure.[41,42] A retrospective study[44] of 86 Medicare patients admitted to the hospital with pneumonia attempted to determine what percentage of patients ultimately diagnosed with pneumonia could reasonably be expected to have the diagnosis made within 4 hours of presentation. The results substantiated concern regarding a 4-hour target, because the investigators determined that 22% of the patients presented in an atypical manner such that even with high quality of care, it would have been unlikely that a diagnosis of pneumonia could have been made and antibiotics delivered, within 4 hours. Another frequently mentioned concern about the 4-hour timing measure was the possibility that the increased attention to patients with pneumonia might lead to less timely care for patients in the emergency department with more acutely life-threatening conditions.

Based on concerns about inappropriate antibiotic use as a result of the 4-hour measure, the antibiotic timing measure was changed to 6 hours in 2008. The current IDSA/ATS CAP guidelines[11] do not mention a specific goal for the timing of antibiotics, but state that they should be given while the patient is in the emergency department to minimize delays. Although the CMS pneumonia technical expert panel considered adopting this measure instead of a specific timing measure, there was concern that in many hospitals patients often stay in the emergency department for 12 to 24 hours before being transferred to the hospital floor, so that antibiotic treatment could be unduly delayed, yet still satisfy the measure by being given in the emergency department.

Antibiotic selection

Of the many processes of care that have been used or proposed as performance measures, it seems likely that the use of guideline-adherent antibiotics would be the most important contributor to patient outcomes. Antibiotic guidelines are based on several concepts: the recognition that most antibiotic treatment of CAP is empiric; the need to cover both sensitive and resistant strains of *Streptococcus pneumoniae*, the most common cause of CAP; the recognition that the atypicals cause a substantial percentage of CAP; observational data showing improved outcomes associated with dual antibiotic coverage in severely ill patients; and the need for specific antibiotic coverage in patients at risk for *Pseudomonas* pneumonia.[11] None of these rationales is based on high-quality randomized data. Nonetheless, a large body of observational data support the use of 2 antibiotics in severely ill patients[45,46] and antibiotics active against atypical agents[47,48] (although there is evidence that much of the observed benefit related to these issues derives from nonantibacterial effects of macrolides, which are often the second antibiotic[49,50]). Based on these data and the ATS/IDSA[11] antibiotic recommendations, the current antibiotic selection performance measure (**Table 4**) requires atypical coverage for all patients and 2 antibiotics for patients admitted to the ICU within 24 hours of presentation. For the rare patient with CAP with risk factors for *Pseudomonas* infection, specific antipseudomonal coverage may be used. The trend in adherence to the antibiotic selection measure is shown in **Table 2**. Most cases of nonadherence to this measure result from monotherapy with a fluoroquinolone in patients with CAP admitted to the ICU. Although some analyses have questioned the benefits of atypical coverage,[51,52] there has been minimal opposition in the United States to the current antibiotic measures.

Process Measures: Prevention

Tobacco cessation counseling, pneumococcal vaccination, and influenza vaccination

Tobacco cessation counseling for patients hospitalized with pneumonia has lost its endorsement by the NQF as a performance measure, because of limited evidence of benefit of single contact counseling at the time of discharge. Although the vaccination measures are currently applied only to patients admitted with pneumonia, they will soon be applied to all admitted patients (with specific exceptions). Because of the frequent difficulty in determining vaccine status, and the financial incentives associated with these measures, hospitals frequently err on the side of vaccinating if vaccination status cannot be determined. Anecdotes regarding patients being vaccinated 2 or 3 times in a season are commonly heard. A study performed before public reporting of hospital-based vaccination rates found that 18% of hospital-based influenza vaccination led to inappropriate duplicate vaccination.[53] Although there is minimal likelihood of patient harm from duplicate influenza vaccination, this finding certainly represents a waste of time and resources. Because pneumococcal vaccination status is even more

Table 4
Medicare National Pneumonia Project recommended antibiotics

Patient Type	Antibiotic Recommendation
Non-ICU patient	β-lactam (IV or IM) + macrolide (IV or PO) or antipneumococcal quinolone monotherapy (IV or PO) or β-lactam (IV or IM) + either doxycycline (IV or PO) or tigecycline (IV) or if less than 65 y old with no risk factors for drug-resistant *Pneumococcus* Macrolide monotherapy (IV or PO) β-lactam = ceftriaxone, cefotaxime, ampicillin/sulbactam, ertapenem (ceftaroline effective January 1, 2012) Macrolide = erythromycin, clarithromycin, azithromycin Antipneumococcal quinolones = levofloxacin,[a] moxifloxacin, gemifloxacin
Non-ICU patient with pseudomonal risk	These antibiotics are acceptable for non-ICU patients with pseudomonal risk only: antipneumococcal/antipseudomonal β-lactam (IV) + antipseudomonal quinolone (IV or PO) or antipneumococcal/antipseudomonal β-lactam (IV) + aminoglycoside (IV) + either antipneumococcal quinolone (IV or PO) or macrolide (IV or PO) The following antibiotics are only acceptable for non-ICU patients with β-lactam allergy and pseudomonal risk: aztreonam (IV or IM) + antipneumococcal quinolone (IV or PO) + aminoglycoside (IV) or aztreonam[b] (IV or IM) + levofloxacin[a] (IV or PO) Antipseudomonal quinolone = ciprofloxacin, levofloxacin[a] Antipneumococcal/antipseudomonal β-lactam = cefepime, imipenem, meropenem, piperacillin/tazobactam, doripenem Aminoglycoside = gentamicin, tobramycin, amikacin Antipneumococcal quinolone = levofloxacin,[a] moxifloxacin, gemifloxacin Macrolide = erythromycin, clarithromycin, azithromycin
ICU patient	Macrolide (IV) + either β-lactam (IV) or antipneumococcal/ antipseudomonal β-lactam (IV) or antipseudomonal quinolone (IV) + either β-lactam (IV) or antipneumococcal/antipseudomonal β-lactam (IV) or antipneumococcal quinolone (IV) + either β-lactam (IV) or antipneumococcal/antipseudomonal β-lactam (IV) or antipneumococcal/antipseudomonal β-lactam (IV) Aminoglycoside (IV) + either antipneumococcal quinolone (IV) or macrolide (IV) β-lactam = ceftriaxone, cefotaxime, ampicillin/sulbactam, Antipneumococcal/antipseudomonal β-lactam = cefepime, imipenem, meropenem, piperacillin/tazobactam, doripenem Macrolide = erythromycin, azithromycin Antipneumococcal quinolones = levofloxacin,[a] moxifloxacin Antipseudomonal quinolone = ciprofloxacin, levofloxacin[a] Aminoglycoside = gentamicin, tobramycin, amikacin

Abbreviations: IM, intramuscular; IV, intravenous; PO, by mouth.
[a] Levofloxacin should be used in 750-mg dosage when used in the management of patients with pneumonia.
[b] For patients with renal insufficiency.
Dale Bratzler, DO, MPH, Medicare National Pneumonia Project, personal communication, 2011.

difficult to determine than influenza vaccination status, this problem is likely more frequent with hospital-based pneumococcal vaccination.

Outcomes Measures

30-day risk-standardized mortality

Several factors make mortality a desirable outcome for assessing quality of care of pneumonia: it is easy to determine, it is a relatively common outcome, and it is of undeniable importance and relevance to patients. However, before accepting mortality as an appropriate performance measure, there must be credible evidence that quality of care affects mortality. Processes such as timing and choice of antibiotics have been linked to mortality, although generally not with prospective randomized studies. Others, such as assessment of oxygenation and the use of diagnostic testing such as sputum or blood cultures, have not been credibly shown to affect mortality. For this reason, although a logical outcome to report, it is not clear that this measure is easily actionable by hospitals as a base for a quality improvement intervention. With respect to the NQF usability criterion, although a mortality report might be useable by a payer or patient to avoid hospitals with excess mortality, such a report is less clearly usable by the hospital.

Since 2009, CMS has been publicly reporting hospitals' pneumonia risk-adjusted 30-day mortality on the Hospital Compare Web site.[54] Because of the tremendous cost that would be associated with a risk-adjustment methodology that depended on clinical data such as used in the PSI, a risk-adjustment methodology was devised that relies on patient characteristics and diagnosed comorbidities that can be derived from preexisting Medicare claims data.[12] Several implications of this methodology bear mentioning. First, because there is no chart review, there is no adjustment for acute severity of illness in the model. This factor has created concern regarding the validity of the risk adjustment. However, the model output correlates well with the PSI, which is based on both historical and clinical variables. In addition, the complex methodology limits the transparency of the measure; a hospital cannot double check the results for accuracy. There has also been concern that because 30-day mortality is being reported, hospitals are in part being judged on what happens to the patient after discharge. Although this situation is true, there are cogent reasons for using 30-day as opposed to in-hospital mortality. First, doing so avoids introducing a perverse incentive for hospitals to prematurely discharge patients to avoid an in-hospital death. In addition, measuring 30-day mortality provides an incentive for the hospital to avoid discharging patients before they have reached stability, and for smooth transitions in care (ie, effective discharge instructions, effective communication with the physician assuming responsibility for the patient's care, and even avoidance of chronic care facilities with questionable quality of care).

30-day risk-standardized readmission rate

Approximately 17% of Medicare patients discharged from the hospital after an episode of pneumonia and 12% of all patients with pneumonia are readmitted to an acute-care hospital within 30 days.[55] This finding clearly represents a tremendous source of potential patient harm and use of resources. Although there is limited evidence specifically for pneumonia that a large component of these readmissions are preventable, Halm and colleagues[56] reported that discharge of patients with pneumonia who were still unstable was frequently associated with post-discharge death or readmission. Other studies have shown that between 25% and 75% of readmissions overall are potentially preventable. It seems unlikely that pneumonia is an exception to this finding. Medicare intends to limit reimbursement for certain readmissions in the near future.

Not surprisingly, given the tremendous associated cost, readmission rates for individual hospitals are also reported on the Hospital Compare Web site. Like the 30-day risk-standardized mortality, this measure is based on a model derived from claims data.[12] Thus, the issues related to this measure are similar to those noted with the mortality measure.

Potential Future Pneumonia Performance Measures

Because the performance rates for several of the current pneumonia process measures approach 100%, there is ongoing discussion regarding potential new pneumonia performance measures. Potential opportunities for improvement in pneumonia care based on published literature include:

- Decreasing the rate of admission to the hospital of low-risk patients[22,24]
- Decreasing the rate of discharge of patients who are still unstable[56]
- Increasing the rate at which patients are switched from intravenous to oral therapy as soon as they are stable[57–59]
- Increasing the rate at which patients are discharged from the hospital as soon as they are stable.[23,60]

Physicians and hospital administrators should also be aware that payers are developing methodologies to track the cost of pneumonia episodes. By defining episodes of care, payers can hold providers responsible for not only the cost of the inpatient stay but also costs related to ongoing medical care related to that episode of pneumonia. One problem with the use of episodes of care relates to attribution of health care services. If a patient returns to the hospital after being treated for pneumonia, is that readmission attributable to the initial hospital, or to the primary care provider who did not have time to see the patient within a week of discharge?

SUMMARY

Pneumonia is common, costly, and responsible for a large burden of morbidity and mortality in the United States and the world. Based on the burden of disease, pneumonia is an appropriate target for performance measurement and systematic attempts to improve quality.

For more than 12 years, payers and regulatory bodies in the United States have been measuring a variety of processes and outcomes related to the care of patients hospitalized with pneumonia, to facilitate efforts to improve quality of care. Performance results were initially disseminated internally to the hospitals to assist efforts to improve care. Subsequently, public reporting and pay for performance programs have increased the ramifications related to performance measurement. There is no doubt that overall adherence to several processes of care has improved drastically since the inception of the performance measurement program. There have also been profound improvements in pneumonia outcomes over the last decade. The evidence that these improvements in outcomes are related to the measured process improvements must remain empirical, because we will never have trials in which patients are randomized to nonrecommended treatment.

Despite the improvements in pneumonia processes and outcomes, there have been concerns that the measurement program may have led to overuse of certain interventions and even risk of patient harm, as a result of both the lack of high-quality evidence in support of some measures (ie, blood cultures and antibiotic timing) and the application of certain processes of care to inappropriate patients to avoid failing a measure (antibiotic timing and hospital-based vaccination). Based on these concerns and as new evidence has become available, the measures have been modified on a regular basis.

Although any large-scale changes in processes of care will result in unexpected consequences, what is important is ensuring that the benefits outweigh the risks. Overall, it seems that the answer to the question posed by the title of this article should be "Yes, pneumonia quality of care should be measured", but with some caveats. New evidence must continually be evaluated to ensure that the measures are appropriately designed. We must continue to be vigilant in detecting and thoroughly investigating concerns of negative unintended consequences, even if merely anecdotal. The CMS National Pneumonia Project has a strong record of doing just this; many of the studies that prompted changes in the measures were performed by investigators collaborating with the leaders of the National Pneumonia Project. The need to diminish the cost of health care in the United States is creating tremendous pressure to use performance measurement as a method of doing so. Although cost control is an appropriate goal, physicians must do all in their power to fight against the use of measures that assess cost but ignore quality.

ACKNOWLEDGMENTS

The author would like to thank Dale Bratzler, DO, MPH, for his critical review of the manuscript.

REFERENCES

1. McGlynn EA, Asch SM, Adams J, et al. The quality of health care delivered to adults in the United States. N Engl J Med 2003;348(26):2635–45.
2. Committee on Redesigning Health Insurance Performance Measures, Payment and Performance Improvement Programs. Rewarding provider performance: aligning incentives in Medicare. Washington, DC: The National Academies Press; 2007.
3. File TM Jr, Marrie TJ. Burden of community-acquired pneumonia in North American adults. Postgrad Med 2010;122(2):130–41.
4. U.S. Department of Health and Human Services. Hospital Compare. Available at: http://www.hospitalcompare.hhs.gov/. Accessed January 24, 2011.
5. Yende S, Angus DC, Ali IS, et al. Influence of comorbid conditions on long-term mortality after pneumonia in older people. J Am Geriatr Soc 2007;55(4):518–25.
6. Frei CR, Restrepo MI, Mortensen EM, et al. Impact of guideline-concordant empiric antibiotic therapy in community-acquired pneumonia. Am J Med 2006; 119(10):865–71.
7. Mortensen EM, Restrepo M, Anzueto A, et al. Effects of guideline-concordant antimicrobial therapy on mortality among patients with community-acquired pneumonia. Am J Med 2004;117(10):726–31.

8. Ramirez JA. Worldwide perspective of the quality of care provided to hospitalized patients with community-acquired pneumonia: results from the CAPO international cohort study. Semin Respir Crit Care Med 2005;26(6):543–52.

9. Meehan TP, Fine MJ, Krumholz HM, et al. Quality of care, process, and outcomes in elderly patients with pneumonia. JAMA 1997;278(23):2080–4.

10. Campbell SG, Marrie TJ, Anstey R, et al. The contribution of blood cultures to the clinical management of adult patients admitted to the hospital with community-acquired pneumonia: a prospective observational study. Chest 2003;123(4):1142–50.

11. Mandell LA, Wunderink RG, Anzueto A, et al. Infectious Diseases Society of America/American Thoracic Society consensus guidelines on the management of community-acquired pneumonia in adults. Clin Infect Dis 2007;44(Suppl 2):S27–72.

12. Lindenauer PK, Bernheim SM, Grady JN, et al. The performance of US hospitals as reflected in risk-standardized 30-day mortality and readmission rates for Medicare beneficiaries with pneumonia. J Hosp Med 2010;5(6):E12–8.

13. Arnold FW, LaJoie AS, Brock GN, et al. Improving outcomes in elderly patients with community-acquired pneumonia by adhering to national guidelines: Community-Acquired Pneumonia Organization International cohort study results. Arch Intern Med 2009;169(16):1515–24.

14. McCabe C, Kirchner C, Zhang H, et al. Guideline-concordant therapy and reduced mortality and length of stay in adults with community-acquired pneumonia: playing by the rules. Arch Intern Med 2009;169(16):1525–31.

15. Menendez R, Torres A, Zalacain R, et al. Guidelines for the treatment of community-acquired pneumonia: predictors of adherence and outcome. Am J Respir Crit Care Med 2005;172(6):757–62.

16. Frei CR, Attridge RT, Mortensen EM, et al. Guideline-concordant antibiotic use and survival among patients with community-acquired pneumonia admitted to the intensive care unit. Clin Ther 2010;32(2):293–9.

17. Bodi M, Rodriguez A, Sole-Violan J, et al. Antibiotic prescription for community-acquired pneumonia in the intensive care unit: impact of adherence to Infectious Diseases Society of America guidelines on survival. Clin Infect Dis 2005;41(12):1709–16.

18. Aujesky D, Fine MJ. Does guideline adherence for empiric antibiotic therapy reduce mortality in community-acquired pneumonia? Am J Respir Crit Care Med 2005;172(6):655–6.

19. Dean NC, Silver MP, Bateman KA, et al. Decreased mortality after implementation of a treatment guideline for community-acquired pneumonia. Am J Med 2001;110(6):451–7.

20. Dean NC, Bateman KA, Donnelly SM, et al. Improved clinical outcomes with utilization of a community-acquired pneumonia guideline. Chest 2006;130(3):794–9.

21. Capelastegui A, Espana PP, Quintana JM, et al. Improvement of process-of-care and outcomes after implementing a guideline for the management of community-acquired pneumonia: a controlled before-and-after design study. Clin Infect Dis 2004;39(7):955–63.

22. Yealy DM, Auble TE, Stone RA, et al. Effect of increasing the intensity of implementing pneumonia guidelines: a randomized, controlled trial. Ann Intern Med 2005;143(12):881–94.

23. Fine MJ, Pratt HM, Obrosky DS, et al. Relation between length of hospital stay and costs of care for patients with community-acquired pneumonia. Am J Med 2000;109(5):378–85.

24. Marrie TJ, Lau CY, Wheeler SL, et al. A controlled trial of a critical pathway for treatment of community-acquired pneumonia. CAPITAL Study Investigators. Community-Acquired Pneumonia Intervention Trial Assessing Levofloxacin. JAMA 2000;283(6):749–55.

25. Fine MJ, Auble TE, Yealy DM, et al. A prediction rule to identify low-risk patients with community-acquired pneumonia. N Engl J Med 1997;336(4):243–50.

26. Martinez R, Reyes S, Lorenzo MJ, et al. Impact of guidelines on outcome: the evidence. Semin Respir Crit Care Med 2009;30(2):172–8.

27. Grimshaw J, Eccles M, Tetroe J. Implementing clinical guidelines: current evidence and future implications. J Contin Educ Health Prof 2004;24(Suppl 1):S31–7.

28. Bratzler DW, Nsa W, Houck PM. Performance measures for pneumonia: are they valuable, and are process measures adequate? Curr Opin Infect Dis 2007;20(2):182–9.

29. Werner RM, Bradlow ET. Relationship between Medicare's hospital compare performance measures and mortality rates. JAMA 2006;296(22):2694–702.

30. National Quality Forum. Measure evaluation criteria. Available at: http://www.qualityforum.org/docs/measure_evaluation_criteria.aspx. Accessed January 24, 2011.

31. Wilson KC, Schunemann HJ. An appraisal of the evidence underlying performance measures for community-acquired pneumonia. Am J Respir Crit Care Med 2011;183(11):1454–62.

32. Linder JA, Kaleba EO, Kmetik KS. Using electronic health records to measure physician performance for acute conditions in primary care: empirical evaluation of the community-acquired pneumonia clinical quality measure set. Med Care 2009;47(2):208–16.

33. Wachter RM, Flanders SA, Fee C, et al. Public reporting of antibiotic timing in patients with pneumonia: lessons from a flawed performance measure. Ann Intern Med 2008;149(1):29–32.

34. Niederman MS, Mandell LA, Anzueto A, et al. Guidelines for the management of adults with

community-acquired pneumonia. Diagnosis, assessment of severity, antimicrobial therapy, and prevention. Am J Respir Crit Care Med 2001;163(7): 1730–54.

35. Afshar N, Tabas J, Afshar K, et al. Blood cultures for community-acquired pneumonia: are they worthy of two quality measures? A systematic review. J Hosp Med 2009;4(2):112–23.

36. Metersky ML, Ma A, Bratzler DW, et al. Predicting bacteremia in patients with community-acquired pneumonia. Am J Respir Crit Care Med 2004; 169(3):342–7.

37. Yu KT, Wyer PC. Evidence-based emergency medicine/critically appraised topic. Evidence behind the 4-hour rule for initiation of antibiotic therapy in community-acquired pneumonia. Ann Emerg Med 2008;51(5):651–62, 662, e651–2.

38. Houck PM. Antibiotics and pneumonia: is timing everything or just a cause of more problems? Chest 2006;130(1):1–3.

39. Houck PM, Bratzler DW, Nsa W, et al. Timing of antibiotic administration and outcomes for Medicare patients hospitalized with community-acquired pneumonia. Arch Intern Med 2004;164(6):637–44.

40. Waterer GW, Kessler LA, Wunderink RG. Delayed administration of antibiotics and atypical presentation in community-acquired pneumonia. Chest 2006; 130(1):11–5.

41. Kanwar M, Brar N, Khatib R, et al. Misdiagnosis of community-acquired pneumonia and inappropriate utilization of antibiotics: side effects of the 4-h antibiotic administration rule. Chest 2007;131(6):1865–9.

42. Welker JA, Huston M, McCue JD. Antibiotic timing and errors in diagnosing pneumonia. Arch Intern Med 2008;168(4):351–6.

43. Polgreen PM, Chen YY, Cavanaugh JE, et al. An outbreak of severe Clostridium difficile-associated disease possibly related to inappropriate antimicrobial therapy for community-acquired pneumonia. Infect Control Hosp Epidemiol 2007;28(2):212–4.

44. Metersky ML, Sweeney TA, Getzow MB, et al. Antibiotic timing and diagnostic uncertainty in Medicare patients with pneumonia: is it reasonable to expect all patients to receive antibiotics within 4 hours? Chest 2006;130(1):16–21.

45. Baddour LM, Yu VL, Klugman KP, et al. Combination antibiotic therapy lowers mortality among severely ill patients with pneumococcal bacteremia. Am J Respir Crit Care Med 2004;170(4):440–4.

46. Waterer GW, Somes GW, Wunderink RG. Monotherapy may be suboptimal for severe bacteremic pneumococcal pneumonia. Arch Intern Med 2001; 161(15):1837–42.

47. Gleason PP, Meehan TP, Fine JM, et al. Associations between initial antimicrobial therapy and medical outcomes for hospitalized elderly patients with pneumonia. Arch Intern Med 1999;159(21):2562–72.

48. Martinez JA, Horcajada JP, Almela M, et al. Addition of a macrolide to a beta-lactam-based empirical antibiotic regimen is associated with lower in-hospital mortality for patients with bacteremic pneumococcal pneumonia. Clin Infect Dis 2003;36(4):389–95.

49. Metersky ML, Ma A, Houck PM, et al. Antibiotics for bacteremic pneumonia: improved outcomes with macrolides but not fluoroquinolones. Chest 2007; 131(2):466–73.

50. Brown RB, Iannini P, Gross P, et al. Impact of initial antibiotic choice on clinical outcomes in community-acquired pneumonia: analysis of a hospital claims-made database. Chest 2003;123(5):1503–11.

51. Mills GD, Oehley MR, Arrol B. Effectiveness of beta lactam antibiotics compared with antibiotics active against atypical pathogens in non-severe community acquired pneumonia: meta-analysis. BMJ 2005; 330(7489):456.

52. Shefet D, Robenshtok E, Paul M, et al. Empirical atypical coverage for inpatients with community-acquired pneumonia: systematic review of randomized controlled trials. Arch Intern Med 2005;165(17): 1992–2000.

53. Metersky M, Ho SY, Petrillo MK. Does hospital-based influenza vaccination result in unintended revaccination? Am J Med 2004;116(12):854–5.

54. Statistical methods used to calculate rates. U.S. Department of Health and Human Services. Available at: http://www.hospitalcompare.hhs.gov/staticpages/for-professionals/ooc/statistcal-methods.aspx. Accessed January 24, 2011.

55. Lindenauer PK, Normand SL, Drye EE, et al. Development, validation, and results of a measure of 30-day readmission following hospitalization for pneumonia. J Hosp Med 2011;6(3):142–50.

56. Halm EA, Fine MJ, Kapoor WN, et al. Instability on hospital discharge and the risk of adverse outcomes in patients with pneumonia. Arch Intern Med 2002; 162(11):1278–84.

57. Ramirez JA, Vargas S, Ritter GW, et al. Early switch from intravenous to oral antibiotics and early hospital discharge: a prospective observational study of 200 consecutive patients with community-acquired pneumonia. Arch Intern Med 1999;159(20):2449–54.

58. Hagaman JT, Yurkowski P, Trott A, et al. Getting physicians to make "the switch": the role of clinical guidelines in the management of community-acquired pneumonia. Am J Med Qual 2005;20(1):15–21.

59. Oosterheert JJ, Bonten MJ, Schneider MM, et al. Effectiveness of early switch from intravenous to oral antibiotics in severe community acquired pneumonia: multicentre randomised trial. BMJ 2006; 333(7580):1193.

60. Fishbane S, Niederman MS, Daly C, et al. The impact of standardized order sets and intensive clinical case management on outcomes in community-acquired pneumonia. Arch Intern Med 2007;167(15):1664–9.

Prevention of VAP: Is Zero Rate Possible?

Stijn Blot, MNSc, PhD[a], Thiago Lisboa, MD[b],
Roser Angles, MD, PhD[c], Jordi Rello, MD, PhD[d],*

KEYWORDS

- Safety • Infection control • Care bundles
- Intensive care unit • Prevention
- Ventilator-associated pneumonia

Patients in intensive care units (ICUs) are identified as targets for quality-of-care and patient-safety improvement strategies. Approximately 1.7 errors per patient occur in the ICU daily, and nearly half of these errors were attributable to the physician and nursing staff.[1] The cost of adverse events in the ICU is substantial, not only because almost 150,000 life-threatening errors occur annually in teaching hospital ICUs[2] but also because the economic cost of 1 adverse event is approximately $4000.[3]

Critically ill patients are at high risk for complications because of the complex and invasive nature of critical care treatments and procedures, the severity of their medical conditions, and the use of immunosuppressive drugs. Reports estimate that there were an average of 178 activities per patient per day in the ICU, and the rate for all adverse events was 80.5 per 1000 patient days, but preventable in only 36.2 per 1000 patient days.[2] The factors that were associated with elevated odds for adverse events were any organ failure, a higher intensity in level of care, and time of exposure.[4]

Many ICU patients have severe acute and chronic illnesses that may be reversed.[5,6] This subset of patients is also at a high risk for infection or medical errors that are current targets for quality-improvement strategies.[7–9]

The World Health Organization defined patient safety as reducing the risk of unnecessary harm associated with health care to an acceptable minimum. An acceptable minimum refers to the collective notions of given current knowledge, resources available, and the context in which care was delivered weighed against the risk of nontreatment or other treatment.[10]

A safer environment is generated by the prevention of errors and their adverse effects.[11,12] Acknowledging the potential for errors and creating strategies for reducing errors at every stage of clinical practice are fundamental in the safety-promotion process.[13,14] Its importance is recognized in the Institute of Medicine report "To Err is Human,"[15] which provides relevant data regarding quality of care and patient safety in the United States.

Strategies to improve outcomes in ICU patients include safety tools, such as a rapid response team, daily goal sheet, checklists, and the development of care bundles with implementation measures. The most important change, however, is cultural, emphasizing that errors should be considered a failed system rather than a people failure. Harm is often the result of a cascade of broken systems.[16] A safety program in critical care should provide a practical and goal-oriented

Supported in part by FIS 07/90960 and AGAUR 09/SGR/1265.
a General Internal Medicine & Infectious Diseases, Ghent University Hospital, De Pintelaan 185, 9000 Ghent, Belgium
b Critical Care Department, Hospital de Clinicas, Rua Ramiro Barcelos, 2350 Rio Branco, Porto Alegre, Brazil
c Quality Department, Vall D'Hebron Institut of Research, Vall d'Hebron University Hospital, CIBERES, Universitat Autonoma de Barcelona, Annexe General 5a, Paseig Vall d'Hebron 119-129, Barcelona 08035, Spain
d Critical Care Department, Vall D'Hebron Institut of Research, Vall d'Hebron University Hospital, CIBERES, Universitat Autonoma de Barcelona, Annexe General 5a, Paseig Vall d'Hebron 119-129, Barcelona 08035, Spain
* Corresponding author.
E-mail address: jrello.hj23.ics@gencat.cat

set of tools to implement a culture of safety to prevent errors and their consequences.[13]

Shulman and Ost[17] discussed the connection between patient safety concepts and infection prevention and how measurable interventions impact patient safety and improve the quality of care and patient outcomes. Although lowering the incidence of nosocomial infections would be an important quality-improvement measure and improve patient safety, misleading interpretations of this process may confound concepts, such as safety-related adverse events and unavoidable complications of critical care. Furthermore, an appropriate interpretation of quality-improvement strategies relies on the ability to measure their effects. Unfortunately, the ability to measure and evaluate the effect of interventions related to health care–associated infection prevention, and more specifically ventilator-associated pneumonia (VAP), is severely limited by the lack of diagnostic sensitivity and specificity.

Significant questions and concerns have been raised regarding reporting rates of nosocomial infections: Are all nosocomial infections an adverse event and a medical error? Are all of these infections preventable? Patient safety strategies are clearly able to reduce the risk of infectious complication, but is a zero-infection rate a feasible endpoint for VAP and other nosocomial infections? Are predefined thresholds of VAP rates and other infections an appropriate quality-of-care indicator?

Infection-prevention measures, and specifically VAP prevention, have been proposed as quality-of-care indicators for ICU patients. This article reviews recent evidence regarding ICU safety promotion and the adequacy of this approach.

INFECTION CONTROL IN THE ICU: THE ROLE OF CARE BUNDLES AND THEIR IMPACT ON PATIENT SAFETY

Nosocomial infections are the most common complications affecting hospitalized patients and have significant morbidity and mortality.[18] VAP is the most frequent and costly infectious complication in ICU patients, which has been estimated to cost at least $40,000 per patient as estimated in 3 matched cohort studies.[19] Currently, infection control is a critical element of patient care and many nosocomial infection episodes are considered potentially preventable. The idea that most infections are unavoidable and some could be preventable has been changed to "all infections are potentially preventable unless proven otherwise."[20] Unfortunately, valid data on the proportion of unpreventable episodes

in different ICU settings are not available, although it is clear that some types of infection, such as catheter-associated bloodstream infections, are easier to prevent than other infections, such as pneumonia.[21]

Using a system-approach model to evaluate factors that contribute to infection development might allow for better identification of risk groups and potential interventions for prevention.[20,22] Jain and colleagues[23] used this strategy to reduce nosocomial infection rates. A set of 4 interventions were employed to obtain improvement: (1) multidisciplinary rounds; (2) daily reevaluation of the indication for continuing critical care; (3) using care bundles for VAP, urinary tract infection, and catheter-related bloodstream infection; and (4) change in safety culture (although this effect could not be accurately measured). These process interventions resulted in a 58% reduction of VAP incidence, a 48% decrease in catheter-related bloodstream infections, and a 37% reduction in the incidence of urinary tract infections. Although it was not possible to identify the most relevant interventions in this study, the change in the perceptions of safety or culture change appeared to be a key factor for success. Yet, patient safety culture is a complex concept that has been defined as "the product of individual and group values, attitudes, perceptions, competencies, and patterns of behavior that determine the commitment to, and the style and proficiency of, an organization's health and safety management that include personnel's safety attitudes, beliefs and knowledge."[24] Important aspects were the conditions that facilitate implementation and adherence to the recommended protocols and processes of care; identifying evidenced-based interventions that improve the outcome; selecting the interventions that impact outcomes; developing measures to evaluate reliability; measuring the baseline situation; ensuring that patients received evidence-based interventions; and a combination of reminders and continuing education, augmented with an audit and feedback system.[25,26]

The factors that are important in this process are awareness of the problem, understanding the pathogenesis, and knowledge of evidence-based guidelines. Lack of knowledge is commonly recognized as a crucial hurdle to adhering to the guidelines. Surveys evaluating the knowledge of ICU nurses about evidence-based guidelines for the prevention of VAP found overall poor test scores, suggesting that low knowledge levels could contribute to limited adherence to infection-prevention guidelines.[27–29] In addition to basic insights and knowledge, skills, attitudes, and social and organizational context will determine the level of success in reducing infection rates.

Because it is multifactorial the result of many factors, overall adherence to evidence-based interventions is highly variable and often at a disappointing level.[30] It is clear that a new paradigm of nosocomial infection prevention should be based on a multidisciplinary and evidence-based effort with an agenda focused on patient safety promotion and quality improvement. A cornerstone of this approach is the Institute for Health Improvement (IHI) initiative, which incorporates a limited number of effective interventions into a bundle that is both conceptually simple and feasible.[31]

Prevention strategies based in care bundles aim to translate the best available evidence into clinical practice by allowing for a more uniform management of patients. By comparison, implementation of individual interventions might improve patient care, but the implementation of several simple measures simultaneously, as a bundle, has a greater likelihood of improving outcome.[32,33] This approach aims to facilitate the implementation of best practice, ensuring a uniform application of the procedures and therapies to all patients. Catheter-related bloodstream infection and VAP are 2 examples of the successful application of prevention and care bundle in the ICU setting.

VENTILATOR-ASSOCIATED PNEUMONIA

VAP is the most common nosocomial infection in ICUs and represents 25% of all ICU infections.[34,35] VAP cost is reported to be as high as $10 billion per year.[36] While the attributable mortality of VAP is controversial, it certainly does prolong mechanical ventilation and the length of stay in the ICU.[36,37] Because of its importance and impact on morbidity in ICU patients, VAP prevention was included in the IHI campaign to save 100,000 lives.[31] This campaign is expected to save 100,000 lives through the implementation of safety measures, specifically through the use of the ventilator bundle to reduce VAP incidence. The bundle included 4 simple measures (**Box 1**). Although not all interventions could directly affect VAP pathogenesis (eg, deep vein thrombosis prophylaxis), a significant reduction in VAP incidence was reported in most centers participating in the campaign.[38–40]

Although several studies described numerous effective interventions for VAP prevention, most of them are not routinely performed. Available evidence suggests that VAP prevention has not translated to clinical practice. What is the cause of this gap between best evidence and practice? In a systematic review,[41] Collard and colleagues

---

Box 1
Ventilator bundle from the Institute for Health Improvement

Stress bleeding/peptic ulcer prophylaxis

Deep vein thrombosis prophylaxis

Semirecumbent position: head of bed elevation at least 30°

Sedation vacation with daily weaning trial

Chlorhexidine oral care

Data from Resar R, Pronovost P, Haraden C, et al. Using a bundle approach to improve ventilator care process and reduce ventilator-associated pneumonia. Jt Comm J Qual Patient Saf 2005;31:243–8.

---

identified the following effective interventions to prevent VAP: a semirecumbent position, use of sucralfate in a low-moderate risk for gastrointestinal bleeding prophylaxis, subglottic secretions drainage, and the use of kinetic beds. However, implementation of these interventions has not been uniform. Causes of medical and nursing staff nonadherence have been assessed,[42–44] suggesting a need for educational interventions that stimulate adoption of these effective measures.

Salahuddin and colleagues[45] found a 51% reduction in VAP incidence through an educational program for VAP prevention. The program was a selection of recommended VAP prevention measures, and its benefit was persistent for 12 months. Educational strategies for reinforcement of prevention practices may be effective to reduce VAP rates. Use of care bundles to improve compliance with prevention measures was also studied in VAP. Resar and colleagues[32] found a reduction of 45% in VAP incidence with the implementation of a care bundle for VAP prevention. Moreover, reduction in VAP incidence was correlated to the degree of adherence to the bundle. Again, it is important to note that successful compliance with infection-control bundles will depend on having sufficient and well-educated staffing in the ICU. Moreover, Crunden and colleagues[46] found a significant reduction in ICU length of stay (LOS) from 13.7 days to 8.36 days, and a reduction in ventilation duration from 10.8 to 6.1 days. Interestingly, Cocanour and colleagues[40] demonstrated in trauma patients that isolated implementation of the ventilator bundle was not enough, and VAP rates decreased only when compliance with the ventilator bundle was improved. This finding, however, underscores the need for an approach that goes beyond the sum of the individual items of the VAP bundle, but also takes into account targeted education, attitudes, and optimizing the organizational context. Additional support is needed to obtain true quality improvement, especially in care aspects that are perceived as unpleasant and difficult, such as oral hygiene in intubated patients.[44] Further studies should also evaluate other endpoints, such as antibiotic use, that should decline if VAP is being prevented.

Although care-bundle implementation appears to be associated with the successful reduction in VAP rates, there should be a cautious interpretation of their benefit. Misinterpretation of prevention study results and of the pathophysiology of VAP may lead to an erroneous idea that a zero-VAP rate is feasible. Studies on the prevention by care bundles are encouraging. Yet, pathophysiologic aspects of VAP, such as differences between early and late-VAP episodes,[35,47,48] and risk factors that differ between trauma and medical patients,[40,49] were not considered in the current version of bundles which limit their ability to prevent all episodes of VAP. In addition, the inaccuracy of VAP diagnoses limits the interpretation of these data, as discussed later. Appropriate staffing levels may be a major influence on the LOS in the ICU, duration of mechanical ventilation, and the development of VAP, presumably because of the maintenance of infection-control standards.[50–53] Lapses in basic infection-control measures, such as hand washing, are more likely with increased workloads for nurses and increased reliance on less-trained health care personnel to deliver care.[54,55] Educational reinforcement and opportunities for ICU staff to participate in mandatory training aimed at hospital-acquired pneumonia/VAP prevention is also important to improve safety and to optimize VAP prevention.[39,56]

A last important aspect for the implementation of a care bundle is that there be a consensus about which items to include in the bundle. As long as a critical number of staff members remains reluctant to implement some preventive measure, successful implementation and favorable adherence is highly unlikely. Preventive measures that appear to be less labor intensive, for example semirecumbent positioning, or the use of innovative devices, such as endotracheal tubes with an ultrathin[57] tapered shape cuff,[58] may be chosen over a strict oral hygiene protocol, which can be perceived as time consuming. Throughout the democratic process to develop a care bundle, the available evidence of the individual preventive measures must remain a major consideration, despite the differences in evidence available for some measures,[59] as well as ongoing controversies about the efficacy of some prevention efforts.[60]

SHOULD VAP BE USED AS A QUALITY INDICATOR FOR SAFETY IN THE ICU?

Initiatives to stop paying hospitals for care made necessary by preventable complications,[61] including nosocomial infections, may have both desirable and unintended consequences.[62] Preventable complications, such as vascular-catheter–associated infections, will no longer be reimbursed by Medicare in the United States. Other ICU infections, such as VAP, may follow.[62] The plan has been criticized for penalizing hospitals that admit frail and other high-risk patients.[63] In addition, an undesirable effect of the plan might be to encourage institutions to underreport nosocomial infections. Linking accreditation and compensation to the incidence of VAP is problematic because there is a considerable uncertainty in making a VAP diagnosis. Controversies regarding this issue are summarized in **Box 2**.

Physicians' ability to diagnose VAP is often poor, and several pulmonary diseases may present with similar clinical signs. Clinical signs of pneumonia (fever, pulmonary infiltrates, and purulent pulmonary secretion) present in ICU patients are caused by VAP in only 30% to 40%.[64,65] Using a quantitative culture of respiratory samples has been advocated as a measure to improve the accuracy of VAP diagnosis. However, no study to date has demonstrated any effect on reducing antibiotic use, rates of superinfection, or improvement in outcomes associated with such a diagnostic strategy.

In addition, the presence of positive cultures of respiratory secretions is only moderately specific for VAP.[64,66] In fact, some of these patients may have purulent tracheobronchitis or ventilator-associated tracheobronchitis (VAT), which is defined as the presence of clinical signs or symptoms of infection and purulent sputum and an endotracheal aspirate with a pathogen having moderate to heavy growth on semiquantitative culture or greater than 10^6 organisms/mL on

---

Box 2
Controversies and issues in using VAP as a quality indicator in ICU

Poor ability to definitely diagnose VAP

Absence of a gold standard for VAP diagnosis

Differences between surveillance and clinical definitions for VAP

Case-mix variation in different institutions

Risk of underreporting of VAP episodes because of the pressure of public reporting

quantitative culture, but no new infiltrate on a chest radiograph.[67,68] VAT may be a precursor to VAP, and antibiotic treatment appears to prevent VAP and improve patient outcomes.

Interpretation of chest infiltrates on chest radiographs is difficult and may be improved with the use of computed tomography (CT) lung scans, but availability of CT scans for these patients may be limited and difficult to carry out. Furthermore, there can still be infiltrates suggestive of VAP that are difficult to confirm or to find consensus among blinded readers, especially in patients with prior diffuse infiltrates, pleural effusions, prior surgery or chest trauma, congestive heart failure, or adult respiratory distress syndrome (ARDS).[69] In a recent study, the accuracy of the chest radiograph reading was compared with high-resolution CT (HRCT) scans in 47 patients with suspected community-acquired pneumonia.[70] HRCT identified all 18 cases of pneumonia apparent on chest radiographs, as well as 8 additional cases that were not diagnosed. The data suggest that HRCT would be a more sensitive and specific tool for diagnosing VAP in critically ill patients. Although this would be more expensive, if used, it would likely improve diagnostic accuracy, but may also have a greater limitation for diagnosing or excluding VAP, especially in patients with ARDS or severe congestive heart failure.

Therefore, the standard definition used to measure VAP rates is based on several nonspecific clinical signs with the addition of microbiologic criteria needed to improve specificity, but may be severely limited by lack of sensitivity and specificity of chest radiographs used to evaluate most ICU patients.

VAP should be accurately diagnosed before relevant and definite recommendations for prevention can be developed.[71] Difficulty in making an accurate diagnosis of VAP makes it an unreliable basis for quality control or interhospital benchmarking of quality of care. Differences between surveillance strategies and the clinical definition of VAP are fundamental. For example, the incidence of VAP may be up to 2 times higher in patients diagnosed by qualitative or semiquantitative secretion cultures compared with quantitative cultures of lower respiratory tract secretions.[35,72] Overemphasizing quantitative culture results in the application of surveillance strategies as a means to improve homogeneity in diagnostic criteria may be misleading because factors, such as previous antibiotic exposure, affect the results of microbiologic techniques. Surveillance including only core data or VAP rates would be unreliable because it would not consider variability in diagnostic criteria.

A clinical definition of VAP, based on clinical and microbiologic data, would probably be the most reliable approach; however, heterogeneity in evaluation of these criteria represents an important limitation for the interinstitutional benchmarking of quality based on VAP rates. Perhaps a uniform interhospital surveillance system would allow a more accurate comparison of VAP rates.[73] By doing so, the denominator problem of reporting VAP rates can be overcome. In a medical ICU, the influence of the denominator used to calculate the occurrence rate of VAP was evaluated.[74] In a cohort of 106 patients with VAP, depending on the denominator used, the occurrence rate changed from 22.8 VAPs per 1000 ICU days (95% confidence interval [CI] 18.7–27.6), to more than 35.7 VAPs per 1000 ventilator days (95% CI 29.2–43.2), to 44.0 VAPs per 1000 ventilator days at risk (95% CI 36.0–53.2). From this information, it is clear that not only uniform definitions but also uniform reporting of surveillance results are of the utmost important.

Moreover, Hurley[75] described the effect of design factors on VAP incidence reported in prevention studies and found a high variation in control groups in different studies. Almost 30% of control groups, in antimicrobial methods for VAP prevention studies, were classified as having a high outlier incidence of VAP. Additionally, as pointed by Klompas and colleagues,[76] if VAP rates are used in determining hospitals' compensation or affect their public reputation, the rate of diagnosis may decline simply because of a shift in the interpretation of subjective criteria, such as a change in secretion character or a worsening gas exchange. Absence of objective and specific diagnostic criteria for VAP compromises reproducibility and makes the comparison of VAP rates among different ICUs impossible to interpret.

Diagnosis is not the only issue of concern for using VAP as quality indicator. Significant differences in surveillance strategies among centers are well described and might constitute a serious confounding factor when comparing data.[73] Another important limitation is case mix and what adjustment can or should be made. VAP incidence and ability to prevent episodes may be variable in different populations. Patient differences in age, disease severity, origin (eg, traumatic, surgical, or medical), comorbidities, or immunosuppressive status may affect results. Thus, hospitals admitting and caring for high-risk patients would be penalized. Nonetheless, specialized units, such as trauma, neurosurgery, or postsurgical ICUs, handle specific patients with different risk factors for VAP. Comparisons performed among these units would be inappropriate. Case mix is difficult to assess but is needed to avoid inaccurate comparisons. Indeed, it has been demonstrated that large (academic) centers have higher nosocomial infection rates compared with smaller hospitals (odds ratio [OR] 1.97, 95% CI 2.90–1.33), but once adjusted for dissimilarities in case-mix, the difference was no longer significant (OR 1.31, 95% CI 2.05–0.84).[77]

An alternative to reporting VAP incidence rates might be to assess the use of risk-reduction measures for VAP as process-quality indicators. Process-quality indicators are likely to be more reliable and cost-effective than the measurement of VAP rates. Comparison of process-improvement measures (eg, compliance with each item in a care bundle for VAP prevention) would be both patient- and center-independent, more cost-effective, and easier to observe than a VAP incidence that may vary according to case mix and individual patient comorbidities and definitions. Uçkay and colleagues[73] describe several risk factors that could be used as potential quality indicators (**Table 1**).

Table 1
Selected potential quality indicators in VAP

Factor Associated	Impact on VAP Prevention
Length of hospitalization[33]	++
Existence of surveillance system[69]	+++
Feedback surveillance results[69]	+++
Education to staff[69]	+++
Alcohol-based hand rub for hand hygiene[69]	+++
Endotracheal suction systems[69]	++
Heat and moisture exchangers[33,69]	++
Sedation policy[33]	++
Weaning protocol[33]	++
Short duration of ventilation[33,70]	+++
Frequent ventilator circuit changes[69]	++
Endotracheal tube cuff pressure[33,71]	++
Supine head position[33,72]	++
Subglottic secretion drainage[33,73]	+++
Compliance with hand hygiene[33,69]	+++
Oral hygiene[42]	++
Stress ulcer prophylaxis[20]	?
Deep venous thrombosis prophylaxis[20]	?
Selective digestive decontamination[74,75]	+?
Oral decontamination[75]	+?
Silver-coated endotracheal tube[76]	++?

+, of concern; ++, important; +++, very important.
Data from Uçkay I, Ahmed Q, Sax H, et al. Ventilator-associated pneumonia as a quality indicator for patient safety? Clin Infect Dis 2008;46:557–63.

SUMMARY

Quality-of-care and safety improvement should be a priority in intensive care. The prevention of nosocomial infections should be a cornerstone in this process, and significant advances have been made.[75,76,78–84] Effective design and implementation requires a multidisciplinary approach, taking into account barriers as well as facilitators. Indeed, design of newer care bundles for VAP prevention based on evidence[85] represents a significant step forward. Implementation of care bundles for prevention seems to be an effective way to improve patient safety. However, some nosocomial infections, such as tracheobronchitis and pneumonia, are not always preventable.

REFERENCES

1. Donchin Y, Gopher D, Olin M, et al. A look into the nature and causes of human errors in the intensive care unit. Qual Saf Health Care 2003;12:143–8.
2. Rothschild JM, Landrigan CP, Cronin JW, et al. The critical care safety study: the incidence and nature of adverse events and serious medical errors in intensive care. Crit Care Med 2005;33:1694–700.
3. Kaushal R, Bates D, Franz C, et al. Cost of adverse events in intensive care units. Crit Care Med 2007; 35:2479–83.
4. Valentin A, Capuzzo M, Guidet B, et al. Patient safety in intensive care: results from the multinational Sentinel Events Evaluation (SEE) study. Intensive Care Med 2006;32:1591–8.
5. Cullen DJ, Sweitzer B, Bates DW, et al. Preventable adverse drug events in hospitalized patients: a comparative study of intensive care and general care units. Crit Care Med 1997;25:1289–97.
6. Winters B, Dorman T. Patient-safety and quality initiatives in the intensive care unit. Curr Opin Anaesthesiol 2006;19:140–5.
7. Pronovost PJ, Goeschel CA, Wachter RM. The wisdom and justice of not paying for "preventable complications". JAMA 2008;299:2197–9.

8. Fung CH, Lim YW, Mattke S, et al. Systematic review: the evidence that publishing patient care performance data improves quality of care. Ann Intern Med 2008;148:111–23.

9. Dougherty D, Conway PH. The "3T's" road map to transform US healthcare: the "how" of high quality. JAMA 2008;299:2119–21.

10. Wold Health Organization. Conceptual framework for the International Classification for Patient Safety. Version 1.1. Available at: http://www.who.int/patientsafety/taxonomy/icps_full_report.pdf. Accessed December 06, 2010.

11. Pronovost PJ, Thompson DA, Holzmueller CG, et al. Defining and measuring patient safety. Crit Care Clin 2005;21:1–19.

12. Vincent C. Understanding and responding to adverse events. N Engl J Med 2003;348:1051–6.

13. Rodriguez-Paz JM, Dorman T. Patient safety in the intensive care unit. Clin Pulm Med 2008;15:24–34.

14. Leape LL. Error in medicine. JAMA 1994;272:1851–7.

15. Kohn KT, Corrigan JM, Donaldson MS. To err is human: building a safer health system. Washington, DC: National Academy Press; 1999.

16. Pronovost P, Miller M, Wachter R. Tracking progress in patient safety. An elusive target. JAMA 2006;296:696–9.

17. Shulman L, Ost D. Managing infection in the critical care unit: how can infection control make the ICU safe? Crit Care Clin 2005;21:111–28.

18. Burke JP. Infection control – a problem for patient safety. N Engl J Med 2003;348:651–6.

19. Kollef MH. What is ventilator-associated pneumonia and why is it important? Respir Care 2005;50:714–21.

20. Gerberding JL. Hospital-onset infections: a patient-safety issue. Ann Intern Med 2002;137:665–70.

21. Harbarth S, Sax H, Gastneier P. The preventable proportion of nosocomial infections: an overview of published reports. J Hosp Infect 2003;54:258–66.

22. Eggimann P, Pittet D. Infection control in the ICU. Chest 2001;120(6):2059–93.

23. Jain M, Miller L, Belt D, et al. Decline in ICU adverse events, nosocomial infections and cost through a quality improvement initiative focusing on teamwork and culture change. Qual Saf Health Care 2006;15:235–9.

24. Sexton JB, Helmreich RL, Neilands TB, et al. The safety attitudes questionnaire: psychometric properties, benchmarking data, and emerging research. BMC Health Serv Res 2006;6:44–54.

25. Pronovost PJ, Berenholtz SM, Needham DM. Translating evidence into practice: a model for large scale knowledge translation. BMJ 2008;337:a1714.

26. Sinuff T, Cook D, Giacomini M, et al. Facilitating clinician adherence to guidelines in the intensive care unit: a multicenter, qualitative study. Crit Care Med 2007;35:2083–9.

27. Labeau S, Vandijck DM, Claes B, et al. Executive board of Flemish Society for Critical Care Nurses. Critical care nurses' knowledge of evidence-based guidelines for preventing ventilator-associated pneumonia: an evaluation questionnaire. Am J Crit Care 2007;16:371–7.

28. Blot S, Labeau SS, Vandijck D, et al. Executive board of Flemish Society for Critical Care Nurses. Evidence-based guideline for the prevention of ventilator-associated pneumonia: results of knowledge test among intensive care nurses. Intensive Care Med 2007;33:1463–7.

29. Labeau S, Vandijck D, Rello J, et al. Evidence study investigators. J Hosp Infect 2008;70:180–5.

30. Warren DK, Zack JE, Mayfield JL, et al. The effect of an education program on the incidence of central venous catheter-associated bloodstream infection in a medical ICU. Chest 2004;126:1612–8.

31. IHI. Prevent ventilator-associated pneumonia. Available at: http://www.ihi.org/IHI/Programs/Campaign/VAP.htm. Accessed November 8, 2010.

32. Resar R, Pronovost P, Haraden C, et al. Using a bundle approach to improve ventilator care process and reduce ventilator-associated pneumonia. Jt Comm J Qual Patient Saf 2005;31:243–8.

33. Eggimann P, Harbarth S, Constantin MN, et al. Impact of a prevention strategy targeted at vascular-access care on incidence of infections acquired in intensive care. Lancet 2000;355:1864–8.

34. Kollef MH, Shorr A, Tabak YP, et al. Epidemiology and outcomes of health-care-associated pneumonia: results from a large US database of culture-positive pneumonia. Chest 2005;128(6):3854–62.

35. The American Thoracic Society and the Infectious Diseases Society of America Guideline Committee. Guidelines for the management of adults with hospital-acquired, ventilator-associated, and healthcare-associated pneumonia. Am J Respir Crit Care Med 2005;171:388–416.

36. Rello J, Ollendorf DA, Oster G, et al. Epidemiology and outcomes of ventilator-associated pneumonia in a large US database. Chest 2002;122:2115–21.

37. Muscedere JG, Martin CM, Heyland DK. The impact of ventilator-associated pneumonia on the Canadian health care system. J Crit Care 2008;23:5–10.

38. Craven D. Preventing ventilator-associated pneumonia in adults: sowing seeds of change. Chest 2006;130:251–60.

39. Babcock HM, Zack JE, Garrison T, et al. An educational intervention to reduce ventilator-associated pneumonia in an integrated health system: a comparison of effects. Chest 2004;125:2224–31.

40. Cocanour CS, Peninger M, Domonoske BD, et al. Decreasing ventilator associated pneumonia in a trauma ICU. J Trauma 2006;61:122–9.

41. Collard HR, Saint S, Matthay MA. Prevention of ventilator-associated pneumonia: an evidence-based systematic review. Ann Intern Med 2003; 138:494–501.

42. Rello J, Lorente C, Bodi M, et al. Why do physicians not follow evidence-based guidelines for preventing ventilator-associated pneumonia? A survey based on the opinions of an international panel of intensivists. Chest 2002;122:656–61.

43. Ricart M, Lorente C, Diaz E, et al. Nursing adherence with evidence-based guidelines for preventing ventilator-associated pneumonia. Crit Care Med 2003;31:2693–6.

44. Rello J, Koulenti D, Blot S, et al. Oral care practices in intensive care units: a survey of 59 European ICUs. Intensive Care Med 2007;33:1066–70.

45. Salahuddin N, Zafar A, Sukhyani L, et al. Reducing ventilator-associated pneumonia rates through a staff education programme. J Hosp Infect 2004;57:223–7.

46. Crunden E, Boyce C, Woodman H, et al. An evaluation of the impact of the ventilator care bundle. Nurs Crit Care 2005;10:242–6.

47. Trouillet JL, Chastre J, Vuagnat A, et al. Ventilator-associated pneumonia caused by potentially drug-resistant bacteria. Am J Respir Crit Care Med 1998;157:531–9.

48. Valles J, Pobo A, Garcia-Esquirrol O, et al. Excess ICU mortality attributable to ventilator-associated pneumonia: the role of early vs late onset. Intensive Care Med 2007;33:1363–8.

49. Hedrick TL, Smith RL, McElearney ST, et al. Differences in early and late-onset ventilator-associated pneumonia between surgical and trauma patients in a combined surgical or trauma intensive care unit. J Trauma 2008;64:714–20.

50. Cho SH, Ketefian S, Barkauskas VH, et al. The effects of nurse staffing on adverse events, morbidity, mortality and medical costs. Nurs Res 2003;52:71–9.

51. Needleman J, Buerhaus P, Mattke S, et al. Nurse staffing levels and the quality of care in hospitals. N Engl J Med 2002;346:1715–22.

52. Marelich GP, Murin S, Battistella F, et al. Protocol weaning of mechanical ventilation in medical and surgical patients by respiratory care practitioners and nurses: effect on weaning time and incidence of ventilator-associated pneumonia. Chest 2000; 118:459–67.

53. Blot S, Llaurado M, Koulenti D, et al. Patient-to-nurse and risk ventilator-associated pneumonia in critically ill patients. Am J Crit Care 2011;20(1):e1–9.

54. Fridkin SK, Pear SM, Williamson TH, et al. The role of understaffing in central venous catheter-associated bloodstream infections. Infect Control Hosp Epidemiol 1996;17:150–8.

55. Pittet D, Mourouga P, Perneger TV. Compliance with hand washing in a teaching hospital. Ann Intern Med 1999;130:126–30.

56. Zack JE, Garrison T, Trovillion E, et al. Effect of an education program aimed at reducing the occurrence of ventilator-associated pneumonia. Crit Care Med 2002;30:2407–12.

57. Poelaert J, Depuydt P, De Wolf A, et al. Polyurethane cuffed endotracheal tubes to prevent early postoperative pneumonia after cardiac surgery: a pilot study. J Thorac Cardiovasc Surg 2008; 135:771–6.

58. Dave MH, Frotzler A, Spuielmann N, et al. Effect of tracheal tube cuff shape on fluid leakage across the cuff: an in vitro study. Br J Anaesth 2010;105: 538–43.

59. Lorente L, Blot S, Rello J. Rational on measures for the prevention of ventilator-associated pneumonia. Eur Respir J 2007;30:1193–207.

60. Lorente L, Blot S, Rello J. New issues and controversies in the prevention of ventilator-associated pneumonia. Am J Respir Crit Care Med 2010; 182:870–6.

61. Edwards JR, Peterson KD, Andrus ML, et al. National Healthcare Safety Network (NHSN) Report, data summary for 2006. Am J Infect Control 2007; 35(5):290–301.

62. Lisboa T, Kollef MH, Rello J. Prevention of VAP: the whole is more than the sum of its parts. Intensive Care Med 2008;34(6):985–7.

63. Rosenthal MB. Nonpayment for performance? Medicare's new reimbursement rule. N Engl J Med 2007; 357(16):1573–5.

64. Klompas M. Does this patient have ventilator-associated pneumonia? JAMA 2007;297:1583–93.

65. Meduri GU, Mauldin GL, Wunderink RG, et al. Causes of fever and pulmonary densities in patients with clinical manifestations of ventilator-associated pneumonia. Chest 1994;106:221–35.

66. Klompas M, Platt R. Ventilator-associated pneumonia – the wrong quality measure for benchmarking. Ann Intern Med 2007;147:803–5.

67. Nseir S, Favory R, Jozefowicz E, et al. Antimicrobial treatment for ventilator-associated tracheobronchitis: a randomized, controlled, multicenter study. Crit Care 2008;12(3):R62.

68. Craven DE. Ventilator-associated tracheobronchitis: questions, answers and a new paradigm. Crit Care 2008;12(3):157.

69. Winer-Muram HT, Rubin SA, Ellis JV, et al. Pneumonia and ARDS in patients receiving mechanical ventilation: diagnostic accuracy of chest radiograph. Radiology 1993;188:479–85.

70. Syrjala H, Broas M, Suramo I, et al. High-resolution computed tomography for the diagnosis of community-acquired pneumonia. Clin Infect Dis 1998;27:358–63.

71. Craven D. Prevention of hospital-acquired pneumonia: measuring effect in ounces, pounds, and tons. Ann Intern Med 1995;122:229–31.

72. Bonten MJ, Bergmans DC, Stobberingh EE, et al. Implementation of bronchoscopic techniques in the diagnosis of ventilator-associated pneumonia to reduce antibiotic use. Am J Respir Crit Care Med 1997;156:1820–4.

73. Uçkay I, Ahmed Q, Sax H, et al. Ventilator-associated pneumonia as a quality indicator for patient safety? Clin Infect Dis 2008;46:557–63.

74. Eggimann P, Hugonnet S, Sax H, et al. Ventilator-associated pneumonia caveats for benchmarking. Intensive Care Med 2003;29:2086–9.

75. Hurley JC. Profound effect of study design factors on ventilator-associated pneumonia incidence of prevention studies: benchmarking the literature experience. J Antimicrob Chemother 2008;61: 1154–61.

76. Klompas M, Kuldorff M, Platt R. Risk of misleading ventilator-associated pneumonia rates with use of standard clinical and microbiological criteria. Clin Infect Dis 2008;46:1443–6.

77. Sax H, Pittet D. Swiss-NOSO Network. Interhospital differences in nosocomial infection rates: importance of case-mix adjustment. Arch Intern Med 2002;162:2437–42.

78. Tablan O, Anderson L, Besser R, et al. Guidelines for preventing health-care associated pneumonia, 2003: recommendations of CDC and the Healthcare Infection Control Practices Advisory Committee. MMWR Recomm Rep 2004;53:1–36.

79. Kress J, Pohlman A, O'Connor MF, et al. Daily interruption of sedative infusions in critically ill patients undergoing mechanical ventilation. N Engl J Med 2000;342:1471–7.

80. Rello J, Sonora R, Jubert P, et al. Pneumonia in intubated patients: role of respiratory airway care. Am J Respir Crit Care Med 1996;154:111–5.

81. Drakulovic MB, Torres A, Bauer TT, et al. Supine body position as a risk factor for nosocomial pneumonia in mechanically ventilated patients: a randomized trial. Lancet 1999;54:1851–8.

82. Valles J, Artigas A, Rello J, et al. Continuous aspiration of subglottic secretions in preventing ventilator-associated pneumonia. Ann Intern Med 1995;122: 179–86.

83. Dodek P, Keenan S, Cook D, et al. Evidence-based clinical practice guideline for the prevention of ventilator-associated pneumonia. Ann Intern Med 2004;141:305–13.

84. Krueger WA, Lenhart FP, Neeser G, et al. Influence of combined intravenous and topical antibiotic prophylaxis on the incidence of infections, organ dysfunctions, and mortality in critically ill surgical patients: a prospective, stratified, randomized, double-blind, placebo-controlled clinical trial. Am J Respir Crit Care Med 2002;166:1029–37.

85. Rello J, Cornaglia G, Lode H. A European care bundle for prevention of ventilator-associated pneumonia. Intensive Care Med 2010;36:773–80.

Index

Note: Page numbers of article titles are in **boldface** type.

A

Adamantane(s), for influenza, 454–455

Adenovirus, 457

Aerosolized antibiotics
  clinical effects of, 563–564
  in ICU, **559–574**
    central and distal concentrations delivery by, 562–563
    described, 559–560
    effect on emergence of bacterial resistance compared with systemic antibiotics, 568
    for VAT or VAP, 564–565
      RCTs of, 565–568
    instillation of, 562–563
    jet nebulizer delivery of, 563
    rationale for, 561
    uncertainties related to, 561–562
    vibrating mesh technology for, 563

Antibiotic(s)
  aerosolized, **559–574.** See also *Aerosolized antibiotics.*
  for pneumonia, timing of, quality of care related to, 583–584
  in bronchiectasis management, 540
  systemic, aerosolized antibiotics vs., in emergence of bacterial resistance, 568

Antiinflammatory drugs
  in bronchiectasis management, 540–542
  nonsteroidal, in bronchiectasis management, 542

B

Bacterial pneumonia(s)
  hospital-acquired, antibiotic pharmacodynamics in, optimization of, **439–450.** See also *Hospital-acquired bacterial pneumonia (HABP), antibiotic pharmacodynamics in, optimization of.*
  ventilator-acquired, antibiotic pharmacodynamics in, optimization of, **439–450.** See also *Ventilator-acquired bacterial pneumonia (VABP), antibiotic pharmacodynamics in, optimization of.*

Bacterial superinfection, viral pneumonia and, 452

Biomarkers
  in evaluation of de-escalation therapy in VAP management, 520
  in optimization of antibiotic therapy for pneumonia due to multidrug-resistant pathogens, **431–438**
    C-reactive protein, 434
    procalcitonin, 431–434
    TREM-1, 434–435
  in pneumonia severity, 473–474

Bocavirus, 461

Bronchiectasis, **535–546**
  causes of, 536–537
  diagnosis of, 537–538
  management of, 538–542
    antibiotics in, 540
    antiinflammatory drugs in, 540–542
    bronchodilators in, 540
    corticosteroids in, 541–542
    general supportive therapy in, 538–539
    macrolides in, 542
    mobilization of airway secretions in, 539–540
    NSAIDs in, 542
    surgery in, 542
    underlying causative conditions–related, 539
    vaccinations in, 539
  pathogenesis of, 536–537
  prevalence of, 535–536
  prognosis of, 542–543

Bronchodilator(s), in bronchiectasis management, 540

C

Care bundles, effect on VAP prevention in ICU, 592–593

Colistin, aerosolized, for VAP, 564–565

Community-acquired pneumonia
  causal microorganisms in, stratification of patients in prediction of, 491–492
  described, 491
  outcomes of, impact of guidelines in, **491–505**
    adequacy of antibiotic treatment recommended by, 492–495
    rationale for implementation of, 496
    timing of antibiotics in, 495–496

Corticosteroid(s), in bronchiectasis management, 541–542

C-reactive protein, in optimization of antibiotic therapy for pneumonia due to multidrug-resistant pathogens, 434

Cytomegalovirus pneumonia, 460–461

Clin Chest Med 32 (2011) 601–604
doi:10.1016/S0272-5231(11)00072-4

Moving?

Make sure your subscription moves with you!

To notify us of your new address, find your **Clinics Account Number** (located on your mailing label above your name), and contact customer service at:

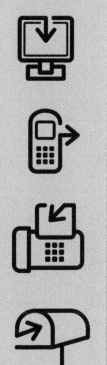

Email: journalscustomerservice-usa@elsevier.com

800-654-2452 (subscribers in the U.S. & Canada)
314-447-8871 (subscribers outside of the U.S. & Canada)

Fax number: 314-447-8029

Elsevier Health Sciences Division
Subscription Customer Service
3251 Riverport Lane
Maryland Heights, MO 63043

*To ensure uninterrupted delivery of your subscription, please notify us at least 4 weeks in advance of move.

Printed and bound by CPI Group (UK) Ltd, Croydon, CR0 4YY

03/10/2024

01040360-0017